FOURTH EDITION

MANAGEMENT STRATEGIES

in

ATHLETIC TRAINING

FOURTH EDITION

MANAGEMENT STRATEGIES
in
ATHLETIC TRAINING

ATHLETIC TRAINING EDUCATION SERIES

Richard Ray, EdD, ATC
Hope College

Jeff G. Konin, PhD, ATC, PT, FACSM, FNATA
University of South Florida

• • •

David H. Perrin, PhD, ATC, FNATA
Series Editor
University of North Carolina at Greensboro

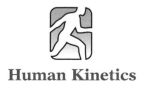

Human Kinetics

Library of Congress Cataloging-in-Publication Data

Ray, Richard, 1957-
  Management strategies in athletic training / Richard Ray, Jeff Konin. -- 4th ed.
    p. ; cm. -- (Athletic training education series)
  Includes bibliographical references and index.
  ISBN-13: 978-0-7360-7738-5 (hard cover)
  ISBN-10: 0-7360-7738-3 (hard cover)
  1. Athletic trainers. I. Konin, Jeff G. II. Title. III. Series: Athletic training education series.
  [DNLM: 1. Physical Education and Training--organization & administration. 2. Sports. QT 255]
  RC1210.R38 2011
  617.1'027--dc22

                          2011006562

ISBN-10: 0-7360-7738-3 (print)
ISBN-13: 978-0-7360-7738-5 (print)

Copyright © 2011 by Richard Ray and Jeff Konin
Copyright © 2005, 2000, 1994 by Richard Ray

The web addresses cited in this text were current as of April 26, 2011, unless otherwise noted.

Acquisitions Editor: Loarn D. Robertson, PhD; **Series Developmental Editor:** Amanda S. Ewing; **Developmental Editor:** Amanda S. Ewing; **Assistant Editors:** Kali Cox and Rachel Brito; **Copyeditor:** Joyce Sexton; **Indexer:** Nancy Ball; **Permissions Manager:** Dalene Reeder; **Graphic Designer:** Bob Reuther; **Graphic Artists:** Bob Reuther and Tara Welsch; **Cover Designer:** Keith Blomberg; **Photographer (cover):** © Human Kinetics; **Photo Asset Manager:** Laura Fitch; **Photo Production Manager:** Jason Allen; **Art Manager:** Kelly Hendren; **Associate Art Manager:** Alan L. Wilborn; **Illustrations:** © Human Kinetics; **Printer:** Edwards Brothers

Printed in the United States of America   10   9   8   7   6   5

The paper in this book is certified under a sustainable forestry program.

Human Kinetics
Website: www.HumanKinetics.com

United States: Human Kinetics
P.O. Box 5076
Champaign, IL 61825-5076
800-747-4457
e-mail: humank@hkusa.com

Canada: Human Kinetics
475 Devonshire Road Unit 100
Windsor, ON N8Y 2L5
800-465-7301 (in Canada only)
e-mail: info@hkcanada.com

Europe: Human Kinetics
107 Bradford Road
Stanningley
Leeds LS28 6AT, United Kingdom
+44 (0) 113 255 5665
e-mail: hk@hkeurope.com

Australia: Human Kinetics
57A Price Avenue
Lower Mitcham, South Australia 5062
08 8372 0999
e-mail: info@hkaustralia.com

New Zealand: Human Kinetics
P.O. Box 80
Torrens Park, South Australia 5062
0800 222 062
e-mail: info@hknewzealand.com

E4651

This book is dedicated to all my teachers, but especially to
Mom and Dad, my first teachers, with devotion and thanks.
To Lindsy McLean and Otho Davis, with respect and pride.
To my students, with hope for the future.
To Carol, with love and joy.

RICH RAY

My contributions to this book are dedicated to Dad, whose brief
time on earth composed of struggles is a constant reminder of
why my bucket list will not wait to be fulfilled.

JEFF G. KONIN

CONTENTS

INTRODUCTION TO THE ATHLETIC TRAINING EDUCATION SERIES

The six titles of the Athletic Training Education Series—*Core Concepts in Athletic Training and Therapy, Examination of Musculoskeletal Injuries, Therapeutic Exercise for Musculoskeletal Injuries, Therapeutic Modalities for Musculoskeletal Injuries, Management Strategies in Athletic Training,* and *Developing Clinical Proficiency in Athletic Training*—are textbooks for students of athletic training and references for practicing certified athletic trainers. Other allied health care professionals, such as physical therapists, physician's assistants, and occupational therapists, will also find these texts to be invaluable resources in the prevention, examination, treatment, and rehabilitation of injuries to physically active people.

The rapidly evolving profession of athletic training necessitates a continual updating of the educational resources available to educators, students, and practitioners. The authors of the six books in the series have made key improvements and have added information based on the most recent version of the NATA *Athletic Training Educational Competencies* before publication.

- *Core Concepts in Athletic Training and Therapy,* which replaces *Introduction to Athletic Training,* is suitable for introductory athletic training courses. Part I of the text introduces students to the idea of prevention. It also addresses the pre-participation exam (PPE), introduces aspects of fitness testing and conditioning in athletes, looks at the nutrition aspects of health and performance, examines how the environment affects athletic participation, looks at the protective devices used in various sports, and introduces methods of taping and bracing. Part II covers clinical examination and diagnosis, including injury mechanism and classification; the principles of primary and secondary surveys; injuries and

conditions that affect the upper and lower extremities, spine, head, neck, thorax, and abdomen; and general medical conditions. Part III covers acute and emergency care, including planning for emergency situations, immediate care for emergency situations, moving and transporting injured athletes, creating an emergency care plan, and obtaining consent for emergency care. Part IV covers therapeutic interventions, including rehabilitation and healing, therapeutic treatment modalities used in athletics, therapeutic exercise parameters and techniques, and pharmacology in athletic training. Part V introduces topics related to health care administration, including information on management functions and insurance. Part VI covers advanced concepts, such as pathophysiology of tissue injury, psychology of sport injury, and evidence-based practice in athletic training. *Core Concepts in Athletic Training and Therapy* fills the need for a text that covers myriad topics at an introductory level. It sets the stage for the other books in the series, which delve much deeper into specific topics.

- In *Examination of Musculoskeletal Injuries,* new information about sensitivity and specificity strengthens the evidence-based selection of special tests, and an increased emphasis on clinical decision making and problem solving and the integration of skill application in the end-of-chapter activities are now included.

- Two new chapters have been added to *Therapeutic Exercise for Musculoskeletal Injuries.* Chapter 16 focuses on arthroplasty, and chapter 17 contains information regarding various age considerations in rehabilitation. This text also provides more support of evidence-based care resulting from a blend of research results and the author's 40 years of experience as a clinician.

- The new edition of *Developing Clinical Proficiency in Athletic Training* contains 26 new modules, and embedded within it is the NATA *Athletic Training Educational Competencies.* The concepts of progressive clinical skill development, clinical supervision and autonomy, and clinical decision making are introduced and explained. The nature of critical thinking and why it is essential to clinical practice are also discussed.

- The third edition of *Therapeutic Modalities for Musculoskeletal Injuries* continues to provide readers with information on evidence-based practice and includes recent developments in the areas of inflammation and laser therapy.

- The fourth edition of *Management Strategies in Athletic Training* continues to help undergraduate and graduate students master entry-level concepts related to administration in athletic training. Each of the 10 chapters is thoroughly updated, and new material is presented on topics such as evidence-based medicine, professionalism in athletic training, health care financial management, cultural competence, injury surveillance systems, legal updates, and compensation for athletic trainers.

The Athletic Training Education Series offers a coordinated approach to the process of preparing students for the Board of Certification examination. If you are a student of athletic training, you must master the material in each of the content areas delineated in the NATA *Athletic Training Educational Competencies.* The Athletic Training Education Series addresses each of the competencies sequentially and thoroughly. The series covers the content areas developed by the NATA Executive Committee for Education of the National Athletic Trainers' Association for accredited curriculum development. The content areas and the texts that address each content area are as follows:

- Risk management and injury prevention *(Core Concepts* and *Management Strategies)*

- Pathology of injury and illnesses *(Core Concepts, Examination, Therapeutic Exercise,* and *Therapeutic Modalities)*

- Orthopedic assessment and diagnosis *(Examination* and *Therapeutic Exercise)*

- Acute care *(Core Concepts, Examination,* and *Management Strategies)*

- Pharmacology *(Core Concepts* and *Therapeutic Modalities)*

- Conditioning and rehabilitative exercise *(Therapeutic Exercise)*

- Therapeutic modalities *(Core Concepts* and *Therapeutic Modalities)*

- Medical conditions and disabilities *(Core Concepts* and *Examination)*

- Nutrition aspects of injury and illness *(Core Concepts)*

- Psychosocial intervention and referral *(Therapeutic Modalities* and *Therapeutic Exercise)*

- Administration *(Core Concepts* and *Management Strategies)*

- Professional development and responsibilities *(Core Concepts* and *Management Strategies)*

The authors for this series—Craig Denegar, Peggy Houglum, Richard Ray, Jeff Konin, Ethan Saliba, Susan Saliba, Sandra Shultz, Ken Knight, Kirk Brumels, Susan Hillman, and I—are certified athletic trainers with well over a century of collective experience as clinicians, educators, and leaders in the athletic training profession. The clinical experience of the authors spans virtually every setting in which athletic trainers practice: high schools, sports medicine clinics, universities, professional sports, hospitals, and industrial settings. The professional positions of the authors include undergraduate and graduate curriculum director, head athletic trainer, professor, clinic director, and researcher. The authors have chaired or served on the NATA's most prominent committees, including Professional Education Committee, Education Task Force, Education Council, Research Committee of the Research and Education Foundation, Journal Committee, Appropriate Medical Coverage for Intercollegiate Athletics Task Force, and Continuing Education Committee.

This series is the most progressive collection of texts and instructional materials currently available to athletic training students and educators. Several elements are present in most of the books in the series:

- Chapter objectives and summaries are tied to one another so that students will know and achieve their learning goals.

- Chapter-opening scenarios illustrate the relevance of the chapter content.

- Thorough reference lists allow for further reading and research.

To enhance instruction, various ancillaries are included:

- All of the texts (except for *Developing Clinical Proficiency in Athletic Training*) include instructor guides and test banks.
- *Therapeutic Exercise for Musculoskeletal Injuries* includes a presentation package plus image bank.
- *Core Concepts in Athletic Training and Therapy, Therapeutic Modalities for Musculoskeletal Injuries,* and *Examination of Musculoskeletal Injuries* all include image banks.
- *Examination of Musculoskeletal Injuries* includes an online student resource.
- *Core Concepts in Athletic Training and Therapy* includes a web resource.

Presentation packages include text slides plus select images from the text. Image banks include most of the figures, tables, and content photos from the book. Instructors can use these images to create their own presentations and to enhance lectures and demonstration sessions. Other features vary from book to book, depending on the subject matter; but all include various aids for assimilation and review of information, extensive illustrations, and material to help students apply the facts in the text to real-world situations.

The order in which the books should be used is determined by the philosophy of each curriculum director. In any case, each book can stand alone so that a curriculum director does not need to revamp an entire curriculum in order to use one or more parts of the series.

When I entered the profession of athletic training over 30 years ago, one text—*Prevention and Care of Athletic Injuries* by Klafs and Arnheim—covered nearly all the subject matter required for passing the Board of Certification examination and practicing as an entry-level athletic trainer. Since that time, we have witnessed an amazing expansion of the information and skills one must master in order to practice athletic training, along with an equally impressive growth of practice settings in which athletic trainers work. You will find these updated editions of the Athletic Training Education Series textbooks to be invaluable resources as you prepare for a career as a certified athletic trainer, and you will find them to be useful references in your professional practice.

David H. Perrin, PhD, ATC, FNATA
Series Editor

PREFACE

Athletic training has evolved through the years. Our predecessors early in the 20th century were little more than clubhouse helpers for a select population of college and professional athletes. Following the establishment in 1950 of the National Athletic Trainers' Association (NATA), however, credentialing and professional education standards helped create a growing demand for our services. Athletic trainers are now allied health care professionals who provide injury prevention and management as well as other health care services for the public. This book describes "athletes" in many ways—as physically active people, clients, and patients—and presents them in real-world settings, including traditional college and high school athletic training programs, sports medicine clinics, hospitals, professional teams, and industrial settings. As athletic trainers' employment settings and clientele have expanded, their need for administrative knowledge and skills has also expanded.

WHY THIS TEXT IS NEEDED

The days when an athletic trainer could get by without significant administrative expertise are gone. The financial assets entrusted to the contemporary athletic trainer require prudent, thoughtful management. Athletic trainers can acquire some of the organizational knowledge and skill they need through on-the-job experience, but many entry-level athletic trainers will not get the information they need that way. The primary purpose of this book is to provide a standard for the kinds of knowledge and skills that every athletic trainer entering the field should master. Because entry-level athletic trainers will confront administrative problems that are growing in number and complexity, they can use this book as a reference to help them cope with such problems while they provide high-quality services to their clients.

This text is also intended to enhance the administrative ability of athletic trainers already in practice. It offers a variety of topics and insights that many athletic trainers past the entry level don't consider in managerial or administrative terms. Practicing athletic trainers will learn to apply management theories to the administrative problems they have faced for years and to craft creative solutions to these problems.

This book brings together the body of knowledge about health care administration and applies it to the profession of athletic training. Credentialing boards of national and state athletic training organizations can use this book as a source of valid questions for credentialing examinations. The administrative challenges that athletic trainers face and the employment settings in which they work are expanding every year. The text considers these developments and provides the greatest depth and breadth of information on athletic training available in a single source.

WHO THIS TEXT WILL BENEFIT

The three primary audiences for this text are

- undergraduate students preparing for credentialing by states and the national Board of Certification,
- graduate students either preparing for state and national credentialing or working toward an advanced degree in athletic training, and
- practicing athletic trainers who are already credentialed but who wish to develop or update their knowledge and skill in athletic training administration.

HOW THIS TEXT IS ORGANIZED

This book presents theories underlying the management principles that athletic trainers have historically been forced to learn through experience. Anecdotes, practical suggestions, and case studies illustrate how management theory applies to the work of athletic trainers. An opening case begins each chapter, and the content of the chapter relates to the opening case. Each chapter concludes with at least two case studies that require readers to apply the theories presented in the chapter to real-world situations.

SPECIAL FEATURES

The following pedagogical aids are intended to help instructors and students master the content.

- **Chapter objectives.** Each chapter opens with a list of expected learning outcomes. These objectives are broad enough to form the behavioral objectives for an entire course in athletic training administration.

- **Key words.** Key words and important phrases appear in bold face to help readers determine the most important concepts at a glance.

- **Glossary.** Readers will find a glossary of important terms at the end of the book.

- **Sample forms.** Each chapter includes sample forms for reference. Readers can modify these forms for their own use.

- **Case studies.** Each chapter begins with an opening case study and concludes with at least two more. Each case includes a hypothetical scenario that will help students understand more fully the relationship between the theory and the application of various concepts discussed in the chapter. The cases at the ends of the chapters are accompanied by a series of questions that require students to synthesize the information presented in the chapter and to develop alternative responses to each scenario. The analysis questions are open-ended and encourage students to be creative in developing possible solutions. The number of right or wrong answers is not fixed.

- **Running review statements.** Summaries of the key points of each major section appear in blue text in the margins to help readers focus on the most important material.

- **Key concepts and review.** The most important concepts are summarized at the end of each chapter. This element is formatted to parallel the chapter objectives for easier review.

- **Bibliography.** A complete reading list, which includes all the references used to develop the chapters, guides students to sources for additional information on any given topic.

- **Index.** An index of the entire text by author and subject facilitates easy reference.

WHAT'S NEW IN THE FOURTH EDITION

Management Strategies in Athletic Training has been significantly improved in this fourth edition. Like the previous three editions, this edition is part of the Athletic Training Education Series, a collection of six textbooks, published by Human Kinetics, designed to meet the bulk of the discipline-specific content for an entry-level athletic training curriculum. Each of the 10 chapters from the third edition of *MSAT* has been updated. New material, like the rest of the information from the third edition, flows from the "Health Care Administration" portion of the NATA *Role Delineation Study* and includes the following:

- Evidence-based medicine
- Ambulatory health care facility accreditation
- Professionalism in athletic health care
- Employment and graduate school decision making
- Whistle-blowing as a method of ensuring accountability
- Advances in patient charting
- Updated preparticipation physical examination standards
- Health care financial management
- Cultural competence
- Methods of referral
- Theories of informed consent
- Providing legal testimony and deposition
- Purchasing and maintenance systems for durable medical equipment
- Marketing a sports medicine practice
- Emergency action planning
- Injury surveillance systems
- Updates on ethical practice in sports medicine
- Advice for employee selection
- Communication and listening skills
- Private-sector sports medicine facility planning
- Updated legal standards
- Updated state regulatory board contact information

- Tips for finding a job
- Athletic trainer compensation
- Negotiating skills for accepting a job
- Employment settings for athletic trainers
- National Athletic Trainers' Association position statements
- Updates on reimbursement for athletic training services
- Updates to the Fair Labor Standards Act
- OSHA requirements for health care facilities
- NCAA Sports Medicine Guidelines Audit
- Updates on continuing education
- Expansion of information management in athletic training clinical and administrative settings
- Updated information on reimbursement for athletic training services, including the athletic training CPT codes
- Updated forms
- Updated advice on job hunting and interviewing skills

NOTE TO INSTRUCTORS

If you are an athletic training educator, you might be wondering how you can most effectively use this book as part of a course on athletic training administration. In our experience, students learn this material best when they can apply it to the things they have seen in their short, but interesting, careers. Don't lecture from this book. Allow students to read the material and develop questions about how they should or could apply the information to real-life problems they've encountered or heard about. Use the questions and exercises in the case studies at the end of the chapter to start class conversations about the material. Keep in mind that the time you have with your students in the classroom is brief compared with the amount of time that they have on their own. We recommend that you use the time students have on their own for "first-exposure learning." One of the authors of this text (R.R.) requires his students to read the assigned chapter and complete the chapter worksheet before coming to class. When they arrive, all he has to do is ask, "Any questions?" and an hour later class is finished. Students typically spend the entire hour talking about, reinforcing, clarifying, and explaining the concepts that they found difficult in their reading. This method has proven far more effective than lecturing in this kind of course.

Several ancillaries are also available to help you present the material in the text.

- The instructor guide is loaded with useful instructional aids. Included in the instructor guide are extra case studies, course projects, chapter worksheets, and sample examination questions. For instructors who are still uncertain about how to develop their course, a sample syllabus—the one that we suggest using as a template—is provided.
- The test package includes more than 130 questions you can use to generate quizzes or tests.
- The image bank includes most of the photos, figures, and tables from the text. Images are grouped first within chapter folders, with art, photo, and table files provided in jpg format. You may reuse the images within your own PowerPoint templates to create your own custom presentations. To help you create your own presentations, we have also provided a blank PowerPoint template.

You can access these ancillaries by going to www.HumanKinetics.com/ManagementStrategiesIn AthleticTraining.

NOTE TO STUDENTS

If you are a student using *Management Strategies in Athletic Training, Fourth Edition,* in an athletic training administration course, you might be wondering if you should use this book just as you would all the textbooks you've been assigned in your other courses. We wouldn't recommend it, and here's why: experience. This book was written to help you experience, through reading and doing, what it is like to be an athletic trainer faced with administrative problems. You'll be introduced to fictional athletic trainers at the beginning of each chapter, and their stories will guide you through the material. Ask yourself how the concepts in the book can or should be applied in a real-life setting as you read the text. How do they apply to the case in the book? How do they apply to the athletic training program at your college or university? As you read each chapter, we recommend that you use the margin of the book to write notes to yourself. "Why did the athletic trainer in this chapter go over his AD's head? Wasn't that dangerous? Is that something I would have done under the

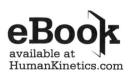

circumstances?" "The book recommends the use of bidding when purchasing supplies. Why doesn't the athletic trainer at our school do this?" Use the questions you develop to guide your participation in class. If you use this approach and aren't afraid to ask questions in class based on your reading, we think you'll find that your athletic training administration class will be one of the most interesting and exciting courses you take on your way to becoming a certified athletic trainer.

FINAL WORD

Athletic trainers of our generation were forced to learn how to become administrators through the school of hard knocks. Our experiences have likely been similar to those of many of our colleagues around the country who came of age in the 1970s and early '80s. We have massaged our management principles and styles through trial and error. We wrote this book so that athletic trainers of the new millennium could better prepare themselves to deal effectively with the many administrative and managerial problems they are likely to face in an increasingly complex health care environment. We hope that after they have read through and experienced the material in this book, they will find themselves prepared for the real world they are about to enter. After all, at the end of the day, athletic training will require not only expansion and growth as they pertain to clinical skills; it will also necessitate managerial leadership at national and local levels that will lead to overall professional enhancement on the health care stage.

ACKNOWLEDGMENTS

We are grateful to have had the opportunity to work together on this fourth edition. Both of us have grown as individuals from the wisdom of our partnership, and we hope that our efforts will be passed on to the next generation of athletic training students.

We are indebted to many people who gave their time and expertise to help make this book possible. We especially want to thank the professionals at Human Kinetics, who not only offered many suggestions to improve the book but also were kind and patient throughout the process. The Athletic Training Education Series editor, Dave Perrin, was a fine team leader in helping to organize this work. We also want to thank Loarn Robertson, PhD, senior acquisitions editor for Human Kinetics, for his patience and understanding; Mike Colello, ATC, for his expert review of the drug-testing section; Rene Revis Shingles, PhD, ATC, for her guidance on cultural competence; and Cameo Scott for her assistance with reviewing websites.

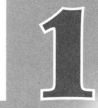

Theoretical Basis of Management

OBJECTIVES

After reading this chapter, you should be able to do the following:

1. Define the concepts of power, authority, and leadership.
2. Understand the historical trends in management and how they might apply to athletic training.
3. Understand the various managerial roles that athletic trainers assume.
4. Understand the various strategies that athletic trainers can employ to improve their managerial effectiveness.

▶ The staff meeting went just about as badly as Sharon Johnson had been afraid it might. The athletic trainers she supervises (in the sports medicine clinic of which she is a part owner) are angry. Sharon is also an athletic trainer, brought in by a physician and a physical therapist to help establish sports medicine services in a struggling outpatient physical therapy practice. When Sharon hired her staff of three certified athletic trainers, her partners required that they contribute a percentage of their health insurance premiums. They assured Sharon that the arrangement would be temporary—three years at most—until they were confident that the expansion into sports medicine was going to pay off. Sharon's athletic trainers were upset because after three years they were still required to contribute to their health insurance costs, even though the clinic's physical therapists didn't contribute a penny. Sharon agreed with the athletic trainers' position. She thought that they ought to be treated like the other professional staff. The problem she faced was that the physical therapist partner wanted to maintain the status quo, whereas the physician was wavering between the two positions.

Sharon finally decided to call a partners' meeting, at which she threatened to pull out of the business unless the issue was resolved in favor of the athletic trainers. The vote was two to one in favor of Sharon's position. Unfortunately, Sharon's cordial working relationship with her two partners deteriorated in the process. The physical therapist became coldly formal, and the physician was upset that Sharon had used a threat to get what she wanted.

Being powerful is like being a lady.
If you have to tell people you are, you ain't.

—JESSE CARR

Athletic trainers often experience elements of Sharon's dilemma, whatever the employment setting. Most athletic trainers have had to suffer through the tension that results from a power play in their organization. Although they typically lack formal education or training in management theory, athletic trainers need to be conversant with major theories of organizational behavior to make maximum use of the power, authority, and leadership that are normal components of their personal and professional profiles.

FOUNDATIONS OF MANAGEMENT

Athletic trainers are often responsible for managing programs with large budgets and staffs. Until recently, intuition and on-the-job experience have been athletic trainers' only tools for attempting to solve administrative problems. Formal study of the principles underlying sound management practice should help athletic trainers perform their jobs better.

The emphasis on the conceptual and theoretical aspects of management is important. Too often, athletic trainers who assume management roles continue to behave like health care providers and neglect to behave like managers. This role confusion is understandable. After all, if you have been a practitioner for 10 years and suddenly take a new position with new responsibilities, you have to make an adjustment. Managerial responsibilities are different from patient care responsibilities. When you take care of a patient, your only responsibility is to the patient. Managerial duties, on the other hand, require you to consider the needs of not only the patients but also the employees, the department, and the organization. You must consider the needs of various external stakeholder groups. In short, you will need to expand your worldview and begin thinking like a manager. An understanding of the major theories of management will help athletic trainers make the transition.

Athletic trainers can perform their managerial responsibilities best when they exercise leadership with the authority provided by their superiors. Both leadership and authority represent a certain kind of power that all athletic trainers have as a benefit of their position and expertise.

In some cases, schools employ just one athletic trainer, immediately thrusting the individual into a managerial role. It is not uncommon for recent athletic training graduates and newly certified athletic trainers with no previous employment experience to accept such positions. More often than not, a staff athletic trainer who has shown himself to be the most effective clinician, whether in a college or university setting or a clinic-based environment, is asked to serve as the head athletic trainer or director of sports medicine and to assume the administrative and managerial responsibilities for the program. He may have no previous formal or informal training for this role. This phenomenon is referred to as the "Peter Principle." The Peter Principle states that in a hierarchy, every employee tends to rise to his level of incompetence (Peter and Hull 1969). While promotion of an athletic trainer to managerial leadership does not in and of itself mean the person will fail as a leader, taking on a position that requires a very different set of skills—and that tends to affect a greater number of staff members—is a challenge that can easily be underestimated.

The Peter Principle states that in any organizational hierarchy, an individual will rise to his level of incompetence. This means that taking on additional responsibilities may come about in the absence of appropriate preparatory training and education.

Power

Scholars who devote their careers to the study of power cannot agree on a precise definition, but the definition most inclusive of the research done on the subject was put forth by Bass (1990). **Power** is the potential to influence.

Why is it important for students of athletic training administration to be able to define, recognize, and use power? Power is the glue that binds persons or groups in a relationship. It is the basis for both authority and leadership. Athletic trainers have significant power in their relationships with coaches, administrators, clients, and other health care professionals. Sharon's case illustrates an athletic trainer who recognizes her potential to influence others and acts on it. Sharon exercised power.

Athletic trainers can exercise power over those above them, below them, and at the same level in an organization. The two primary modalities for the exercise of organizational power are **position power** and **personal power**.

Position Power

Athletic trainers, by virtue of their positions, have resources they can use to influence the behavior of others in their organizations. Someone who supervises athletic training students, for example, can influence their behavior through the use of rewards and punishments, such as grades, financial aid, work–study money, desirable team assignments, and internship placements. In an organization that follows a medical chain of command, the athletic trainer can use the power provided by that policy to change the behavior of a coach who may desire to usurp the athletic trainer's medical authority.

The ability to influence the behavior of a superior has been termed **counterpower** (Yukl 1981). Counterpower is a tool that most athletic trainers need because they are typically viewed as support personnel who are less important than other organizational decision makers. Without counterpower, athletic trainers would be little more than technical consultants to more powerful coaches and athletic administrators, unable to influence the actions of those two important groups.

One of the ways athletic trainers can effectively use position power is by controlling the flow of information (Pettigrew 1972). By controlling information, athletic trainers can influence the perceptions and attitudes of their subordinates. For example, assistant athletic trainers often learn of changes in departmental policy through their head athletic trainers. And athletic training students depend largely on instructors and supervisors to inform them of changes in the profession.

Athletic trainers can also make superiors reliant on them for certain types of information. For example, in the draft systems of professional sports, potential draftees are examined by both physicians and athletic trainers. How the results are passed on to decision makers can significantly influence whether an athlete is drafted or not. Ultimately, the athletic trainer exercises influence through providing or withholding information.

Personal Power

The athletic trainer's ability to influence others in the organization often depends more on personal characteristics and personality attributes than it does on formal authority. Indeed, athletic trainers who use charisma and personal appeal to influence others in their organizations are more likely to receive acceptance and support for their ideas. Coercive power and authoritarian methods, on the other hand, are more likely to produce mere compliance, decreasing satisfaction and performance levels among the staff members whom these athletic trainers supervise (Yukl 1981).

One of the most effective elements of athletic trainers' personal power is their reputation as experts. People are likely to follow the recommendation of someone they perceive as an expert (French and Raven 1959). Athletic trainers make judgments every day based on their expertise in sports medicine. Athletes and other physically active patients who follow the treatment plan outlined by an athletic trainer probably have faith in the athletic trainer as an expert. When they fail to follow their treatment and rehabilitation plans, they may have lost faith in the expertise of the athletic trainer supervising their programs. In these cases, the athletic trainer must resort to position power as the basis for achieving compliance. Unfortunately, using the external motivators of position power is rarely as effective as using the internal motivators of personal power.

It should also be noted that one's expertise in health care is often influenced by one's "bedside manner" and interpersonal skills. It has been said that "people do not care how much you know, until they know how much you care." This statement can be directly applied to an athletic training setting. That is, if an athletic trainer is extremely knowledgeable with her assessment and rehabilitation skills but is abrupt and curt with a client, the client may not place trust in the interaction and may not be motivated toward compliance. On the other hand, if an athletic trainer is courteous, does not appear to be rushed, and finds time to allow the client to ask questions regarding his injury, the client will likely place a higher level of trust in the athletic trainer and comply with whatever advice he receives. We see these types of exchanges whenever we visit a physician's office. Regardless of the prestige displayed by wall plaques in a medical office, the provider–client exchange will likely determine the client's level of satisfaction and the client's ultimate perception of the provider's expertise.

Authority

Authority is the aspect of power, granted to either groups or individuals, that legitimizes the right of the group or individual to make decisions on behalf of others. Implicit in this definition is the notion that authority is a subset of the broader construct of power. Although some authors disagree with this proposition (Friedrich 1963; Kahn 1968), most evidence clearly identifies authority as a type of power (Burns 1978; Dejnozka 1983; Good 1973; Jacobs 1970; Katz and Kahn 1966; King 1987; Lasswell and Kaplan 1950; Organ and Bateman 1986). If power is the glue that binds persons or groups together in a relationship, then authority is the applicator through which power is exercised. Without authority, athletic trainers would lack position power.

Central to the meaning of authority is the concept of legitimacy. Authority is legitimate by its very nature (Good 1973; Hollander 1978; Karelis 1987; Weber 1962). **Legitimacy** is a check on the scope of an athletic trainer's authority. Consider Sharon's case at the beginning of this chapter. Although she might have wanted to grant the request of her staff members, she didn't have the authority to do so without the consent of her partners. Any decision made without her partners' consent would have lacked legitimacy.

Legitimacy is an especially important concept for athletic trainers who supervise the work of others. Barnard (1938) postulated that each person has a **zone of indifference**. People typically accept requests or orders within this zone without conscious questioning because they view them as appropriate given the status of the person making the request. Orders or requests outside the zone, however, lack legitimacy, and people often refuse to comply with them. Athletic trainers who supervise assistants or students should be cautious about asking them to do things outside the zone of indifference. Asking an athletic training student to wash a whirlpool may be legitimate, but don't expect enthusiastic support if you ask the same student to wash your car!

Another property implicit in this definition of authority is that it involves decision making and is therefore action oriented. Like its parent, power, authority can be observed only when it is exercised. If Sharon had not acted on the vote of her partners in the health insurance case, she would have abrogated her authority in the matter. Athletic trainers are called on to make many administrative decisions during the course of a typical day: Should I order more tape? How should I arrange the team physician's injury clinic schedule? How many athletic trainers will I need to cover the wrestling tournament? Athletic trainers exercise the authority that they have been granted when they answer these questions with action. Indeed, many of their administrative problems stem from hesitation to use their authority.

One notable exception exists to the action orientation normally associated with authority. Some situations call for the athletic trainer to exercise authority by making a conscious decision *not* to act. Let's consider Sharon's dilemma as an example. Suppose that instead of being neutral, her physician partner was against Sharon's point of view on the health insurance issue and in favor of the position of the physical therapist partner. In that case, Sharon would know that calling a vote on the matter would likely result in a formal company position against full compensation of health insurance benefits for staff athletic trainers. The only prudent action she could take in this circumstance would be no action at all, other than to continue to try to convince her partners to support her. To request a vote would be counterproductive. The important point is that Sharon's inaction would be goal oriented. She would be letting the issue lie for the moment so she would be able to fight another day.

The athletic trainer's use of her authority can be a powerful tool to prompt task accomplishment. Authority provides a new athletic trainer an immediate power base to help her accomplish tasks. This circumstance is sometimes referred to as the **honeymoon effect**. Newly hired people in athletic training programs are often granted more authority to make decisions than they would be six months or a year after arrival. The honeymoon effect is an important factor in rejuvenating programs. Without it, new athletic trainers would have less effect because they wouldn't be able to implement new ideas as easily.

Several problems can develop when athletic trainers overuse their authority to accomplish tasks in athletic training programs. Athletic trainers who rely too heavily on their authority are likely to find that their staff respond with mere compliance and minimal effort (Organ and Bateman 1986). The athletic trainer who constantly reminds his assistants that he is the boss might be successful in extracting a modest amount of work from the assistants, but he is also likely to experience a high rate of turnover. Athletic trainers who rely heavily on authority are also likely to find that their subordinates try to avoid them. The threat, perceived or real, that an authoritarian supervisor will impose negative sanctions against subordinates is a common theme, even for athletic trainers who have no rational basis for their perceptions.

Leadership

Leadership is the process of influencing the behavior and attitudes of others to achieve intended outcomes. Like authority, it is a subset of the broader construct of power (Burns 1978). There are nearly as many definitions of leadership as there are scholars who have studied the topic—over 130 distinct definitions exist (Burns 1978). One of the few common denominators among this host of definitions is the assumption that leadership involves an intentional influence process by a leader over followers (Yukl 1981). In addition, leadership is success oriented. If a "leader" attempts an action and doesn't gain the support of followers, has leadership really taken place?

Why is a discussion of leadership important for athletic trainers? The exercise of leadership is the keystone of managerial success. Without the ability to influence attitudes and behaviors toward some predetermined goal, the athletic trainer is an ineffective agent for change in his organization. Unfortunately, we often think of leaders as persons on the national or international stage. Churchill, Gandhi, and Roosevelt were certainly effective leaders. The more common form of leadership, however, is a local phenomenon. Leaders surround all of us in our homes, churches, and communities and in the sports medicine settings in which we work. Without leadership, the organizations that employ us would stagnate and cease to be effective in providing needed services to clients.

Athletic trainers can better appreciate the importance of effective leadership and the effect it can have on their managerial success by understanding the two types of leadership found in most social structures, including organizations that employ athletic trainers. Burns (1978) contends that leadership takes two distinct forms: transactional and transformational. **Transactional leadership** involves the simple exchange of one thing for another in a relationship between two people. An athletic trainer pays her assistants in exchange for work. An athletic director agrees to send an athletic trainer to a conference in exchange for covering a state high school basketball tournament. Most administrative activities in organizations in which athletic trainers work involve the transactional form of leadership. This book is devoted primarily to principles and techniques intended to improve the athletic trainer's ability to be a transactional leader. Transactional leadership is the stuff of management.

Nevertheless, a program or organization in which only transactional leadership takes place will probably not thrive. Organizational renewal and program improvement require transformational leadership. **Transformational leadership** transcends the day-to-day administrative requirements of operating an athletic training program by elevating standards through the creative use of change and conflict. The athletic trainer who can successfully prepare budgets, hire staff, purchase supplies, and schedule personnel is an effective transactional leader. The athletic trainer who recognizes the need to reduce the incidence of eating disorders among his athletes and who implements programs that successfully accomplish this task exhibits transformational leadership.

Transformational leadership usually involves change in the organization. This change is likely to engender some degree of conflict. Consider the example of setting up an eating disorders program. Such programs cost money. Instructional materials must be developed or purchased. Group facilitators and therapists must be contracted for. Funding either will have to come from existing programs or be raised specifically for the project. Making decisions about these issues often brings athletic trainers into conflict with coaches and athletic administrators who are in competition for scarce financial resources. The athletic trainer who is a skilled transformational leader will be able to manage the conflict to meet the needs of coaches, athletic administrators, and athletes with eating disorders. As you can see, the transformational aspect of leadership is both challenging and essential if an athletic training program is to meet the changing needs of its clients.

A BRIEF HISTORY OF MANAGEMENT

Although basic concepts of organizing the labor of others toward a common goal date back to the ancient past, the study of management techniques is a more recent phenomenon. What follows is a brief description of some of the prominent management ideas that have been developed over the past 100 years.

Scientific Management

The **scientific management** movement began in the early 1900s. Widely acknowledged as the father of modern management, Frederick Taylor introduced the idea of division of labor and management whereby workers should be viewed as parts of a large machine whose function was to produce a product. He believed that money was the sole motivating force that would induce workers to perform their jobs well. One of Taylor's major contributions was the time and motion study, a method of breaking down a worker's job into discrete tasks

Management is an old concept. Its study and practice have changed over the years. Early 20th-century managerial theories include scientific management and human relations management. Management theories developed in the later half of the century include Field Theory, MacGregor's Theory X and Theory Y, and Deming's Total Quality Management.

and mathematically analyzing each task for maximum efficiency. Taylor's contribution to managerial science resulted in more efficient industrial practices in an environment where the self-esteem needs of employees were largely ignored because they were not thought to be important. An efficiently designed athletic training room or sports medicine clinic where the staff can serve the maximum number of athletes or other physically active patients with the least amount of movement between stations is an example of the influence of Taylor's thinking applied to athletic training.

The primary concept driving the development of scientific management was a desire for greater efficiency. Another early theorist in the scientific management movement who helped to define the methods necessary to achieve efficiency was Harrington Emerson. Emerson was an engineer who believed that strict compliance with his 12 principles would lend greater efficiency not only to specific jobs within a company but also to the entire business. Although Emerson designed his principles with the railroad industry in mind, he was convinced that they had application to any enterprise in which predictability of results was desirable. These principles are summarized in the following sidebar.

Henri Fayol was another early pioneer in the push for greater efficiency through scientific management. Although many of his ideas were similar to those of Taylor and Emerson, Fayol believed in a principle he called **unity of command**. Whereas Taylor thought that efficiency was enhanced by having the work of an employee directed by several foremen, each with his own area of responsibility, Fayol was convinced that maximum efficiency was possible only when orders were issued by a single boss. If Fayol had been an athletic trainer, he likely would have argued in favor of the appointment of a head athletic trainer who would oversee the entire athletic medicine program—a concept that is in widespread use today.

Human Relations Management

The 1920s and 1930s saw the rise of the human relations school of managerial theory. The two primary thinkers in this tradition were Mary Parker Follett, a social worker, and Elton Mayo, a Harvard professor. Follett advocated a departure from the strict authoritarianism of Taylor and the other proponents of scientific management. She believed that employees at all

---

■ Emerson's 12 Principles of Efficiency

1. **Ideals:** Develop clearly defined goals.
2. **Common sense:** Ensure that goals contribute to the improvement of the enterprise.
3. **Competent counsel:** Seek advice from those who know more than you do.
4. **Discipline:** Ensure that employees know their jobs, and establish a system for recruiting and selecting good employees.
5. **The fair deal:** Provide fair wages and good working conditions.
6. **Records:** Document and analyze the work process in order to make good decisions.
7. **Dispatching:** Plan the work schedule for maximum efficiency.
8. **Standards and schedules:** Establish standards for work through proper placement of employees.
9. **Standardized conditions:** Optimize the work setting.
10. **Standardized operations:** Develop a consistent process for the performance of tasks.
11. **Standardized practice instructions:** Teach all employees to perform tasks in the same manner.
12. **Efficiency reward:** Provide financial incentives for excellent performance.

levels of an organization should cooperate to develop approaches to accomplishing goals. This democratization of the workplace was a significant departure from the hierarchical structure advocated by scientific management theorists, who thought that the employee's job was simply to implement the orders of his superior. Follett taught that cooperation between managers in various departments and between managers and workers was an important motivating element that would lead to greater improvements in meeting organizational goals. In addition, she believed that managers should vary their actions depending on the situation. Managers, she thought, should "take orders" from the situation. The notion of a head athletic trainer who makes all managerial decisions would be anathema to Follett. She would advocate frequent discussions among all members of the sports medicine staff to make policy and solve problems jointly.

Elton Mayo is associated with one of the best-known industrial studies of the modern era. The Hawthorne studies were a series of experiments designed to test the effect of manipulating various working conditions on the production of telephone relay switches. Mayo's experimental design involved informing, and in some cases consulting, the employees being studied regarding the conditions to be manipulated and the variables to be measured. The experiments lasted several years. In most cases, irrespective of the working condition being manipulated, the workers' productivity rose dramatically, even when conditions were adjusted to be less favorable. Three primary lessons emerged from the Hawthorne studies:

1. Involvement of employees in workplace decisions can result in improvements in productivity.
2. Factors other than environmental conditions are most important in influencing worker production.
3. Experimental research—especially research involving human behavior—should employ a control group so that comparisons between groups can be attributed to the effect of the independent variable.

The **Hawthorne effect** occurs when subjects in an experiment change their behavior simply because they know they are being studied. Like Follett, Mayo would encourage athletic trainer-managers to involve everyone on the sports medicine staff in collaborating and providing input on decisions about the operation of the program. Although this approach seems to be common sense to most of us in the 21st century, it was radical thinking in the early part of the 20th century.

Modern Management Theories

Since the 1950s, many theorists have devoted their entire careers to the study of management. One such theorist was Kurt Lewin (Gillies 1994). His Field Theory of human behavior posits that employee actions in the workplace are the product of three interacting variables: employee personality, work-group structure, and sociotechnical climate. Lewin believed that influencing employees to change their behavior (and thereby improve productivity and efficiency) involved three phases: unfreezing (creating motivation for a change in behavior, either by applying pressure or by reducing threats associated with the change), changing (modifying behavior by either mimicking a role model or learning new behaviors through a discovery process), and refreezing (integrating the new behavior into the workplace with constant reinforcement from others).

Imagine a situation in which a relatively young and inexperienced university athletic trainer repeatedly made the mistake of leaving the athletic training students assigned to him in unsupervised situations. As this athletic trainer's supervisor, you would be responsible for enforcing the program policy of requiring supervision of students at all times. Using Lewin's theories, you might employ a three-stage strategy to make sure that this happened.

First, you would attempt to unfreeze the athletic trainer's behavior. You might accomplish this in several ways, including education and familiarization with institutional and accrediting agency rules. You could also employ threats of sanctions. ("Student supervision is one of your most important jobs. I can't recommend a raise or a favorable performance review if you continue to leave the students unsupervised.")

Next, you would attempt to change the athletic trainer's behavior by providing him with a copy of the institutional and accrediting agency rules. You might also ask him to shadow you for a day in your work environment so that he can learn how you successfully integrate your clinical and educational roles. The final step in the process would be to refreeze the appropriate behavior by praising the athletic trainer when you see him providing supervision of student clinical activities. Better yet, you might ask a few of the students to thank him for sharing his time and expertise.

In 1960, Douglas McGregor proposed a new conception of human nature in the workplace with his Theory X and Theory Y. Theory X represented the traditional view of humans at work. Under Theory X, workers were assumed to be inherently lazy, avoiding work whenever possible. Theory X assumes that workers prefer to be directed by others and that their primary concern is financial reward rather than self-improvement. Because of these qualities, Theory X postulates that workers must be coerced to perform their jobs well. Theory Y, on the other hand, holds that work is a natural activity and is as necessary as rest or play. If a person is committed to a task, she will require little direction to accomplish her goals. The belief that workers naturally learn to seek out and accept responsibility is also a tenet of Theory Y. Finally, Theory Y hypothesizes that most people have the capacity to solve organizational problems and that this ability is not the sole province of managers. Most of us can probably think of supervisors we have worked for who were from either the Theory X or the Theory Y school of thought. Athletic trainers who anticipate moving into a management role should contemplate which set of assumptions they agree with most closely. If your management style is predominantly Theory X and your supervisees are predominantly Theory Y, workplace friction is likely to be a problem. Similarly, if you are new to your supervisory role and your staff was previously led by a supervisor with a contrasting set of assumptions about the nature of work and workers, you should expect a difficult period of transition.

The most interesting and important trend in management theory and practice in modern times is the application of W. Edwards Deming's management principles to the industrial workforce in post-World War II Japan. Deming's ideas form the cornerstone of the **Total Quality Management (TQM)** movement, which is still popular in organizations all over the world. Deming taught the importance of a clear focus on the mission of an organization and the need for management to demonstrate continuous commitment to this mission and to communicate it to everyone in the organization. He believed that trust and rewarding innovation were two important elements of organizational improvement. Education and self-improvement for people at every level of an organization are fundamental. Total Quality Management is a popular management philosophy in health care organizations. Athletic trainers who work in hospitals are likely to find themselves involved in TQM at an early stage in their careers.

The Japanese took Deming's ideas and integrated them with the particular characteristics of their culture to create one of the most powerful, efficient, and productive workforces in history. Six concepts are central to the Japanese managerial philosophy (Gillies 1994). First, the primary trait desired in potential employees is the quality of their character. The training they will need to perform their jobs can be delivered in-house. Second, employees develop a close personal identification with the organization because they are employed for life. Although lifelong employment as a national norm is eroding in Japan, the concept of making an employee feel part of an organizational family is a sound one. Third, the Japanese believe that career progress should be steady but slow. Employees should work in many different departments before moving into managerial positions. Fourth, decision making in Japanese companies is a collective process. Members of the work group all have input into organizational decisions. The group is more valued than the individual. Fifth, a culture of continuous improvement based on the needs of clients is of overriding importance. Finally, Japanese companies practice the Asian cultural tradition of saving face by supporting and moving unproductive employees around the organization until they become successful.

THREE MANAGEMENT ROLES

Management is that element of the leadership process that involves planning, decision making, and coordinating the activities of a group of people working toward a common goal. Athletic trainers' regular management activities include scheduling, purchasing, hiring, evaluating, developing programs, accounting, and many others. In his classic text on the science of management, Fayol (1949) defined the following five elements of management: (1) planning, (2) organizing, (3) command, (4) coordination, and (5) control. Gulick and Urwick (1977) added staffing, directing, reporting, and budgeting to Fayol's original list. Dale (1965) thought that innovation and representation were also important management functions.

Mintzberg (1973) described three major roles that all managers, including athletic trainers, assume from time to time:

1. Interpersonal roles
2. Informational roles
3. Decisional roles

> Athletic trainers in managerial positions have to assume three roles as part of their jobs: interpersonal, informational, and decisional roles. Each of these roles is complex and has multiple components.

Interpersonal Roles

Every athletic trainer who manages a department or program will probably be forced to assume three different **interpersonal roles** at one time or another. The first is the **figurehead role**. As the person who has been granted formal authority for a particular program, the athletic trainer will be called on to perform certain routine functions such as providing signatures, public speaking, and answering requests for information. The figurehead role is often the most visible managerial task that the athletic trainer will undertake. Although it is probably not as vital to the long-term health of the program as other managerial roles, the figurehead role is important because of the public relations value that it can yield.

The second managerial role the athletic trainer must assume is that of a leader. We have already discussed transactional and transformational leadership.

The third managerial role the athletic trainer must assume is that of liaison. The **liaison role** is an important part of the athletic trainer's success or failure as a manager. Athletic trainers must work with a variety of people to run a successful athletic training program (see figure 1.1). Although vertical liaison with coworkers above and below him in the organization is commonly understood to be a function of the athletic trainer, horizontal liaison with professional peers is vital to developing and maintaining goodwill between the athletic training program and other departments of the organization and between the program and outside entities. Mintzberg (1973) hypothesized that social equals tend to interact with one another more often than they do with superiors or subordinates. Thus, athletic trainers need to develop relationships with athletic trainers at other institutions, health professionals in the community, coaches, consulting physicians, and parents. All these people will have an effect on the athletic trainer's managerial success.

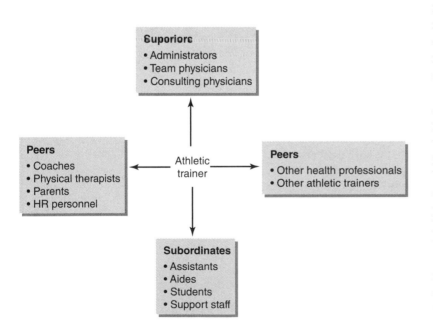

▶ **Figure 1.1** Liaison relationships of the athletic trainer.

Informational Roles

The first **informational role** an athletic trainer plays is that of both a **monitor** and a **disseminator** of information. The athletic training program is constantly bombarded by information from a variety of sources on a variety of topics. Journals and trade publications present news of technological advances in preventing and treating athletic injuries. Newsletters and memoranda route organizational news and policy changes. Progress reports and clinical notes arrive in the mail from team and consulting physicians. The first response of the effective athletic trainer-manager is to filter the information. Is it appropriate to share this memo with the staff? Who needs to know about the complications of Rick's knee surgery? Athletic trainers in a variety of employment settings decide these and similar questions daily.

After deciding what information should be passed along and to whom it should be passed, the athletic trainer must decide how to deliver it in a timely, efficient, and effective manner. Some items can be posted on a **bulletin board** where the staff can scan the information at their leisure. Other items require more explanation and documentation and should therefore be put in writing and delivered individually. This process is especially important if the information is confidential or if it is necessary to document that the information was actually passed along. For example, if an athletic trainer is not performing up to the standards set by the organization, it would be important to communicate these concerns in writing to keep them confidential and to document that the institution had warned the athletic trainer of dissatisfaction with her work.

Oral Communication

To be effective in the role of monitor and disseminator of information, the athletic trainer must both understand and be skilled at communicating with everyone in the organization. Oral communication is one of the primary modes of disseminating information in an organization. Three elements influence the process of oral communication (Drafke 1994):

1. The meaning of the sender
2. The meaning of the receiver
3. Interference between the sender and receiver

Unfortunately, these three elements often interact in a way that impedes effective communication. How often have you said something to someone only to learn that the person was offended either by the way you said it or by the context in which the message was delivered? Sharon's case in the opening scenario demonstrates the importance of *how* and *where* something is said rather than just *what* is said. Sharon made a statement to her partners in a tension-filled environment where she knew that conflict existed. If she had delivered the same message in a different manner in a different setting, perhaps the outcome would have been more positive. Her oral tone, along with the potentially hostile mind-set of her partners, probably skewed the meaning of most of what she had to say.

Interference in the communication process is a common problem. Noisy or distracting work environments can cause interference. Interference is also inherent in the methods used to transmit a message from one person to another. For example, because a written message does not usually allow for immediate feedback or clarification, the potential for interference using that method is quite high. Face-to-face communications, on the

---

■ Methods for Effective Communication

As a monitor and disseminator of information, you need to use appropriate communication tools. Keep in mind important issues such as efficiency, necessity for documentation, and confidentiality when choosing a method. Several methods of communication can be effective:

- Bulletin boards
- Staff meetings
- Individual meetings
- Letters or memos
- Newsletters
- Telephone calls
- Electronic mail
- Text message alerts
- Web pages

other hand, allow for greater interaction between the parties and therefore have a much lower potential for interference. Information filtered through a third party is the method most likely to result in corruption of the original message, because it is subject to interference at more than one step of the process. Because of the potential for altered meaning due to interference in various communication methods, Drafke (1994) ranks the following methods in terms of their effectiveness:

1. Face-to-face communication
2. Telecommunication
3. Written communication
4. Communication through a third party

A note on Drafke's ranking is appropriate. As previously mentioned, written communication serves an important purpose in helping to document that communication actually occurred. Although sitting down with a colleague to discuss an issue in a quiet, calm environment has certain advantages, much of the benefit of this method is lost if the environment becomes noisy or uncomfortable. Written communications also have the advantage of allowing the sender to make careful choices about the words used to convey the message. Sharon's case provides a useful example. She used words in her partners' meeting that she thought of and delivered when she was upset. Had she taken time to compose her thoughts in writing and to edit the document over the course of several days while allowing herself to detach from the issue emotionally, she might have been more effective.

Listening Skills

Active listening requires one to provide undivided attention to the messenger without having a preconceived thought about what one wants or expects to hear.

An important aspect of successful two-way communication involves what is referred to as "active listening." Athletic trainers spend abundant amounts of time listening to others: coaches, athletes, and staff. Active listening involves a total effort and attention given to a message (Konin 1997). Of greatest significance is that the listener does not have a preconceived outcome for the verbal exchange and instead approaches the conversation with an open mind. One key to verifying successful active listening skills is to simply repeat back a portion of the conversation to the other party. For example, if an athlete asks you if you think he will be ready to return to play within the next week, you can respond by saying, "Do I think you will be ready to play within the next week? There is a good possibility that if your healing continues at the pace it has been going thus far, and you remain compliant with your exercises, you may be able to play before the end of the week." If your response was merely, "I'm not sure," the athlete may not feel as though you listened or even cared about what he was saying. Smith (1975) has described different levels of listening skills that can be adapted for athletic trainers to use as a guide for improved communication. Different circumstances may warrant the use of different approaches and techniques for active listening.

One level often used by athletic trainers is **analytical listening**. This happens every time an athletic trainer takes a medical history from a patient and listens for specific kinds of information to be conveyed. For example, if you were taking a medical history from a soccer player who recently injured her knee, you would be listening for key words such as "pop" or "twist" and associate such words with a ligament or meniscus injury. This is not preconceived listening, because you may also hear other words such as "grinding" or "squeaking," and you might associate such terms with a patellofemoral malalignment. Therefore, you are technically being open-minded in your listening approach.

Levels of Listening

1. **Analytical.** Listening for specific kinds of information
2. **Directed.** Listening to answer specific questions
3. **Attentive.** Listening for general information to obtain an overview
4. **Exploratory.** Listening due to one's own interest
5. **Appreciative.** Listening for pleasure
6. **Courteous.** Listening as a result of feeling obligated
7. **Passive.** Not listening in an attentive manner

Nonverbal Communication

The most important modifiers of an intended message are usually nonverbal elements of that message. Mehrabian (1981) concluded that 55% of any given message is nonverbal. Nonverbal cues can function in a variety of ways to alter a message. Gestures and body position can reinforce an oral message, or they can contradict it. If Sharon had opened the meeting by saying, "I'm glad to see both of you this morning" while smiling and looking directly at each of her partners, her message would have been quite different than if she had scowled and avoided eye contact. Sharon could have helped control or regulate the meeting by leaning forward, raising her hand, or acting as if she was about to speak as a way of indicating that she had something to say. If Sharon had lost the vote, she would have subverted her actual message ("No problem. I understand and accept your decision.") if she staring coldly at her partners for a few moments and then spoke in a flat monotone. See the sidebar for a list of nonverbal communication cues that you should be aware of (Drafke 1994).

The **spokesperson role** is the third informational role that athletic trainers assume. Mintzberg (1973) points out that effective managers must keep two important groups informed. The first group includes the organizational decision makers, also known as **internal influencers**. Internal influencers are people who either are members of or have close ties to an organization and who have the power to help shape policy and practice. Table 1.1 shows examples of internal influencers in various settings where sports medicine programs operate.

The second group an athletic trainer should communicate with in his role as spokesperson is the organization's public. Like internal influencers, the members of the sports medicine program's public will vary by setting. Common to each setting are clients (physically active patients, athletes, student-athletes), suppliers, community supporters (members of booster clubs, parents, fans, members of alumni groups), consulting health professionals, and the news media. The athletic trainer will communicate with each of these groups from time to time, taking on the role of the organization's expert in sports medicine. The expert spokesperson role is a source of considerable personal power for the athletic trainer.

■ Nonverbal Communication Cues

1. **Clothing and grooming.** Neat, well-fitting clothes and grooming that conforms to cultural norms often send a message of competence and control.

2. **Territoriality.** Maintain a culturally accepted distance (usually 24 to 40 inches [60 to 100 centimeters] in the United States) when addressing a colleague. Meetings that take place in the manager's office are often intended to be more formal, serious, or important.

3. **Posture and facial expression.** Crossed arms or a body orientation facing away from a person indicates anger, impatience, or boredom. A fixed gaze with a scowl indicates anger or disagreement. Avoiding eye contact often indicates guilt or embarrassment. Long, uncomfortable stares may be seen as intimidating.

4. **Gestures.** Finger tapping expresses boredom. A closed fist or a pointing index finger can indicate anger. A polite handshake indicates receptiveness.

TABLE 1.1 Internal Influencers in Common Athletic Training Settings

Type of setting	Influencers
High school	Coaches, team physicians, athletic directors, principals, central office administrators, board of education members
College and university	Coaches, athletic administrators, other university administrators, team physicians, trustees
Clinic	Clinic owners, hospital administrators, referring physicians, hospital trustees, supervisors
Professional athletics	Coaches, general managers, other club administrators, owners, team physicians

Decisional Roles

The last group of roles that athletic trainers must assume as part of their managerial responsibilities is probably the most important; it is made up of **decisional roles**. Decisional roles require the athletic trainer to use both personal and position power by exercising authority. The effective athletic trainer-manager will also use decisional roles to exercise transformational leadership by planning strategies to serve clients better.

The first decision-making role assumed by the athletic trainer is an **entrepreneurial role**. Although most of us envision an entrepreneur as someone who creates new businesses, the term refers here to an athletic trainer who designs and initiates changes for her programs and organizations. If the athletic trainer fails in this entrepreneurial role, the sports medicine program will probably stop improving. One of the ways athletic trainers can become entrepreneurs for the sports medicine program is by focusing on small, solvable problems and new opportunities and initiating improvements in both areas. All athletic trainers could probably come up with a list of 10 to 15 concrete steps that would improve their programs. Athletic trainers could also improve their programs by taking advantage of some of the opportunities they face. The key is the ability to make decisions about which changes to implement based on what is feasible.

Being entrepreneurial does not require one to possess a master of business degree (MBA). Individuals possessing entrepreneurial-like skills can be described as having the "five Ds": desire, diligence, (grasp of) details, determination, and discipline. Furthermore, generally speaking, entrepreneurs are generally highly competitive, tend to possess a liking for social environments, and believe strongly in organization and planning. A strong argument can be made that these same characteristics are necessary for success in any athletic training setting.

The second decision-making role involves the athletic trainer as **disturbance handler**. Disturbances requiring the attention and intervention of the athletic trainer usually revolve around conflict. The role of conflict manager is often a difficult and uncomfortable one for athletic trainers for several reasons. First, conflict usually involves change. Indeed, some scholars have defined the term *conflict* as change (Burns 1978). Controlled change is a necessary ingredient for healthy program and organizational growth. Unfortunately, such change often occurs with some human costs attached.

Blake and Mouton (1984) have identified eight traditional methods managers should consider to resolve a conflict. Each is most effective under specific circumstances, and many cases may require a combination of two or more approaches.

1. Cooperation by edict. This approach is the most frequently attempted and least frequently successful. The method requires that the athletic trainer have a high degree of control over subordinates, and its effects diminish rapidly. "My way or the highway" is a poor conflict management technique for most complex situations. By walking into the meeting, banging the table with her fist, and demanding a change in the benefits policy, Sharon got her way, but she might have permanently fractured the relationship with her partners.

2. Negotiation. Negotiation between the two parties may resolve surface issues, but deep-seated conflict often remains unresolved because neither side gets everything desired. Negotiation often ends up destroying old precedents and establishing new ones, so it should be used with caution. If Sharon had used a negotiation strategy, she might have suggested that the clinic raise the money needed to pay the full cost of the athletic trainers' medical insurance by eliminating or reducing a benefit that all employees now receive, such as continuing education funding. Although this solution may have met the athletic trainers' insurance needs, no one would have felt good about the loss of continuing education funding.

3. Leadership replacement. Leadership replacement is a common technique when conflict resolution fails at one level and rises to the next level of the organization. Although new leaders can bring fresh perspectives to a problem, they lack a sense of the history and culture of the organization. In essence, this is the strategy that Sharon proposed to resolve the issue in the opening case. "If you don't respect me enough to take my advice on this matter," she said, "then find someone else."

4. Personnel rotation. Although this may be an effective conflict resolution method for a small staff, it is unlikely to change large-group norms. Changes because of personnel rotation are usually temporary in large groups. The other two partners in Sharon's practice might have decided to bring in a new partner had Sharon resigned. This wouldn't have resolved the conflict between the athletic trainers and the partners, but it would have demonstrated the partners' resolve to stick to their position and eased interpartner conflict.

5. Organizational structural changes. Such changes are often attempted to ameliorate conflict. Unfortunately, if the nature of the work remains the same, so does the conflict. If the two partners had decided to allow Sharon to purchase the part of the practice involving the athletic trainers and lease their services back to the parent company, they would have been applying this strategy. Sharon could then have implemented the personnel policies she desired without continued conflict with her partners.

6. Liaison persons. Liaison persons are often appointed or elected to represent the parties in a conflict. Although this method can be beneficial, it can slow communication by adding another layer to the organizational structure. If the relationship between Sharon and her physical therapist partner was strained to the point that an impasse was unavoidable, Sharon might have been wise to ask one of the physical therapist employees who agreed with her position to speak with the partner and act as a go-between.

7. Flexible reporting relationships. Using flexible reporting relationships can be an effective way to manage interpersonal conflict, especially if the conflict is between the program head and one of the subordinate staff. Having the staff member report to another staff member instead of the program head can often insulate the two players from each other. For example, if a clinic employee who reports to Sharon is acknowledged by all to be a good and capable professional but this employee has a problem with Sharon's management style, it might be wise to rearrange the reporting relationship so that the employee reports to one of the other partners.

8. Mediation and arbitration. These conflict resolution techniques are the last resort because they involve bringing in a third party from outside the organization to impose binding solutions that both parties may accept but that neither party is likely to desire or feel ownership in. If Sharon and her partners cannot agree on the medical benefits issue, they might submit to a mediation process whereby they would bring a third party, perhaps an attorney or another mediation specialist, into the case. The mediator would listen to all the facts and attempt to lay out a strategy that all the parties could agree to.

Thomas and Kilmann (1974) described five more general approaches to conflict resolution. To help resolve conflicts in the sports medicine unit, athletic trainers could choose one of the following methods.

1. Competition. Competing resolves conflict between two or more members of the sports medicine unit through confrontation. Central to the concept of competition is the notion that one athletic trainer's position power will be imposed to the exclusion of others'. This method is similar to cooperation by edict. In Sharon's case, she was the "winner" and her two partners were the "losers." Sharon was able to exert her will over that of her partners. Unfortunately, the relationship she enjoyed with them then deteriorated.

2. Accommodation. Accommodating involves conceding to the other party in the conflict. The physical therapist and physician in the opening case accommodated Sharon by conceding to her wishes in the matter.

3. Avoidance. Avoiding involves bypassing a conflict to prevent the unpleasant consequences normally associated with confrontation. Unfortunately, this method resolves nothing, and conflict is almost certain to reappear at some point. Avoidance is one of the most frequent methods employed by managers in all kinds of settings. If Sharon had failed to confront her partners she would have been practicing avoidance. The medical insurance question would continue to hound her, but she would maintain the relationship with her partners.

4. Collaboration. Collaborating is the method most likely to result in lasting conflict resolution. With this approach, parties to a conflict attempt to solve the problem together by investigating various possible alternatives. Collaboration requires creative solutions that typically meet the needs of both parties. It would have been ideal if Sharon could have collaborated with her partners to find a creative solution in the opening case. Collaboration becomes difficult, however, once emotions become part of a dispute and positions harden. After Sharon demanded that her partners change the benefits policy, it would have been surprising if the three partners had been able to collaborate on that issue.

5. Compromise. Compromise is similar to collaboration in that it attempts to meet the needs of both parties. The major difference is that compromising resolves the conflict by defining a position somewhere between those of the two parties, whereas collaboration develops new positions previously not considered by either party. Compromise is the result of negotiation. The swap of medical benefits for continuing education mentioned earlier is a good example of the kind of compromise that results from negotiation.

The third decision-making role played by an athletic trainer is **allocator of resources**. The athletic trainer generally has formal authority to determine how time, money, supplies, equipment, and personnel should be deployed. If the athletic trainer-manager does not have this authority, frustration and managerial apathy are likely to result. Sharon's case is a good example. Although she wanted to allocate company funds toward full compensation of the athletic trainers' health insurance costs, she was unable to do so unless her partners granted formal authority. This circumstance frustrated not only Sharon but also the staff athletic trainers.

The final managerial role that an athletic trainer assumes is the role of **negotiator**. The athletic trainer negotiates on behalf of the organization he represents. Thus, the negotiator role is a combination of several roles, including the figurehead, the resource allocator, and the spokesperson (Mintzberg 1973). Although someone closer to the top of the organizational structure usually ratifies most arrangements negotiated by the athletic trainer on behalf of the organization, the athletic trainer must be granted enough authority to enter into meaningful discussions with another party. Typical arrangements negotiated by athletic trainers include prices for supplies and services, sponsorship for various activities, involvement with development and fund-raising efforts, and grants for specific programs.

IMPROVING MANAGERIAL EFFECTIVENESS

Leaders usually, but not always, exercise authority by making legitimate requests. In response, staff might commit, comply, or resist. Athletic trainers can use many methods to decrease the likelihood of resistance and increase the possibility of commitment (Yukl 1981). When making requests of subordinates, athletic trainers should take the following positive steps to ensure commitment.

■ **Be courteous and respectful.** Avoid emphasizing differences in status, intelligence, financial responsibility, and other factors related to rank. If Sharon was having trouble with one of her employees, she would be unlikely to gain that employee's commitment by saying "I'm the boss. You work for me. Do it or else." The employee might comply, but that would be the best Sharon could hope for.

■ **Radiate confidence.** If the leader communicates doubt through verbal or nonverbal cues, the staff is unlikely to comply with enthusiasm. The athletic trainers who came to Sharon for redress of their medical benefits complaint would probably feel better about the situation if Sharon approached the issue with confidence, saying, "Don't worry. I'll get this mess straightened out."

Successful athletic trainer-managers will be able to elicit commitment from their subordinates and coworkers if they are courteous, confident, and open-minded. Athletic trainers must also use simple language, make reasonable requests, and explain their requests. Finally, they must use their authority regularly, especially to confirm task accomplishment.

■ **Use simple language.** When instructions must necessarily be complicated, check to be sure that subordinates understand them. If Sharon is communicating a complex treatment plan to a new staff member, she would do well to use the simplest language possible, ask the staff member to restate the instructions, and check later to make sure that the staff member is carrying out the instructions. Inexperienced leaders often make the mistake of using excessively technical terminology as a way of demonstrating their position power.

■ **Make reasonable requests.** Test requests for legitimacy by consulting with coworkers above you or at the same level in the organization. Referring to formally approved policies, rules, and negotiated agreements can help legitimize requests. Sharon might have strengthened her position with her partners in the opening case if she had taken the time to get some advice on the reasonableness of her position. If she could have referred to formal company documents, such as the employee handbook, she might have been able to make a stronger case.

■ **Provide rationale.** Providing reasons for your request will help reduce the perceived status gap between you and your staff. If Sharon circulates a memo to all clinic staff that informs them that employee parking fees are about to double, she had better explain the reasons for the price increase. If she doesn't, the employees are free to attribute any false motive they can think of to account for the increase. If she does explain the increase, the employees still won't like it, but they have a better chance of understanding it and complying.

■ **Use the chain of command.** Following established lines of communication decreases the possibility of message distortion. Make requests in writing whenever possible. If one of the clinic's employees bypasses her supervisor and takes her concern directly to Sharon, all three parties will be in a difficult position. Sharon and the employee now have information that the supervisor doesn't have. This lack of information will certainly lead to trouble at some point in the future.

■ **Use authority regularly.** If you make legitimate requests regularly, your staff will be less likely to resist. If Sharon continuously backs away from issues that require her to make decisions based on her authority as a partner in the company, her employees will grow accustomed to that mode of decision making. When the day comes that Sharon does exercise her authority, the employees are likely to resent her for doing so.

■ **Exercise authority to confirm task accomplishment.** If you do not demand compliance for legitimate requests, future noncompliance is more likely. If Sharon asks one of her employees to do something, the employee doesn't do it, and Sharon doesn't take any action, all employees will soon figure out that Sharon is a pushover and a weak leader.

■ **Be open-minded.** Staff members who consider their leader a heartless automaton with no concern for their ideas or feelings are unlikely to respond to requests with enthusiasm. If Sharon listens to her employees' concerns with genuine interest and acts on those concerns whenever possible, she is much more likely to gain the trust and respect of those employees.

APPLICATIONS TO ATHLETIC TRAINING: THEORY INTO PRACTICE

The following two case studies will help you apply the concepts in this chapter to situations that you may face in actual practice. The questions at the end of the case studies are open-ended; many correct solutions are possible. A working knowledge of the injury evaluation skills you learned from the Athletic Training Education Series text *Therapeutic Exercise for Athletic Injuries* is especially useful for case study 1.

During the second half of an National Collegiate Athletic Association (NCAA) Division III tournament soccer game, the goalkeeper of the host team was involved in a collision and fell to the ground in pain. Julie Raferty, the school's athletic trainer, evaluated the injury on the field and determined that the goalkeeper, who was unable to run or cut and could walk only with a pronounced limp, had suffered a grade 2 ankle sprain. Julie decided to remove the player from the game based on three factors: The athlete could not perform without significant dysfunction; the team had another game in a few days and the athletic trainer wanted to begin immediate treatment in preparation; and the team was winning the game by two goals and appeared to be in control.

As Julie helped the goalkeeper from the field, the coach jogged out to meet them and asked the athlete how he felt. When he replied that his ankle was injured but not too badly, the coach said it was the athlete's decision whether to keep playing. Julie interjected, telling the coach that she thought further play would jeopardize a rapid recovery. The coach looked again at the athlete and said that the decision was his. The athlete replied that he would try to continue. Julie again tried to express her opposition, but the athlete was already limping back to the goal and the coach was leaving the field.

Julie was confused, upset, and incensed that the coach would usurp her authority in the matter. The athletic department had a medical chain-of-command procedure that clearly authorized the team physician, or the athletic trainer in the physician's absence, to make decisions about playing status for injured athletes. Julie wasn't sure what she could have done to change the outcome.

QUESTIONS FOR ANALYSIS

1. How do the concepts of power and authority apply to this case? Who had power, and how was it used? What was the basis for this power? Who had authority, and how was it used?

2. What might Julie have done differently (either before or during the incident) to avoid the situation?

3. What should Julie do now? Which conflict resolution methods are most appropriate for this case? Is there only one correct solution, or do several possibilities exist?

After interviewing for a job in a large Texas high school, Jim Hoopes, a certified athletic trainer with 17 years of experience, decided he would accept a job offer there. His primary reason for accepting the job was that he was burned out in NCAA Division I athletics. He thought that the high school position would give him contact with athletes, an aspect of his work that he enjoyed, without the headaches of running a major university sports medicine program.

Jim arrived in Texas in June to allow plenty of time to organize his new program before the athletes came back in August. During the first week on the job, Jim began to realize that he should have asked a few questions during his interview. Although the sports medicine program had an adequate budget, Jim could not order any equipment or supplies without written permission of his athletic director. When Jim presented a list of supplies needed for the next year, the AD approved only half the items. In addition, he told Jim that he would have to purchase them from the local sporting goods dealer. Jim complained that he needed all the items on the list and that if he purchased everything from the local vendor, the sports medicine budget would be spent before Christmas.

Another problem Jim faced during the first few weeks concerned a drug and alcohol education program he proposed for student-athletes. Jim wanted to involve all the coaches and team captains in a preliminary workshop and then develop programs for individual teams. When he presented his plan, the AD smiled and said, "That kind of thing has been tried before and it didn't work then. I don't see why it would work now. Besides, we don't have any serious problems like that in our school."

When the athletes arrived in August, Jim quickly gained a reputation as a caring and competent athletic trainer. Injured athletes came to know him as someone who would take good care of them and who could help them return to action as soon as possible. The coaches also appreciated Jim's talents and expertise. They liked the way he communicated with them and appreciated his hard work in keeping their teams healthy.

QUESTIONS FOR ANALYSIS

1. In what ways did the honeymoon effect work for Jim in his new job? In what ways didn't it work?

2. Which of Jim's early leadership actions were transactional? Which were transformational?

3. Which management roles did Jim assume during his first few months on the job? Which were most important in helping him establish relationships with the various groups at his new school?

4. Jim is obviously having trouble working with his new athletic director. Which conflict management strategies should he consider in attempting to work out his differences? Given the personality style of the AD, what are some likely outcomes of Jim's conflict management attempts?

5. If you were in Jim's position, would you have handled anything differently? What alternative actions would you have taken?

SUMMARY

The role of the athletic trainer in a health care arena requires a skill set beyond one that incorporates only a clinical knowledge base. Athletic trainers in all practice settings need to understand the concept of leadership and the principles associated with power and authority. Athletic trainers will often take on managerial-type roles and tasks in the absence of prior formal preparation or training. Strategies that include timely and effective communication, efficiency, and attention to detail can contribute to an athletic trainer's managerial style. Communication is a critical part of ensuring teamwork and productivity. Rapidly changing technology has enhanced the options available for communication. Additionally, interpersonal skills remain important for both verbal and nonverbal human interactions. How one communicates as a leader and a manager can be just as important as the content of the message itself. Being an effective manager and leader also requires the ability to plan, organize, and coordinate multiple tasks simultaneously. Ultimately, an athletic training manager possesses the responsibility for decision making that determines the outcomes of circumstances. Athletic training managers should make such decisions while incorporating a reliable foundational process, taking into considering all stakeholders that would be affected by any managerial decision.

KEY CONCEPTS AND REVIEW

1. Define the concepts of power, authority, and leadership.

Power is the potential to influence. Athletic trainers have two forms of power: personal and position. Authority is that aspect of power, granted to either groups or individuals, that legitimizes the right of the individual or group to make decisions on behalf of others. Leadership is the process of influencing the behavior and attitudes of others to achieve intended outcomes. Leadership takes two forms: transactional and transformational. Transactional leadership involves the exchange of one thing for another between two people in a relationship. It makes up the majority of managerial tasks that athletic trainers perform. Transformational leadership raises the standards of the program or organization through the creative use of conflict and change. It is essential for the ongoing health and development of a sports medicine program.

2. Understand the historical trends in management and how they might apply to athletic training.

At least three distinct trends in management theory occurred in the 20th century. The primary goal of scientific management was to increase productivity. The human relations school of management theory emphasized involving individuals in every level of an organization in decision making for goal accomplishment. Modern management theories include Field Theory, McGregor's Theory X and Theory Y, and Deming's Total Quality Management.

3. Understand the various managerial roles that athletic trainers assume.

Management is the element of the leadership process that involves planning, decision making, and coordinating the activities of a group of people working toward a common goal. Athletic trainers play many managerial roles, which can be generalized into three groups: interpersonal, informational (which includes elements of both verbal and nonverbal communication), and decisional roles.

4. Understand the various strategies that athletic trainers can employ to improve their managerial effectiveness.

Athletic trainers can improve their managerial effectiveness by using nine techniques: making polite requests, making requests in a confident tone, making clear requests, making legitimate requests, explaining the reasons for the request, using proper channels, exercising authority regularly, insisting on compliance, and being responsive to concerns of subordinates.

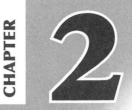

Program Management

▶ Janet Horton arrived at work one morning to find a note on her desk from the director of rehabilitation services requesting her presence at a meeting later that morning. She wasn't sure why the director would want to meet with her. She had been doing a good job since arriving at the hospital two years earlier. Still, she was apprehensive as she walked down the hallway to the meeting.

"Janet," the smiling director said, "you have been doing a fine job here at Memorial Hospital. As the only certified athletic trainer in the department, you are playing an important role in helping us establish our niche in the sports medicine market. Our physically active patients appreciate having an athletic trainer on staff who can work with them during their rehabilitation. I want you to take on a very important project. The hospital administration and I think we need to be more aggressive in marketing our sports medicine program. We want you to begin an outreach program to the three Ashton County high schools to help attract patients to our hospital. School doesn't start for a few months, so you have plenty of time to get organized. Thanks a lot and keep up the good work."

Janet had mixed emotions about the new assignment. On one hand, she was pleased that the director trusted her with this new responsibility. On the other hand, she had no experience with community outreach programs. She didn't know where to begin.

The best is the enemy of the good.

—VOLTAIRE

The predicament Janet finds herself in is a common one, because all organizations change over time. Whether you are employed in a high school, college, professional, industrial, corporate, or clinical setting, you are bound to face organizational changes at some point in your career. These changes force us to examine our sports medicine programs from time to time to see if they are still consistent with both the needs of our clients and the mission of the institution that employs us. The concepts discussed in this chapter will help athletic trainers plan, implement, and evaluate sports medicine programs, as well as make the necessary and timely changes required to effectively manage a program.

VISION STATEMENTS

The first step an athletic trainer must take when planning sports medicine programming is to develop a brief, succinct description of what the program should eventually become—a **vision statement**. The vision statement should be both ambitious and compelling (Block 1987). It should spell out the athletic trainer's hopes and aspirations for the program. For her community outreach program, Janet might consider a vision statement that looks like this:

> The Memorial Hospital Sports Medicine Outreach Program shall provide injury prevention, care, and rehabilitation services of recognized excellence to the high school students of Ashton County. Memorial Hospital is committed to becoming the leader in sports medicine services in the Ashton County area.

The vision statement contains four distinct elements. First, the statement identifies the provider of the service: Memorial Hospital. Second, it identifies the service to be provided: injury prevention, care, and rehabilitation. Third, it identifies the target clients: the high school students of Ashton County. Finally, the statement includes a quality declaration that identifies aspirations for how internal and external audiences will receive the program. Although these elements might seem self-evident, they are important because of the way they function in

A vision statement is the first step in planning for a new sports medicine program or the improvement of an existing one.

the next step—the mission statement. The vision statement should become the ultimate standard by which the program is judged. Without a clearly articulated vision statement, developing the program mission and evaluating the effectiveness of the program become much more difficult. As programs evolve over time, managers must consider modifying the goals associated with the program's vision statement, or in some cases changing the vision statement to adapt to necessary changes in the program.

> ### ■ Four Elements of the Sports Medicine Program Vision Statement
>
> 1. Name of the service provider
> 2. Description of the service to be provided
> 3. Identification of the target clients
> 4. Quality declaration

MISSION STATEMENTS

After the athletic trainer has explored and identified her vision for the sports medicine program, she should expand on this vision and create a mission statement. Pearce (1982) has defined the **mission statement** as "a broadly defined but enduring statement of purpose that distinguishes a business from other firms of its type and identifies the scope of its operations in product and market terms." Gibson, Newton, and Cochran (1990) have suggested the following components of a mission statement. Adapted for a sports medicine program, they include

- the particular services to be offered, the primary market for those services, and the technology to be used in delivery of the services;
- the goals of the program;
- the philosophy of the program and the code of behavior that applies to its operation;
- the "self-concept" of the program based on evaluation of strengths and weaknesses; and
- the desired program image based on feedback from internal and external stakeholders.

The mission statement for a sports medicine program should help an athletic trainer accomplish three things (Gibson, Newton, and Cochran 1990). First, the mission statement should help the athletic trainer direct resources toward accomplishing specific tasks. This aspect is especially important because athletic trainers are often called on to perform a variety of tasks for a divergent group of supervisors. Athletic trainers need a framework within which they can make decisions about the relative importance of one task versus another.

The second function of the successful mission statement is to inspire athletic trainers to do a good job. The mission statement should communicate that the work they do is important and needed. The athletic trainer should believe in the precepts described in the mission statement. Want (1986) has suggested that successful mission statements help employees, including athletic trainers, understand the values and beliefs of the organization and thereby help establish employee commitment.

Finally, the mission statement should be action oriented and should stimulate a change in behavior. The statement should require the formation of program goals and objectives. Ideally, it should challenge the athletic trainer to conduct a periodic evaluation of the effectiveness of the sports medicine program.

Based on these principles, the mission statement for the Memorial Hospital Sports Medicine Outreach Program might read as follows:

> The Memorial Hospital Sports Medicine Outreach Program delivers traditional athletic training and sports medicine services to the student-athletes of the three high schools located in Ashton County. The services that we will deliver are of three primary types: injury prevention (taping, bracing, padding, orthotics construction), management of athletic injuries, and rehabilitation of athletic injuries. In addition, whenever possible, we will strive to integrate education about athletic injuries so that our clients can learn to lead healthier, injury-free lives. We are committed to

The mission statement of the sports medicine program should serve as a blueprint for every program activity and service. The statement should be comprehensive enough to describe the program but simple enough that everyone knows it well.

using whatever technology is available and affordable in the delivery of these services. We will remain committed to the continuous upgrading of the equipment used in the delivery of sports medicine services so that our clients will receive the most modern care available in the area.

The purpose of the program is fourfold. First, we hope to allow easy access to sports medicine services for high school student-athletes. Second, we hope to encourage a philosophy of sport that places a high value on health and wellness. Third, we hope to enable injured student-athletes to return to their sports as soon as is medically safe. Finally, we hope to achieve a substantial reduction in the risk of athletic injury for high school students in our service area.

The underlying philosophy for the outreach program is the same as that for all other programs of Memorial Hospital; that is, the needs of the patient shall always be the first consideration for all members of the hospital staff. Furthermore, we expect the athletic trainers who will be providing these services to maintain the highest standards of quality consistent with the National Athletic Trainers' Association Code of Professional Practice and the credentialing statutes of this state.

We are committed to ongoing evaluation of our outreach program so that our clients can be assured of the highest quality in sports medicine care. Furthermore, we are committed to addressing problems and concerns in a timely manner so that we can continue to meet the needs of our clients and employees.

Finally, the Memorial Hospital Sports Medicine Outreach Program aspires to be a program of recognized excellence. We intend to support the program with the human and financial resources necessary to accomplish the stated goals of the program. We desire to establish Memorial Hospital as the primary and most outstanding outlet for the delivery of sports medicine services in the area.

PLANNING

The athletic trainer has long been thought of as a jack-of-all-trades. Although athletic trainers' roles have become more specialized since sports medicine clinics began in the late 1970s, most athletic trainers still handle a variety of job-related activities (see figure 2.1). Because the athletic trainer's job has so many aspects, he must develop planning skills.

Planning is an athletic trainer's best hope for accomplishing sports medicine program goals. Without planning, she leaves the ultimate success or failure of the sports medicine program to chance (Castetter 1986). Ackoff (1970) has defined the planning process as a special type of decision making with three characteristics: It takes place before any action occurs; it is needed to produce a future state that would be unlikely to occur without action; and the desired future state results from multiple, interdependent decisions.

The Memorial Hospital case illustrates the need for careful sports medicine program planning. The hospital administration has placed the bulk of the planning responsibility in Janet's lap. The plan she develops, if adopted by the hospital administration, will eventually determine whether the program succeeds or fails. To plan effectively, Janet should break the task into its two component parts: strategic planning and operational planning.

Strategic Planning

Strategic planning is a process that identifies a course of action to be taken to bring about a future state of affairs. Although those at the top of an organizational structure usually conduct it, strategic planning at the program level can have many benefits.

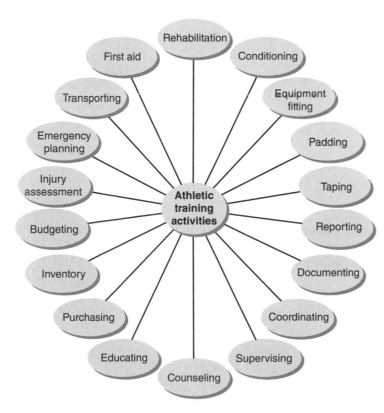

▶ **Figure 2.1** Job-related activities of the athletic trainer.

First, strategic planning requires an athletic trainer to examine the sports medicine program and ask two questions: Why does this program exist? What should the business of this program be? These questions are fundamentally important. Because all organizations and their programs change, the questions must be asked and answered regularly, or athletic trainers might find that their sports medicine programs no longer serve the purposes for which they are most needed.

The second reason for ongoing strategic planning at the sports medicine program level is to determine whether the program is consistent with the overall mission of the institution or organization. This issue is especially important in institutions or organizations subject to rapid change. Sports medicine clinics based in hospitals are especially vulnerable to the shifting missions of their institutions. The mission of a professional athletic team often changes dramatically when a new coach is hired. If the sports medicine program isn't periodically reviewed for mission congruence, problems will arise because the administration might view the purpose of the sports medicine program differently than the athletic trainer does.

The third reason for strategic planning at the sports medicine program level is that it helps build support for the program. Strategic planning is, by definition, a process that involves persons at all levels of the organization. By asking students, staff athletic trainers, coaches, clients, and administrators to take part in the strategic planning process, an athletic trainer will be forging important allies with an increased sense of ownership in the sports medicine program. Furthermore, input from stakeholders can provide a breadth of knowledge compiled from an external perspective that may be overlooked by those directing and implementing a program.

Finally, strategic planning should be a tool for improvement, helping to determine the relative strengths and weaknesses of the program and to transform it positively. In addition, the strategic planning process will help direct operational plans that are more action oriented. Proponents of strategic planning suggest incorporating a strategic planning process that is performed regularly (at least every few years) and involves input from all stakeholders. Some organizations make the mistake of performing a strategic planning process only in the wake of adverse experiences or concerns.

Many conceptual models could be used to develop a strategic plan for the sports medicine program. The model presented in figure 2.2 adapts the process developed by Steiner (1979), but athletic trainers should further modify the methodology to meet the needs of their institutions. In most cases, the combination of institutional mission, needs, and goals will help determine the most appropriate planning methods.

Athletic trainers must do two kinds of planning to help their programs fulfill their mission: strategic and operational. Both are essential if a sports medicine program is to be successful.

Major Outside Interests

The first groups whose interests must be considered when it comes to developing a strategic plan are those outside the institution or organization. Of these groups, the interests of clients should take precedence. Other important interests include those of parents; the local community; vendors; professional associations like the National Athletic Trainers' Association (NATA) and the National Collegiate Athletic Association (NCAA); and local, state, and federal governments. Professionals who manage athletic training education programs must be familiar with the Board of Certification (BOC) requirements and the standards of athletic training education accrediting bodies. In some cases, an athletic trainer will need only simple information

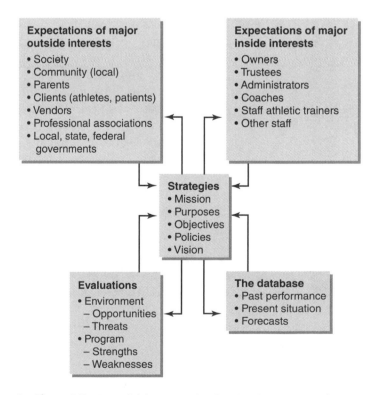

▶ **Figure 2.2** A model for strategic planning in sports medicine.
Adapted with the permission of The Free Press, a Division of Simon & Schuster, Inc., from STRATEGIC PLANNING: What every manager must know by George A. Steiner. Copyright © 1979 by The Free Press.

from one of these groups. For example, if a program is in a state that monitors the credentials of athletic trainers, it is obvious that the program will need to be staffed by athletic trainers with the credentials required by law. Conversely, some of the information that the athletic trainer will need to develop the strategic plan might be more difficult to gather. For example, as important vendors of medical services, local physicians might have a substantial interest in how the sports medicine program is planned. Only by meeting with those physicians and involving them in the planning process can an athletic trainer be assured of their enthusiastic endorsement of the program being planned.

Major professional associations and the government are two important sources of information for assessing what outside interests are necessary to develop the strategic plan for the sports medicine program. Professional associations such as the NATA, the NCAA, and the National Federation of State High School Athletic Associations (NFSH) are important because they are often the source of professional credentials that act as "gatekeepers" for practitioners in sports medicine and they mandate quality standards for sports medicine programs. The NCAA and the NFSH set the rules for each sport, including safety rules that affect athletic trainers and sports medicine programs. Both of these organizations have rules for administering physical examinations that have a marked effect on sports medicine programs.

Clients   The most important group in the strategic planning process is the program's client base. Without patients, athletic trainers and sports medicine programs would be unnecessary. The athletic trainer can incorporate clients' perceptions into the strategic planning process in several ways, including the use of written questionnaires, telephone surveys, and suggestion boxes.

If the athletic trainer needs detailed insight, it might be necessary to involve clients as members of planning committees. Another method for securing detailed feedback from clients on the quality of services and their desire for future services is the focus group technique. This technique involves gathering a group of approximately 10 clients who are representative of the total population of clients. A trained facilitator meets with the group and asks a series of open-ended questions about program quality and the clients' desires for the future. This process is generally repeated with several different groups as a reliability check. The information is then collated and used to help build the strategic plan.

Gathering valid and reliable information from clients is not a task for the untrained. The literature is full of poorly written and poorly analyzed client-based questionnaires. Sampling methods and statistical analysis of the data must meet modern scientific norms. Athletic trainers can turn to several sources of assistance for this phase of the strategic plan. Most colleges and universities have faculty members with expertise in social science research who are willing to consult. Many larger educational institutions have full-time planners available to assist with projects like these. Most large hospitals have either full-time planners or contracts with management consultants to help in the development of the strategic plan. The skill set required to adequately and appropriately collect reliable, valid, and valuable data should not be overlooked. One should be prepared to budget for potential consulting fees if the services of external reviewers or even internal faculty members are used. In any case, the amount of money budgeted on the front end may be well worth the investment as compared to the potential costs associated with less than helpful data compiled as the result of inexperienced planning.

Accreditation   Among the most important outside interests a sports medicine program must consider is standards-setting groups that provide health care organizations or their programs with **accreditation**. Accreditation

Contact the Board of Certification at www.bocatc.org/. For information on accreditation of athletic training education programs, visit the Commission on Accreditation of Athletic Training Education at www.caate.net.

■ Methods for Gathering Feedback From Clients on Sports Medicine Services

- Written questionnaires
- Web-based surveys
- Telephone surveys
- Suggestion boxes
- Involvement on planning committees
- Focus groups
- Exit interviews

is a statement by a standards-setting organization that the sports medicine program meets certain performance standards. Although athletic training service programs associated with high schools, colleges, and universities are generally not accredited (except as part of their institution's overall accreditation by one of the regional educational accrediting agencies), sports medicine programs housed in clinics and hospitals will be subject to the scrutiny of the accreditation process typically associated with those settings. Accreditation is usually voluntary, but strong incentives for a health care organization to become accredited are often in place. In some cases, the state license that an organization needs to operate is dependent on its accreditation status. Access to third-party reimbursement and managed care contracts is often easier if a health care organization is accredited by an appropriate standards-setting body.

Although the process for obtaining accreditation is similar for most standards-setting bodies (see the later section on program evaluation), the important element to remember during the strategic planning process is to build the goals, programs, and practices of the sports medicine program with accreditation standards in mind. Be aware that accreditation standards are usually minimalist in design. In other words, a particular standard usually describes the absolute minimum level of performance the sports medicine unit must achieve to satisfy the requirements of the standard. The danger in building a program around the accreditation standards is that the program might do things well, but at a minimally acceptable level. If outstanding performance is the goal, athletic trainers will have to look well beyond the minimal requirements of most accreditation standards. Those who plan clinic- and hospital-based sports medicine programs should consult two important accrediting agencies: the **Joint Commission on Accreditation of Healthcare Organizations (JCAHO)** and the **Commission on Accreditation of Rehabilitation Facilities (CARF)**.

> For more information about JCAHO programs, write to the Joint Commission on Accreditation of Healthcare Organizations. The JCAHO website address is www.jcaho.org.

The JCAHO is the oldest and largest health care standards-setting body in the nation. It accredits approximately 15,000 health care organizations in the United States and has offered accreditation for ambulatory care facilities, including hospital-based and independent rehabilitation clinics, since 1975. Advantages of JCAHO accreditation include the following:

1. Provides objective evaluation of the program's performance

2. Stimulates quality improvement

3. Enhances community confidence

4. Helps meet Medicare certification requirements

5. Enhances access to third-party reimbursement

6. Helps meet facility licensing requirements

Another accreditation agency that athletic trainers who work in clinics and hospitals should consider as they plan their programs is the Commission on Accreditation of Rehabilitation Facilities. CARF is a nonprofit agency that establishes standards of quality for rehabilitation services. Established in 1966, CARF accredits approximately 38,000 programs. The agency offers accreditation for organizations that typically house sports medicine programs through its Medical Rehabilitation Division. Accreditation by CARF is intended to

1. offer consumer protection and enhance consumer confidence,

2. involve consumers in developing standards for rehabilitation,

3. promulgate common performance standards for rehabilitation programs,

4. identify rehabilitation programs that have met national performance standards,

5. improve government relations with the rehabilitation industry by offering evidence of effective use of public money for rehabilitation purposes, and

6. provide rehabilitation facilities with tools for improvement.

> For more information, write to the Commission on Accreditation of Rehabilitation Facilities. The CARF website address is www.carf.org.

Major Inside Interests

Athletic trainers are not typically found (but are becoming more common) among the top management of an institution or organization. Top managers, including team owners, university administrators and trustees, and boards of education have certain expectations for the sports medicine program, so it is important that the athletic trainer involve a representative sample of these persons as part of the planning team. Without the active support of these groups, the strategic plan for the sports medicine program is likely to fail. Consider the Memorial Hospital case as an example. The director of rehabilitation services asked Janet to plan the sports medicine outreach program by herself. Janet knows two things: First, at least a few, and possibly more, hospital administrators support the program; and second, she isn't sure which direction the program should take. The next logical step for Janet is to identify those administrators who support the concept and include them in the planning process. This approach will have two likely effects: It will strengthen ownership for the program among the people who will eventually have to approve or disapprove it, and it will provide Janet with some fresh ideas about the type of program the hospital wants.

Coaches make up another major inside group. Including coaches in the planning effort is wise, because they have a legitimate need to be involved in, or at least informed about, the health care of their athletes. The success of the team and their success as coaches often depend on the overall health of their athletes. In addition, coaches have a powerful influence on the attitudes and behaviors of the athletes on their teams. If the coaches in the three Ashton County high schools don't have confidence in the expertise and care patterns that Janet will offer them through the outreach program, they are unlikely to be receptive to the advice she offers, and Memorial Hospital is unlikely to receive many referrals. Janet is the hospital's primary marketing tool to these schools, and most of her contacts will be with students and coaches. The final reason coaches should be involved in the planning process is that they are an important power base in any athletic program. A successful coach can become one of the most powerful people in the entire organization. Using such power to build alliances with the sports medicine program makes sense.

The most important inside group to tap in developing the strategic plan is the institution's athletic trainers. They are the professionals inside the organization with the most sports medicine expertise. As such, they are the best sources of information about how to develop the program, but they must be involved in the proper manner. Too often, meetings intended to develop strategic directions for sports medicine programs can become complaining sessions about problems with working conditions, salary, and professional standing in the institution. These issues are important, but if they become the focus of the athletic trainers' roles in the strategic planning process, the resulting plan will be little more than a shopping list of their demands—an outcome that is unlikely to foster administration support or improved care for injured athletes and other physically active patients. Athletic trainers must constantly ask themselves during the planning process, "How can we improve the quality of service to our patients?" Questions that deviate significantly from this are unlikely to have strategic value.

One method of appealing to inside-interest stakeholders is to present information comparing your own sports medicine program to peer sports medicine programs. Peer institutions can be defined in a number of ways. They may be similar to your program in geographical location, thus drawing from a similar clientele. They may be in a different geographical location but serve the same type of client population that your program serves. They may also have a facility similar to yours in size or even care for similar total numbers of athletes and teams. By providing a comparative analysis showing how your organization stacks up against peers, you can often present a compelling case for your program's growth and development. One word of caution: You should be prepared to find that your program fares better than its peers in some categories. While it is a benefit to be aware of such findings and this may even be a positive attribute for internal stakeholders to know about, such information may be interpreted by upper level management as potential reasons not to further invest in your growth.

Benchmarking is the term used to associate a recognized comparison of one's own program to the best in the industry. Different aspects of services, outcomes, and deliverables can be measured in terms of metrics and used to assess a program's overall performance level as well as components of the program. As a result, improvements can be made related to quality of care, timely delivery of services, and perhaps cost savings. Historically, benchmarking for the athletic training profession has been accomplished through informal networking among colleagues. In the future, more formal approaches should be considered to justify athletic training services, outcomes, and costs in the health care arena.

The Database

This portion of the strategic planning model helps athletic trainers devise alternative action plans and estimate their potential value for meeting the goals of the sports medicine program. First, the past performance of the program is analyzed; and trends in patient loads, injury rates, clinic profits or losses, and athletic trainer performance evaluations are considered, along with other information. Next, the program's present situation is analyzed. Data about staffing levels, budget, client population size, number of sports to be served, demands and expectations of outside and inside interests, and any applicable laws that affect the program will be needed. Finally, a forecast for the future is developed. Ammer and Ammer (1984) have defined the term **forecast** as a process of predicting future conditions based on various statistics and indicators that describe the past and present situations. Forecasts are highly informed and educated guesses that should always be backed up with documented evidence. Athletic trainers should consider the predicted rise in the cost of medical goods and services and the future availability of professional staff, support employees, and consulting medical personnel when preparing the forecast. In addition, they should consider advances in technology, because the available technology often drives the practice of sports medicine.

WOTS UP Analysis

The last data collection procedure to be accomplished in the strategic planning process is often referred to as a **WOTS UP analysis** (Steiner 1979). WOTS UP is an acronym for "weaknesses, opportunities, threats, and strengths underlying planning." Because the WOTS UP analysis identifies strengths and weaknesses already present in the sports medicine program, it is most appropriate for programs that are already established (see appendix A). A broad spectrum of participants should conduct the WOTS UP analysis. Interpretation of the data is subject to the biases of the interpreter, so only the involvement of a representative group of both outside and inside interests will yield useful results.

The WOTS UP analysis often reveals important sources of both opportunities and threats for the sports medicine program. In the Memorial Hospital case, a WOTS UP analysis would probably help Janet identify allies she might not have previously considered; many will have a stake in seeing the program succeed. She would also undoubtedly identify sources of opposition to the program that she would need to develop plans to deal with. Many of the techniques used in this strategic planning process can be interchanged with those used in the process of program evaluation. See the section on program evaluation (pp. 56-67) for more information. A WOTS UP analysis has also been referred to as a SWOT analysis, representing the same categories of assessment.

Operational Planning

After developing a strategic direction for the sports medicine program, an athletic trainer must translate the strategies into practice through use of **operational plans.** Whereas strategic plans are meant to provide program direction over a long period, say five years, operational plans define the activities of the program for a much shorter period, usually no more than one or two years. The importance of functioning operational plans for the sports medicine program should not be underestimated. One of the most common pitfalls in every type of organization that undertakes strategic planning is the failure to effectively translate the strategic vision for the program into workable, useful operational plans (Garofalo 1989). Three often misunderstood types of operational plans are policies, processes, and procedures.

Policies

Castetter (1986) has defined **policy** as a plan for expressing the organization's intended behavior relative to a specific program subfunction. By definition, policies are broad statements of intended action promulgated by boards empowered with the authority to govern the operation of the organization.

Policies are not intended to answer detailed questions about how the sports medicine program operates. They are intended as road maps to guide an athletic trainer in developing and operating a sports medicine program in accordance with the desires of the policy board. Athletic trainers will rarely be empowered to dictate policies unless they sit on the governing boards of institutions. They should, however, be consulted in the development or modification of institutional policies that affect the sports medicine program. A well-managed organization with a sports medicine program should have policies in place that express the intended behaviors of the program. The athletic trainer is obviously a crucial ingredient in advising those in authority on the development and implementation of these policies. An example of a policy statement for the Memorial Hospital Sports Medicine Outreach Program might look like the statement below.

Processes

Processes are the next step down from policies on the hierarchy of operational plans. **Processes** are the incremental and mutually dependent steps that direct the most important tasks of the sports medicine program. Each process should relate to at least one, and possibly many, of the policies that govern the program. Each policy will undoubtedly have several supporting processes.

■ Sample Policy Statement

Memorial Hospital acknowledges its role in the following activities:

- Reducing the incidence of injury among high school student-athletes
- Making competent medical care readily and easily available to the student-athletes of Ashton County

In addition, Memorial Hospital recognizes that a program delivering sports medicine services to the three high schools of Ashton County will help it fulfill its mission to be the leader in sports medicine in the Ashton County area. Consequently, the Board of Trustees of Memorial Hospital has established the following policies:

1.0 Provide sports medicine services at the site of athletic practice and competition for the three Ashton County high schools.

1.1 Provide sports medicine coverage using only personnel who have been trained and credentialed as experts in sports medicine, including certified athletic trainers.

1.2 Maintain an injury database to determine the risk of injury to athletic participants.

1.3 Provide hospital-based management of injuries requiring follow-up care.

1.4 Provide education on the prevention of injuries and the development of healthy lifestyles to the students of the three Ashton County high schools.

1.5 Assist in the prevention of athletic injuries by providing physical examinations and screening services for the students of the three Ashton County high schools.

Procedures

Procedures provide specific interpretations of processes for athletic trainers and other members of the sports medicine team. They are not abstract. They should be written in clear and simple language so that different people will interpret them in the same way. Procedures are the lowest level of the planning hierarchy. An example of how policies, processes, and procedures are linked for the Memorial Hospital program is provided below.

Practices

Even the most well-considered procedure often leaves room for an athletic trainer to make professional judgments about how to handle particular administrative tasks. The ways in which administrative tasks are actually accomplished are known as **practices**. Practices should never contradict the directions provided for in the procedure they are intended to support. For example, a sports medicine clinic might have a written procedure requiring that all therapeutic modalities be calibrated and safety inspected once per year. This sound procedure is consistent with professional standards. The athletic trainer-administrator still has several decisions to make. Which vendor will he contact to service the equipment? What time of the year will he choose to have the equipment serviced? Should he send all the equipment out at once, send half of the inventory at one time, or stagger the schedule for each piece of equipment? The decisions he makes are examples of practices. Practices are important because they allow the athletic trainer to make decisions based on changing conditions without violating the letter or spirit of the policies and procedures manual.

The sports medicine program should assess its practices from time to time for congruence and conformity to the procedures they support. In addition, the practices in the sports medicine program must be consistent with professional standards and state and federal laws. For example, sports medicine programs operating in NCAA colleges and universities must use practices consistent with the guidelines included in the *NCAA Sports Medicine Handbook.*

■ Processes of the Sports Medicine Program

- Injury prevention
- Injury recognition
- Injury management
- Injury rehabilitation
- Organization and administration
- Education and counseling

■ Linking Policies, Processes, and Procedures

Policy 1.0

The policy of Memorial Hospital is to provide sports medicine services at the site of athletic practice and competition for the three Ashton County high schools.

Process for the Injury Rehabilitation Subfunction

The sports medicine team, including the physician, athletic trainer, and physical therapist, shall work together to provide student-athletes with a rehabilitation program appropriate for their injuries. Consideration will be given to the location of the rehabilitation program (home, school, or hospital), the equipment required to attain the desired rehabilitative effect, the insurance coverage provided by the student's family, and the insurance coverage provided by the school.

Procedure for Discharge From Rehabilitation

Physical therapists or athletic trainers shall discharge student-athletes from rehabilitation only after consulting with the attending physician. Discharge shall occur when the critical long-term goals, established when the student-athlete was admitted, have been met. All discharged student-athletes shall be given oral and written instructions in the long-term care of their injuries. The names of all discharged student-athletes shall be placed on the mailing list for the Memorial Hospital Sports Medicine Newsletter. All discharged student-athletes shall be called at both six months and one year postdischarge by an athletic trainer to check on the status of their injuries.

Policies, processes, and procedures are usually communicated to employees in the form of a policies and procedures handbook. This document is important. Not only does it educate employees regarding the procedures they are to follow; it also serves as a legal foundation for action if they do not. Poorly written or incomplete procedure handbooks are frequently the basis for employee action against employers because they are often viewed as a kind of contract. It is important to ensure that all parties held accountable for the policies and procedures not only are provided with and asked to read the handbook, but also are asked to sign a document stating that they have in fact read all of the information, understand the policies and procedures, and agree to abide by them.

Large organizations, such as hospitals and universities, commonly have more than one handbook. One contains all of the organization's policies (remember that policies are statements passed by the board in control of the organization). Another contains procedures intended to apply to all employees of the organization, regardless of which department employs them. Human resources procedures are typically codified in procedure manuals of this type (see figure 2.3). The last kind of manual contains procedures specific to a certain subunit or department of an organization. It typically includes procedures that apply only to the kinds of activities that take place in that department. See figure 2.4 for an example of such a manual for a hospital-owned orthopedic and sports medicine clinic. The boxes on pages 33 and 35 contain examples of procedures drawn from two different settings: a dress code from a university sports medicine program and a 10-hour work-shift procedure from a sports medicine clinic.

Topics on Which the NCAA Has Issued Sports Medicine Guidelines

For the most recent versions of these guidelines, see the *NCAA Sports Medicine Handbook* at www.ncaapublications.com.

- Sports Medicine Administration
- Medical Evaluations, Immunizations and Records
- Dispensing Prescription Medication
- Lightning Safety
- NCAA Alcohol, Tobacco and Other Drug Education Guidelines
- Emergency Care and Coverage
- Medical Disqualification of the Student-Athlete
- Skin Infections in Athletics
- Prevention of Heat Illness
- Assessment of Body Composition
- Nutrition and Athletic Performance
- Nontherapeutic Drugs
- Nutritional Ergogenic Aids
- Menstrual Cycle Dysfunction
- Weight Loss—Dehydration
- Blood-Borne Pathogens and Intercollegiate Athletics
- The Use of Local Anesthetics in College Athletics
- The Use of Injectable Corticosteriods in Sports Injuries

- Cold Stress and Cold Exposure
- "Burners" (Brachial Plexus Injuries)
- Concussion or Mild Traumatic Brain Injury (mTBI) in the Athlete
- Participation by Student-Athlete with Impairment
- Pregnancy in the Student-Athlete
- The Student-Athlete With Sickle Cell Trait
- Protective Equipment
- Eye Safety in Sports
- Use of Trampoline and Minitramp
- Mouth Guards
- Use of the Head as a Weapon in Football and Other Contact Sports
- Guidelines for Helmet Fitting and Removal in Athletics
- Catastrophic Incident in Athletics
- Dietary Supplements
- Depression: Interventions for Intercollegiate Athletics
- NCAA Legislation Involving Health and Safety Issues
- NCAA Injury Surveillance System
- Summary
- Banned Drug-Classes

Contents

Procedure Title

Absences, Excused
Absences/Tardiness, Unscheduled
Adoption Assistance
Awards Dinner
Benefit Accrual Hours
Bereavement
Bulletin Boards
Cardiopulmonary Resuscitation (CPR)
Certification
Call-In Compensation, Standby and Emergency
Confidential Information
Confidentiality of Information on Computer Systems
Counseling, Corrective Action
Credit Union
Death in Family
Disability Insurance
Dismissal
Dress Code/Personal Appearance
Dual Relationships between Hospital Employees and Patients
Educational Assistance
Employee Assistance Program
Equal Opportunity
Family and Medical Leave, Unpaid
Fair Treatment
Flexible Staffing
Floating Holiday Time
Gifts and Tips
Health Requirements and Services for Employees
Holidays
Insurance, Life
Insurance, Supplemental Life
Introductory Employees
Job Posting
Jury Duty
Laser Image Identification Badges
Lay-Off Procedure
Leave of Absence
New Employee Orientation
Overtime, Rest and Meal Periods
Paid Time Off
Part-Time Employees
Patient Care, Staff Requests Not to Participate in Aspects of
Pay, Shift and Weekend Premium
Payroll Check Distribution
Payroll Deductions
Performance Reviews
Preemployment Alcohol/Drug Screening
Promotion Guidelines
Recruitment Cash Bonus
Relatives, Employment of
Resignations
Retirement
Seniority
Sexual Harassment
Social Security
Solicitation and Distribution of Literature
Staffing, Supplemental
Time Clocks
Vacation
Weapons
Work Schedule
Workers' Compensation
Workers' Compensation Supplement

▶ **Figure 2.3** Table of contents for a human resource procedures manual for a midsize not-for-profit hospital.
Adapted, by permission, from *Human Resources Procedures Manual,* Holland Community Hospital, Holland, MI.

Dress Code Procedure

All members of the university sports medicine staff shall be professionally attired at all times during their work shift. Staff members and students shall wear a university-approved name badge at all times when on duty. The first badge shall be provided at university expense. The cost of replacement badges is the responsibility of the staff member. Athletic trainers (staff and students) shall wear a uniform shirt approved by the head athletic trainer while on duty. Each staff member will receive two uniform shirts per year. Additional uniform shirts are the responsibility of the staff member. All staff members shall wear a uniform jacket when covering outdoor events during cool weather. The jackets are the property of the university and may be checked out from the clothing locker in the main athletic training room storage room. The following clothing is prohibited at all times, regardless of setting:

- Blue jeans
- Sweatshirts
- Unkempt clothing
- Clothing with holes

Questions regarding this procedure should be directed to the head athletic trainer.

Contents

AUTHORIZATION AND INTAKE

Medical supervision of rehabilitation services

Receiving and processing referrals for rehabilitation services

Prior authorization

Reimbursement

Intake process

DOCUMENTATION AND COMMUNICATION

Communicating the status of the hospital outpatient

Communicating the physical therapy ambulatory and transfer needs of the hospital patient with nursing and other ancillary services

Communicating the status of patients seen under contract

RECORD KEEPING

Patient records—The patient folder

Department records

PATIENT CARE

Assignment of patients

Outpatient registration

Patient scheduling

Priority of care for hospital patients

Dispensing of crutches, braces, and other patient care items

Broken appointments and cancellations

Discharge planning for rehabilitation patients

Quality assurance

Home visit program

Participation of the patient/family in the treatment plan

Assessments of patients

Orientation

Initial assessment

Case management—Neurorehabilitation

Initial team meeting

Individual program plan

Therapeutic progress report

Client referral

Follow-up

Waiting list

Physical aggressive behavior and self-injurious behavior

Recipient rights

Peer review

Input from persons served

Outcomes

Accessibility

Education of clients/care givers regarding universal precautions/infection control

Nonvoluntary discharge

DEPARTMENT MANAGEMENT

Hours of operation

Charging for services

Preventative maintenance

Approval process for new and revised procedures

Pricing for patient charge items

Ordering supplies and equipment

Authorizing/training of vehicle operators

Maintenance/inspection of van

Handling vehicle incidents/accidents

Access to outpatient rehabilitation

Utility management

Robbery emergency plan

Hostage crisis plan

PERSONNEL

Flexible staffing

Dress code

Time, mileage, and productivity logging

Orientation

Continuing education

Comp time for professional salaried exempt employees

Vacations and leaves of absence

Ten-hour shift option

Rehabilitation department staffing

Therapist staffing pool

Verification of credentials

SAFETY

Handling incidents

Handling patient arrests

General safety rules

Emergency plan

Power failure

INFECTION CONTROL

Personnel policies—General information

Contract personnel policies

Three-minute surgical scrub

Debridement

Linen disposal

Wound cultures

Dressing removal

Burn patient management

Special handling of physical therapy equipment

Isolation patients receiving whirlpool

Reusable sterile supplies, Care and storage of

Disposable sterile supplies, Care and storage of

Disinfection of whirlpool tanks

Departmental routine cleaning

Routine cleaning by Environmental Services

Disinfection of bandage scissors

Disinfection of hyperbaric extremity chamber

Treatment protocol for hyperbaric chamber

Management of catheterized hydrotherapy patients

Fluidotherapy

PHYSICAL THERAPY

BAPS

Biofeedback

Compression—Jobst pump

Compression—Wright linear pump

Conditioning—Treadmill

Contrast bath

CPM

Cryotherapy—Cold packs

Diathermy

Electrical stimulation—High voltage

Electrical stimulation—Low voltage

Electrical stimulation—Medium frequency

Electrical stimulation—MENS

Electrical stimulation—TENS

Fluoromethane spray

Gait training

Hot packs

Hydrotherapy—Hubbard tank and whirlpool

Hyperbaric oxygen unit

Hyperstimulation analgesia with pulsed IR laser

Isokinetic testing

Massage

Myofascial release

Paraffin bath

Phonophoresis

ROM splint fitting

Traction—Cervical, manual

Traction—Cervical, motorized

Tilt table

Ultrasound

▶ **Figure 2.4** Table of contents for a procedures manual for a hospital-owned orthopedic and sport medicine clinic.

Adapted, by permission, from *Rehabilitation Services Procedure Manual*, Holland Community Hospital, Holland, MI.

Ten-Hour Work-Shift Procedure

Memorial Hospital offers its employees the option of working either five 8-hour shifts per week or four 10-hour shifts per week. Because each department can accommodate only a certain percentage of its employees on a 10-hour shift, each employee is required to apply for this privilege with his or her supervisor. Interested employees should complete the "Request for 10-Hour Shift" form and submit it to their supervisor. The supervisor shall make every reasonable effort to accommodate the employee's request, consistent with the need to keep the department adequately staffed at all times. The supervisor shall respond in writing to the employee's request within 10 days. Supervisors are instructed to consider the following elements when deciding if an employee should be granted 10-hour shift status:

- The minimum number of employees required to service patients during peak, minimal, and average loads
- The minimum number of employees required to implement the department's emergency plan
- The degree to which the employee requires supervision consistent with hospital policy and state law
- The number of employees already granted 10-hour work-shift status; the number of such employees should not normally exceed 25%

Employees who have questions regarding this procedure should consult with their supervisors.

Other Types of Operational Plans

Policies, processes, and procedures are types of operational plans common to almost every organization. They should be reviewed and modified as appropriate at least once every three years. Other types of operational plans have fixed life spans. Budgets are a type of operational plan that are usually one year in length. (See chapter 4 for an expanded discussion of budgets.) Two additional planning techniques that result in fixed-term operational plans are program evaluation and review technique (PERT) and Gannt charts.

PERT   **PERT** (Penton/IPC Education Division 1982), an acronym for **program evaluation and review technique**, is a useful tool for helping athletic trainers develop plans for implementing programs. It is also useful for evaluating actual outcomes against expected outcomes. PERT is essentially a method of graphically depicting the time line for and interrelationships among different stages of a program. Users depict events as circles and activities as lines or arrows connecting two or more events. One of the advantages of using the PERT planning technique is that it allows athletic trainers to display in diagram form events that occur simultaneously. PERT is most often used with large, complicated projects in business and industry, but it can also be applied to the smaller projects that athletic trainers are often called on to develop and administer (see figure 2.5).

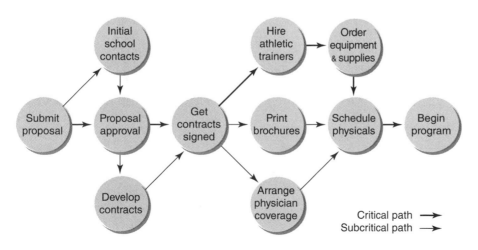

▶ **Figure 2.5**   PERT diagram for a hospital-based sports medicine outreach program.

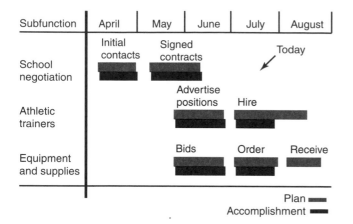

Subfunction	April	May	June	July	August

Figure 2.6 is a Gantt chart showing:
- School negotiation: Initial contacts (April), Signed contracts (May), Today (arrow, July/August)
- Athletic trainers: Advertise positions (June), Hire (July)
- Equipment and supplies: Bids (June), Order (July), Receive (August)

Plan ▬ / Accomplishment ▬

▶ **Figure 2.6** Gannt chart for a new hospital sports medicine outreach program.

Gannt Charts A **Gannt chart** is a graphic planning and control method (Stoner 1982). It has many potential applications in sports medicine because it takes discrete tasks and maps them on a calendar (see figure 2.6). Athletic trainers can use a Gannt chart to demonstrate to their superiors the progress being made on particular projects (Randolph and Posner 1988). When used in this way, a Gannt chart becomes a powerful tool for communicating sports medicine plans to crucial members of the internal and external audience. For example, in the opening case of this chapter, Janet could use a Gannt chart not only to plan the implementation of the sports medicine outreach program but also to provide her superiors with concise, easy-to-understand progress updates.

Both PERT and Gannt charts are challenging for the untrained to construct. Depending on the complexity of the project, the result, graphically illustrating the milestones and critical path of a project, can appear somewhat bizarre. The first few times an athletic trainer attempts these methods, she should use pencil and paper. After gaining expertise, the athletic trainer can use computer software to help create either chart. Many easy-to-use programs designed specifically for this purpose are available.

Communicating and Developing Support for the Plan

Unfortunately, all the effort an athletic trainer expends developing the sports medicine program plan will be wasted unless other people inside and outside the organization accept it. One of the most difficult aspects of planning for the delivery of sports medicine services is developing a sense of ownership in the people who make up the major organizational power bases. Plans developed without such ownership are unlikely to remain politically viable for long. The ability to translate plans into action and develop support for the program is the ultimate measure of political skill. The concept and process of incorporating stakeholders into a form of shared ownership are often referred to as "buy-in." Achieving buy-in for a sports medicine program plan is a key step toward successful implementation.

Types of Organizational Players

Block (1987) has developed a support-building strategy that could be useful to athletic trainers as they attempt to develop ownership for their sports medicine programs. The strategy is based on the **agreement–trust matrix** (see figure 2.7). The first step in the process is to identify people who will have an influence on the eventual success or failure of the sports medicine program. After these people have been identified, they are labeled as explained next.

Allies The **allies** of the athletic trainer exhibit a high level of agreement with the plans for the sports medicine program. In addition, they are people whom the athletic trainer trusts. They not only are supporters of the sports medicine program but also have an established record of honesty and truthfulness. The director of rehabilitation services at Janet's hospital in the opening scenario is a good example of an ally. He has expressed his support for Janet and her work, and his request to have her develop the outreach program demonstrates trust in her judgment.

Opponents **Opponents** of the athletic trainer should not be viewed as enemies. They are persons whom the athletic trainer trusts to give an honest opinion of the sports medicine program or its components, but who have opposing views to those of the athletic trainer. Opponents can often serve a useful purpose—their challenge can lead to critical examination of the sports medicine program, resulting in stronger strategic and operational plans.

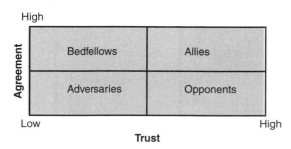

High	Bedfellows	Allies
Agreement	Adversaries	Opponents
Low		High

Trust

▶ **Figure 2.7** Agreement–trust matrix.

One possible opponent from the opening case might be an orthopedic surgeon who serves as an unofficial team physician for one of the Ashton County high schools. Although he might be a trustworthy person with whom Janet has had good relations in the past, he might harbor disagreement with her proposal because it could potentially funnel away a significant number of surgical cases from his practice if Janet or her staff begin acting as gatekeepers for injured high school athletes.

Bedfellows **Bedfellows** are those who agree with the plans of the athletic trainer for the sports medicine program but have a history of untrustworthy behavior. Bedfellows are generally quick to ally themselves with the sports medicine program, but they tend to be manipulative and to operate "behind the back." The vice president for finance at the hospital in the opening case is a good example of a bedfellow. He might be an enthusiastic supporter of the outreach program during the conceptual phase of planning. When the contracts are signed with the high schools and he has to find money in the budget for additional athletic trainers to support the program, however, he might prove to be a less enthusiastic member of the team. Bedfellows are often quick to support ideas in the conceptual stage, but they often fail to deliver when they are asked to contribute to get a program up and running.

Adversaries People with whom the athletic trainer has attempted negotiation that has been fruitless are known as **adversaries**. They not only disagree with the athletic trainer's plan for the sports medicine program but are untrustworthy and dishonest as well. The athletic trainer must be able to distinguish between adversaries and opponents. A common pitfall occurs when opponents who are honest, trustworthy persons with differing viewpoints are labeled as adversaries. Opponents can make the sports medicine program stronger. Adversaries often gain strength through confrontation because that tends to legitimize the alternative vision they have for the sports medicine program. Negotiation will not alter their vision of how the program should function. If an athletic trainer has done a good job of including a wide spectrum of people in the planning effort, the number of adversaries should be relatively small.

The likeliest adversaries Janet will confront are the other sports medicine service providers in the Ashton County area. Clinics that now provide some services to the three county high schools will undoubtedly oppose Janet's plans to create a sports medicine monopoly at the hospital. The clinics and the hospital were in competition before this issue, and the new proposal will only serve to enhance that sense of competition.

Gaining Support From Organizational Players

Block (1987) suggests specific strategies for developing support among the four types of organizational players:

Allies

- Confirm the fact that the person agrees with the sports medicine plan.
- Profess appreciation for the quality of the relationship.
- Admit any faults and shortcomings of the sports medicine plan.
- Request the support and continued counsel of the ally.

Janet might use the following language in a conversation with the director of rehabilitation services to develop his support:

> *Thanks for showing your support for the outreach program at the staff meeting this morning. I appreciate your confidence in me and your support for the program. I know the plan is not complete yet, but I hope to have the holes patched up by next week. As the plan continues to take shape I'll need your support more than ever. Thanks again.*

Opponents

- Profess appreciation for the quality of the relationship. Emphasize the trust and honesty that have characterized the relationship.
- Explain the plan for the sports medicine program along with any arguments that support its implementation.

- Define your interpretation of the opponent's views in a nonthreatening manner.
- Attempt to engage the opponent in a problem-solving process to find common points.

Janet might use the following language in a conversation with the orthopedic surgeon to develop his support:

Dr. Jones, I want you to know how much I've enjoyed working with you since I arrived at the hospital two years ago. You're one of the best surgeons I've ever worked with and you've really taught me a lot. You've read about the outreach program we're planning. Let me take a few minutes to explain why I think it's so important for the high school students of our county. . . . I know you may think that our program might take away some of the business you've developed at the high school. We certainly don't want that to happen. Can you suggest some strategies we might consider as we implement our outreach program that would help us accomplish our goals while helping you maintain what you've worked so hard to establish?

Bedfellows

- Confirm the fact that the person agrees with the sports medicine plan.
- Convey your concern about the person's willingness to be open and honest. Express a willingness to share a portion of the blame and to find a way to improve the trust relationship so that the program can move ahead.
- Clearly state your expectations for the person's behavior toward the sports medicine program. What is it that you want the person to do?
- Ask the person what expectations he or she has for you in order to improve the relationship.
- Attempt to establish a consensus for future working relationships with bedfellows.

Janet might use the following language in a conversation with the vice president for finance to develop his support:

Jim, your support of the outreach program at the senior staff meeting last week was just great. I'm glad that you agree with what we are trying to accomplish with the program. But I'm concerned that as we continue to move ahead with the plan, the financial realities of adding staff are going to confront us in a very real way. If your support breaks down at that point, the program will be in big trouble. I know that you and I have had a few disagreements in the past. I'm sorry we haven't always been the best of colleagues—I'll accept some of the blame for that. But this program is too big and too important to allow our past differences to get in the way. When the budget request comes across your desk in a few weeks, Jim, I really hope you'll be able to approve it. I appreciate the time you've given me to talk to you about this and hope that we'll be able to do this in the future when we have issues that we need to confront together.

Adversaries

- Explain the plan for the sports medicine program with any arguments that support its implementation.
- Define your interpretation of the adversary's views in a nonthreatening manner.
- Explain any actions you have taken or will take to implement the sports medicine plan so that everything is out in the open.
- Avoid making demands that are unlikely to be met.

Janet might use the following language in a conversation with the owner of a competing clinic:

Sally, I wanted you to know that we plan to institute an outreach program for the Ashton County high schools beginning next month. I didn't want this to hit you "out of left field." We think that there are many potential benefits for our county's high school athletes under this plan. I know that you will be concerned that this program will cut into your business. It isn't our intention to hurt your business. We simply have identified a need in the community that we feel a responsibility to meet. Our program will provide the following services.

FACILITY PLANNING

As athletic trainers become more involved in administrative leadership roles and have increasing potential for remuneration for services, the development of sports medicine programs may involve the planning of a facility. Planning a sports medicine facility is not a task for the novice and inexperienced athletic trainer. A number of elements must be considered during the earliest planning stages (Knowles 1997).

Location

Location. Location. Location. As with any property, the geographical location of the property is integral to the usage and accessibility of the sports medicine program. On a college campus where open land space and available room space within an existing facility are rare commodities, options may be limited, and available locations may or may not be the most ideal choice. When building a private practice type of setting, one must consider a number of additional aspects. For example, with the building of any facility, one must adhere to particular zoning guidelines in order for business activities to occur. In a private practice setting, patients drive the business. Therefore, one should research the demographics of the area to ensure that potential client bases are large enough to support the business. Many other questions should also be considered:

- Is the facility easily accessible by car?
- Is the facility near other medical offices, making it convenient for patients to do business in one location?
- Is the facility too close to a competitor that is providing the same type of services?
- Is the facility located in an area of growth or in an area of relative decline?

Name

Naming a business is perhaps one of the most important considerations for a private practice sports medicine setting. Ultimately, the name of the business should become recognizable to the general public so that anyone who hears the name immediately associates it with sports medicine services. There are a number of options when deciding on a name for a business. Regardless of what name is chosen, it must be registered with the appropriate state and federal corporation and tax entities to verify that no business with the same name already exists.

The following is a list of examples that Janet could consider for naming a sports medicine facility in Tampa, Florida:

Owner's Name: Janet's Sports Medicine Center

Location: Tampa Sports Medicine Center

Specialty Identification: Sports Injuries Specialists

Acronyms: Tampa Injury Specialists, TIS

Naming a business is always a risky proposition that should be carefully thought out before any formal operations are planned. The name that is eventually chosen will be branded in such a way that every association with the business will link back to the name. Each of the options just listed for naming a business has strengths and weaknesses. Using a person's name may mean that developing a known identify around town will take some time. However, if the person already has a reputation for expertise in sports medicine, a business title inclusive of the person's name will be beneficial. Use of a subspecialty term in the title to describe the type of expert services provided may draw the attention of clients with like injuries. However, it may give potential clients with other types of injuries the impression that the practice does not have expertise in other areas.

Business Structure

It is a common and recurring theme among health care providers that their services are a essentially a form of business. All business operations must operate under legal structure as typically defined by individual states. Legal structure is essentially a process that regulates the business operations; identifies who the business owner is; and ensures a method for tax collection, employee wages and protection, and fair practice acts. Though individuals may own their own business as a self-proprietor, many register their business as a corporate entity. As a self-proprietor, one assumes all risk and liability associated with the business, and personal assets can be used against any debt or claim against the individual and the business. With corporate status, an individual becomes a corporate officer, and any claim against the business does not affect her personal assets. Different types of corporations involve various leadership and ownership structures.

Taxes and Licenses

All businesses must register with their state for a business license. In some locations, city or county business licenses (or both) are also required. Part of business license registration is a description of the types of services one provides. Health care–related services often fall under "professional regulation." Both state and federal registration of a business are required for the purpose of collecting governmental tax revenue. Various forms of taxes may need to be paid based on the type of tax structure, the number of employees one has hired, and the amount of claimed revenue versus expenses of the business operation. While many consider taxation an undue burden, incentives often are provided to small business owners and minority business owners to encourage business growth and operations.

Business Development Team

No athletic trainer should assume that he knows everything there is to know about starting a private sports medicine practice. Despite the fact that athletic trainers possess creative skills and a strong work ethic, some areas of business development require consultation with experts to ensure a better chance of success. Legal advice can be beneficial to the planning of a new facility with regard to real estate guidelines, business registrations, and contractual document preparation. Accountants can be of assistance in determining what type of tax structure a business should operate under. The process of actually identifying a good location to build a facility can benefit from the use of a real estate agent.

Insurance

Athletic trainers are familiar with liability insurance as health care providers. Operating a facility also entails risk; thus risk management plans should include insurance coverage for the facility. This would include protection against any adverse conditions related to the property or equipment and even financial loss that could ultimately lead to business failure. If the business will employ staff, health insurance offerings will become an expense that must be planned for. Additionally, if third-party reimbursement will be sought for services, contractual relationships will need to be formed with insurance companies.

Equipment

Athletic training students are commonly involved with a school project that requires planning an athletic training room. Planning any facility always involves carefully evaluating space for equipment usage and patient flow. Aside from equipment size and space requirements, electrical outlet and voltage requirements should be assessed. Whirlpools are commonly used in sports medicine facilities and require proper plumbing and electrical planning. Additionally, rest rooms, sinks, and other "wet" areas require appropriate plumbing and flooring.

Utilities

Planning a facility is similar to building a house. All utilities should be considered: water, electric, phone, and any special requirements that may apply to equipment such as whirlpools and rehabilitative equipment. This is a critically important element of the planning process since most of the installation for utilities is done in the early stages of building before the walls and floors are completed. Thus, alterations after building completion tend to be cumbersome and expensive and require the removal of ceiling or flooring material.

MEETINGS AND CONFERENCES

Two important planning subfunctions about which competent athletic trainer-administrators should be knowledgeable are planning for effective meetings and conferences. Every athletic trainer will be involved in meetings from time to time during her professional career. Although the opportunity to plan for conferences comes less often and to fewer athletic trainers, the responsibility to coordinate this activity properly is important because of the expense and the number of people commonly affected by the typical conference.

Planning for Meetings

One of the most common methods for developing and communicating organizational plans is the meeting. Meetings in sports medicine settings can take many forms. The most common is the staff meeting, in which personnel from a work group unit (for example, the athletic trainers employed by the university athletic department or the rehabilitation professionals employed in an outpatient clinic) gather to discuss issues critical to the function of the unit. Athletic trainers can also be involved in other kinds of meetings. For example, Janet, the athletic trainer in the opening scenario, will undoubtedly have to meet—probably more than once—with the staff from the Ashton County schools to organize the hospital's outreach program. Irrespective of the type or setting, meetings are often viewed as exercises in frustration. Many of us have participated in meetings that accomplished nothing. We often walk away afterward fuming, "Did anything useful happen in there? What a waste of time!"

Although dull, unproductive meetings might be the norm, they are not inevitable. Tropman's (1996) research with meeting experts throughout North America revealed that four qualities characterized successful meetings:

1. The group was able to reach decisions in the meetings.
2. The group rarely needed to meet to undo or revise decisions that they had already made; they made high-quality decisions the first time.
3. The decisions made were important and meaningful to the organization.
4. The meetings were enjoyable, and the members felt that they had spent their time well.

The meetings that Janet must organize with the Ashton County schools will be more successful if she can implement the following seven principles of effective meeting management (Tropman 1996).

1. Organize for the Meeting

Although it sounds obvious, many meetings fail because nobody prepares for them. Meetings are like a play—they need a script, actors, props, and practice. The script is the agenda (see figure 2.8). The actors are the meeting participants. Some will have more noticeable roles than others, but all are necessary if the meeting is to be successful. The props are the materials needed to conduct business during the meeting. These usually include various documents and might include equipment such as a blackboard, flip chart, or overhead projector. The last element—practice—is something that most meeting managers disregard. All of us in athletics

Meetings are a necessary and often lamented part of the athletic trainer's managerial life. Athletic trainers can experience more success in their meetings if they organize well, divide the meeting into three parts, control their own meeting behavior, avoid new business and reports, look to the future, and make high-quality decisions. Conference planning, while not central to most athletic trainers' responsibilities, must be done correctly to avoid expensive mistakes. Conference planning involves working with a steering committee, establishing a theme, planning a program, identifying and recruiting speakers, and making space and other physical arrangements.

AGENDA

Sports Medicine Outreach Program Planning Committee Meeting

February 4, 2012

Third-Floor Conference Room

Item	Facilitator
1. Announcements	
a. High school contract negotiations	Janet
b. New supply bid procedures	Bill
2. Decisions	
a. Budget allocations	Tom
b. Staff travel reimbursement	Bill
c. Comp time for ATCs covering night events	Janet
3. Discussion	
a. Which physicians should we recruit?	Janet
b. How should we market the program?	Tom and Janet

▶ **Figure 2.8** Sample meeting agenda.

know the importance of practice. Practice helps eliminate mistakes and prevents random elements from interfering with performance. Practice in the context of a meeting might include checking with several key members of the meeting group to get their read on important issues to be discussed or decided during the meeting. Practice certainly involves the preparation that each participant makes for the meeting by becoming familiar with the items on the agenda. It may be helpful to request agenda items from meeting participants in advance and provide a deadline by which items must be added.

2. Divide the Meeting Into Three Parts

Too often, participants in a meeting play a role that requires them to speak only once. For example, when Janet meets with the department to report on the progress she has made with the outreach program, she'll probably stand up, deliver her report, answer a few questions, and sit down. That might be all she does in this department meeting. Although her involvement was important, she could probably fall asleep after speaking (which happens often at meetings) and no one would miss her input. One method that can be used to organize a meeting and maximize the participants' time and input is to divide the meeting into three parts:

1. Announcements
2. Decisions
3. Discussion

If this formula is rigidly adhered to, all meeting participants will be able to give appropriate input at the right times. Meeting managers who deviate from this formula run the risk of allowing the meeting to stray from its original purpose.

3. Control Your Meeting Behavior

Most people who hate meetings (which is most people) are particularly annoyed because of the behavior of other meeting participants. We are quick to see the faults in others but slow to recognize our own shortcomings. This issue is important for athletic trainers who participate in meetings. Behavior in a group setting is infectious. Optimism or pessimism can sweep through a meeting room if the climate is right. You should carefully analyze your own meeting behavior as a first step toward trying to improve the meeting behavior of others.

4. Avoid New Business

A common item on most meeting agendas is "new business." The intent of the new business section is to allow meeting participants to bring issues or concerns to the table for discussion and decision. The problem with this time-honored practice is that nobody in the room, with the exception of the person who introduced the issue, is prepared to address the topic with any intelligence. New business, therefore, violates the first principle—organize for the meeting. People can't organize for something they don't know anything about. A good rule to follow when conducting a meeting is "discuss everything on the agenda and don't discuss anything not on the agenda."

5. Avoid Reports

Too often, staff members waste valuable time listening to reports in a meeting when the information could more effectively be delivered and analyzed in writing beforehand. Written reports can be referred to in the decisions section or the discussion section of the meeting. If participants receive written reports in advance of the meeting, they have the opportunity to digest the information and formulate well-considered questions at their own pace rather than make snap judgments on a tight time schedule. Written reports should be brief and contain only the most important elements of an issue or proposal. Participants can be referred to reports that are more inclusive if they want more information, but short executive summaries will encourage them to read and prepare for the meeting.

6. Look to the Future

One of the most frustrating aspects of most meetings is the sense of hurried decision making. Most meeting groups gain exposure to issues too late in the decision cycle. Athletic trainers involved in planning meetings can avoid this problem by carving out some time—during either the announcements or the discussion period—for consideration of future issues. This preview helps those in the group prepare their thinking for when the issue is finally presented to them in a formal way. Facilitating informal discussion of issues is a difficult technique to master. The meeting chairperson must be well versed in the organization's issues and be able to package the information for the group so that members can process it appropriately. This future-oriented discussion is different from the new business section discussed earlier. In the new business section of a meeting, one of the participants typically makes a formal motion that will require the group to make a binding decision. Future-oriented discussion is just that—discussion. The group need not make any immediate decisions, although they may choose to brainstorm about the way they might handle future challenges.

7. Make High-Quality Decisions

Making high-quality decisions is difficult. Most meeting groups fail because they cannot make decisions at all—of any quality. They simply fail to decide. Those who do make decisions often have to go back and undo or revise their decisions. The important elements involved in making high-quality decisions in a group setting include gathering and communicating all pertinent information, processing the likely outcomes of various alternatives, developing a list of pros and cons for the alternatives, considering the perspectives of all the stakeholders, and deciding to decide. The chairperson of the meeting is critical in this regard. Decisions do have to be delayed when these elements are not satisfied. If the chair can orchestrate all these elements, however, the time has arrived to make a decision. Revisiting the decision after its implementation to evaluate its effectiveness and learn lessons for the future is important, but this process should not interfere with making a decision in the first place.

Planning for Conferences

One of the most common—and most expensive—continuing education methods for all kinds of professions is the conference or symposium. Every athletic trainer will be involved several times in his career as a participant in conferences, and some will coordinate or serve on conference planning committees from time to time. Conference planning is an important leadership skill that will enhance the administrative skills package of any athletic trainer in any employment setting. The following elements are important steps in planning conferences. Although they are presented sequentially, many will overlap with each other; and depending on the situation, the order of the steps may be modified to meet a specific need.

18 to 24 Months Before the Conference

The following activities are the first to be accomplished in the planning of a conference. Generally, the larger the conference, the earlier this planning should begin.

Appoint the Conference Coordinator   The conference coordinator typically serves as chairperson of the steering committee (see the next section). The following are a few qualities this person should possess.

- **Organized.** The primary duty of the conference coordinator is to coordinate the various members of the steering committee in their work. The conference coordinator must be able to synthesize information from a variety of sources to ensure that critical planning elements are accomplished.

- **Decisive.** The conference coordinator will be expected to make decisions—sometimes with the support and agreement of the steering committee and sometimes on the spur of the moment. When crises arise during the conference—as they usually do—the coordinator must be decisive enough to make good decisions quickly with the information available at the time.

- **Visionary and detail oriented.** The coordinator must be able to keep the goals of the conference in mind at all times and must be able to guide the various subcommittees in their work toward accomplishing those goals. On the other hand, the conference coordinator must also monitor the hundreds of details that are part of a successful symposium and be able to step in and make decisions when required.

- **Flexible.** The coordinator will learn throughout the planning process that many aspects of the plan will undergo change. In some cases, the changes will be unexpected, and in other cases the coordinator will be required to make changes in the conference planning process. It will benefit the coordinator to be prepared to accommodate changes by being flexible and having alternative plans.

Establish the Steering Committee   Planning a conference is usually not a solitary activity—it is a team effort. Conferences have so many elements that they would quickly overwhelm one person, no matter how well organized and efficient. Because most athletic trainers plan conferences on a volunteer basis as part of their professional service activities, or on a paid basis as only one part of their job responsibilities, the work should be spread around so that no one person is excessively burdened. The members of the conference steering committee often serve as the chairpersons of subcommittees charged with one narrow aspect of the conference (for example, marketing and promotions, entertainment, audiovisual, or registration). Only people with the following qualities should be chosen for the steering committee:

- **Knowledgeable.** Each member of the steering committee should have enough experience and expertise to understand the issues involved in the conference. Ideally, steering committee members should have previous experience in conference planning. They should have the necessary skills to carry out the functions that they will manage in planning the conference. For example, the member of the steering committee who chairs the finance subcommittee should have experience in business or in managing budgets. Similarly, the audiovisual subcommittee chair should have computer and similar technical skills.

- **Interested, committed, and available.** Conference planning can take a long time. Some steering committees meet for two years or more before the conference. Even after the conference has ended, details remain to attend to. Steering committee members must be committed to sticking with the project from start to finish. In addition, potential committee members must have enough time to dedicate to their planning responsibilities. All prospective members of the committee should reflect on their commitments during the conference planning time before agreeing to serve to ensure that they will be able to fulfill their responsibilities.

- **Team oriented.** Some people work well in groups. Others don't. The steering committee is a team—a group of people working toward a common goal. Although each member of the steering committee may be responsible for a different aspect of the conference, all these elements are intimately connected. Committee members must be able to communicate and work effectively with others to deliver an effective experience for conference participants. It is likely that areas of planning will overlap between different groups, necessitating team collaboration. Collaboration between committees is essential. For example, audiovisual committee members may choose to include cutting-edge technology to create the best possible presentation images. However, the finance committee members may not approve of this because of budgetary limitations.

- **Responsible and dependable.** The chair of the steering committee will be frustrated and the committee will be demoralized if one or more committee members fail to do the jobs assigned to them. The committee chair should learn as much as possible about prospective steering committee members before extending an invitation to serve. Those with a proven record of responsibility should be further considered. Those who have a reputation for letting people down or leaving tasks uncompleted should be removed from consideration.

Establish the Conference Theme, Objectives, and Target Audience People attend conferences for a variety of reasons, but underlying each of these reasons is the desire or need to learn more about a particular topic. The best conferences have a theme that is supported by a number of objectives. The more narrowly focused the conference theme, the more likely the conference is to appeal to an audience with a specific learning objective. For example, a conference with the theme "Knee Injuries" is much broader than one with the theme "Advances in the Surgical Management of ACL Injuries." The former is likely to attract a larger, more diverse audience but is unlikely to provide as much depth as the latter. Often conference planning for topics considers those that seem to be of greatest interest at the current time. Some conferences by necessity are targeted at large audiences—sometimes with thousands of attendees (for example, the annual conferences of NATA or the American College of Sports Medicine). These conferences usually have broad, nonspecific themes, such as "Athletic Training in the Next Millennium" or "New Horizons in Sports Medicine." Large conferences like these commonly include a number of smaller, more focused sections that cover a single topic or a group of related topics. In any case—whether the conference is large or small, with a broad or a narrow focus—specific learning objectives for the conferees should be established in advance. Each learning objective should relate in some way to the overall conference theme. Learning objectives should be assessed as a way of determining the degree to which the purposes of the conference have been accomplished.

Set a Date and Establish a Time Line The date of the conference is a critical element in its eventual success or failure. The following are a few questions planners should consider when choosing a date:

- **Is this conference traditionally held on a specific date?** Some annual conferences attract the same target audience year after year. People often schedule their yearly calendars around these traditional conference dates. Moving the date of a conference that is traditionally held during a specific week may alienate some members of the target audience, but it may draw in new attendees who have other annual commitments during that time. It is also helpful to have an awareness of when reporting for continuing education credit is due, as typically there will be a fair number of athletic trainers who have not yet met their requirements for recertification or licensure.

- **Are members of the target audience available?** Although predicting the availability of all members of the target audience is impossible, the steering committee should know the audience well enough to avoid obvious conflicts. For example, a conference targeted at high school athletic trainers is unlikely to draw in many attendees if it is held on a Friday evening in the fall. A survey sent to a random sample of the target audience asking for the most convenient dates for the conference is a good way to determine the availability of potential conferees. Holding a conference at the same site and close to the date of another event that large numbers of the target audience will attend is another way to ensure that potential conferees may be available. However, if a large event held locally is of interest to your audience to the point that it detracts from your ability to attract attendees, overall participation may diminish and revenue generation could be affected.

- **Are the facilities available?** If the conference is tied to a specific location, then the date for the conference could be influenced by the availability of the facilities. The earlier the date for the conference is established, the more likely it is that the desired location and facilities will be available. It is also important to keep in mind that earlier booking sometimes translates to higher fees, whereas booking closer to the conference date—before a facility has been rented—provides some leverage for bargaining but is slightly more risky.

Once the date has been established, the steering committee should establish a time line for each of the tasks involved in planning the conference. In addition, each subcommittee should develop its own time line that will allow it to accomplish its duties in a manner consistent with the master time line. See figure 2.9 for a sample time line.

15 to 17 Months Before the Conference

After the planning committee is in place, preparations for the conference begin in earnest. Specific members of the committee should be appointed to manage each of the following functions.

Establish the Program Along with the speakers, the program will be the heart and soul of the conference. The various presentation topics included in the conference should make up a mini-curriculum designed to help attendees accomplish the learning objectives established for the symposium. Several methods are available for delivering the conference curriculum:

- **Lectures.** Traditional format in which a single person or a panel of experts addresses the audience. This method can accommodate a large number of attendees at once.

- **Keynote.** A type of lecture usually delivered to the entire assembly of attendees, often at the beginning of the conference, dealing with a topic central to the conference theme.

- **Workshops.** Sessions led by an instructor, usually involving smaller numbers of attendees, that allow for a higher degree of audience participation.

- **Laboratories.** A kind of workshop that emphasizes hands-on skill building, often using instructional aids, tools, or specimens.

Task	Target date
1. Speaker thank-yous/honoraria sent	Late July
2. Exhibitor request forms sent	Late July
3. Exhibitor prospectus prepared	July/August
4. Exhibitor contract prepared	July/August
5. Tour companies researched and solicited	July/August
6. Speaker database	August
7. Shuttle bus/security proposals solicited	August
8. Speaker and registration gift selection begun	August
9. Advance registration form prepared	September
10. Housing form prepared	September
11. DVDs/CDs sales company proposals solicited if necessary	September
12. Speaker and registration gift selected	September
13. Cancellation insurance application mailed	September
14. Liability insurance application mailed	September
15. Confirm times for free communications and poster presentation sessions	Late September
16. Approve letter that proceeding publisher sends to speakers	Late September
17. Registration flyer preparation	September/October
18. Speaker database to proceeding publisher	Mid October
19. Related organizations letters of program invitation for following year convention	Late October
20. Preliminary program prepared	October/November
21. Shuttle bus company and security selected	November
22. Tour company contract signed	November
23. Exhibitor registration form prepared	November
24. Proceedings publisher to send letters to speakers	November
25. Summary of room block categories prepared	November
26. Exhibitor room block request form prepared	November
27. Room block memo sent to special housing groups	Late November
28. Preliminary program to Marketing Department	December 1
29. Exhibitor registration form to printer	December
30. Brochure sent to vendors	December
31. Speaker registration/housing/AV/speaker forms sent	December
32. Exhibitor forms prepared for confirming packet (registration, housing, etc.)	December
33. Moderator/panelist information letter sent	December
34. Awards lunch menu/catering coordination begun	January
35. Welcome reception menu/catering coordination begun	January
36. Memo and meeting space request form mailed to committee/task force chairs	January
37. Final program preparation begun	January

(continued) ▶

▶ **Figure 2.9** Sample time line for a large international conference.

Courtesy of the National Athletic Trainers' Association.

Task	Target date
38. Shuttle bus contract/security contracted signed	January
39. Memo to next city convention & visitors bureau re: exhibit arrangements for pre-promotion	January
40. DVDs/CDs sales company selected	January
41. Memo to host city convention & visitors bureau re: convention personnel needs for kiosks/city information	January
42. Reconfirm or order if necessary adequate inventory of logo golf-type shirts for office volunteers	January
43. Badge holder order placed	January
44. Ribbon order placed	January
45. Catering planning begun	January
46. Committee/allied groups meeting confirmation mailing	On-going as of January
47. Exhibitor packets mailed	February
48. Exhibit booth assignments begun	February
49. Complimentary exhibit booth invitations and materials mailed	February
50. Host committee dinner arrangements completed	March 1
51. Meeting plans drafted for convention center, hotel(s), decorator	March
52. Reminder memo sent to speakers w/incomplete paperwork	March
53. Rooming lists begun	March
54. Final program to desktop publisher	Mid March
55. Begin production of staff guide	March
56. Obtain AV/speaker release forms sent to speakers	March
57. Convention event tickets ordered	March
58. Final shuttle arrangements determined	March
59. Review and follow-up on items for registration packets	March
60. Moderator meeting and guidelines memos and resumes sent	Late March
61. Invitations and complimentary registration letters sent to liaison organizations and association CEOs	April 1
62. Attendee registration confirmation/information letter sent out	April 1
63. Speakers' names to gift company for imprinting	Early April
64. Final rooming list to housing service	April 1
65. Special event invitations mailed	April
66. On-site registration form prepared and printed	April
67. Security arrangements finalized	April
68. Speaker final arrangements letter sent	April 15
69. Meeting plans sent to convention center, hotel(s), decorator	May 1
70. Convention plant/flower order placed	May
71. Convention materials shipped to convention center	Mid June
72. Post convention pay bills	July
73. Rebates for hotel	July-September

▶ **Figure 2.9** Sample time line for a large international conference. *(continued)*

- **Panel discussion.** Typically follows a series of two or more speakers and is moderated by a facilitator who poses questions to the panelists and directs questions from the participants to the speakers.
- **Point-counterpoint.** Typically involves two speakers with opposing views on a topic. One speaker presents the topic from one point of view, followed by the second presentation from an opposing viewpoint. Point-counterpoints may also be followed by panel discussions.

These teaching methods can be used individually in developing the program or can be combined. For example, a conference might begin with a keynote address, after which conferees can choose between concurrent sessions composed of lectures followed by breakout sessions on topics related to the lecture subject matter. Some conferences are made up exclusively of lectures but offer pre- and postconference workshops, sometimes at additional cost. Conferences that have a small target audience are often delivered exclusively in workshop format. No matter what format is used, adequate time between educational sessions must be planned for meals and breaks.

Establish the Budget Conferences are expensive. After the desired format of the conference has been established, a realistic budget that supports the conference objectives must be created. Several items must be considered in establishing the conference budget:

- **Expenses.** Have all likely costs been included (see the later section on miscellaneous services)? Does the budget include a contingency for cost overruns?
- **Income.** Has the registration fee been established at a level sufficient to pay the costs associated with the conference? If not, have other sources of income, including exhibitor fees and sponsorships, been included at a level that is reasonably achievable? Do the registration, exhibitor, and sponsorship fees represent a reasonable value given the audience resources and content of the conference?

Identify the Location and Secure the Facility Once the target audience has been identified, the program established, and the budget fixed, the location of the conference can be decided. Two critical factors in this decision are geographic location and facility type.

1. **Geographic location.** Several factors influence the choice of a geographic location for a conference:
   - **Nature of the target audience.** If the audience is national or international in scope, the conference will most likely have to take place in or near a city with a large airport. If the audience will be large, a city with a large conference center and many hotels in reasonable proximity to the conference center will be required. Some cities are more expensive places to host conferences than others. The affordability of the city for the target audience is an important consideration in deciding where to host a conference.
   - **Time of year.** Most cities have a peak season and an off-season. Hotel and meeting space costs are higher during the peak season.
   - **Recreation and entertainment.** Some conferences include recreation as an important adjunct to the program. Warm-weather sites or locations with interesting cultural attractions can boost conference attendance or encourage attendees to bring their families.
2. **Facility type.** The two most important considerations in determining the kind of facility in which to host a conference are length of the conference and the number of likely participants. Conferences longer than one day that draw attendees from more than a few hours away require a facility with sleeping rooms and restaurants. Large conferences require meeting facilities with large ballrooms for lectures and a number of smaller rooms for workshops and other breakout sessions. The convention and visitors bureau or the chamber of commerce of the city in which the conference will be held will

provide much information on the facilities available in the area. (These organizations will also provide, often at no charge, other items designed to improve the experience of the conferees.) When conference meetings become larger in scope so that increased meeting space is required and more participants are likely to use hotel rooms for overnight stays, leverage to negotiate lower conference room rental fees, reduced or no costs for rented audiovisual equipment, and other perks may be negotiated with hotel conference managers. The following kinds of facilities are most often used for conferences:

■ Large hotels in urban areas

■ Suburban hotels with conference facilities

■ Conference centers

■ Colleges and universities

12 to 14 Months Before the Conference

The pace of the planning effort picks up significantly about one year before the conference. The conference will begin to take shape after three elements have been planned: speakers, meals and entertainment, and registration.

Recruit Speakers   Although all the elements included in this discussion are crucial to the success of a conference, nothing will have a greater effect on the success or failure of the conference than the quality of the speakers. Establishing and sticking to a reasonable speakers' budget is important, but if the speakers are not good, the conference will fail. For recruiting speakers, Watkins (2003) recommends the following:

■ **Determine the desired outcome of a presentation before choosing a speaker.** Make sure that the speaker understands the objectives the committee has established for his or her presentation, and make sure that the speaker will tailor the presentation to accomplish those objectives. If the speaker has a canned presentation that he or she is unwilling to modify to meet the objectives of the conference, the presentation is unlikely to be effective.

■ **Investigate the speaker's reputation.** Learn as much as possible about a speaker's effectiveness before extending an offer to be part of the program. Websites, articles, and books written by the speaker, and testimonials from those who have heard the speaker, are helpful. Keep in mind that the most expensive or well-known speakers are not always the most effective for a given purpose.

■ **Research the speaker's ability to engage the audience.** Public speaking requires expert content level and delivery at a minimum. However, keeping an audience engaged in learning and sustaining their engagement over an extended period of time often involves a form of entertainment on the part of the speaker. An experienced public speaker takes the time to review course evaluation feedback in order to improve. Over time, incorporating such feedback benefits the speaker's presentations and ultimately the audience's receptiveness to the delivery of the material.

■ **Consider using a speaker's bureau.** Some organizations have a list of speakers who are experts on certain topics. These organizations can often be helpful in identifying the right speaker and arranging for that person to be part of a conference.

■ **Have a backup plan.** A variety of events can conspire to cause a speaker not to show up on time for his or her presentation. Inclement weather, transportation delays, communication errors, illness, and simple irresponsibility are common reasons. Careful planning can minimize the effects of some, but not all, of these circumstances. Develop a risk management plan to minimize the likelihood that a speaker will be a no-show. In addition, try to have a backup speaker available, typically from the local area, who can be ready to step in at short notice. All this is part of the flexibility associated with the planning of meetings.

Speakers who agree to present at the conference should be asked to sign a contract specifying the date, time, location, and topic of their presentation. The amounts of any honorarium and reimbursable travel expenses should be included in the contract.

Plan for Meals and Entertainment   All people, including all conference attendees, need to eat. Most people also like to be entertained. The steering committee must plan for both of these important elements. Several factors must be considered in this part of the conference plan:

- **Time.** Build in enough time for meals and recreation. If conferees are on their own for meals, make sure that an adequate number and variety of restaurants in various price ranges are nearby and that participants have enough time to eat and return to the conference on time.

- **Meal functions.** Meals are sometimes included as part of a conference program. A speaker may be a part of some meal functions, and awards ceremonies are occasionally part of others, depending on the nature of the conference. Meals included as part of the program are usually, but not always, included in the registration price. Most conference facilities that provide food and beverage services require that conferences contract for these services rather than bringing in food or drink from the outside to serve the participants. It is important to know if a contract includes such requirements, as the fees will likely be higher than for external catering.

- **Registration.** Some entertainment or recreational events may require preregistration. A minimum number of participants may be needed to keep costs at prenegotiated levels.

- **Information.** Conferees should be provided with information on local restaurants, entertainment, and recreational venues. This information is usually available from the convention and visitors bureau or the chamber of commerce, sometimes at no charge.

Plan for Registration   The steering committee must decide in advance how it will handle registration for the conference. Most conferences encourage preregistration (and offer discounted prices if people register early) because planners can then allocate resources appropriately. Preregistration also helps cement the prospective attendees' commitment to attend the conference. Additionally, preregistration helps to reduce the number of late or same-day registrations, which can add costs for copying, room space additions, postcontractual meal additions, and so on. The steering committee will have to decide whether it will allow on-site registration, and if so, whether the price will be different from that for attendees who register before a predetermined deadline. The registration form should include all the information the planners will need to accommodate the needs of the attendees and to plan for the proper arrangements for each aspect of the conference (see figure 2.10). A mix of registration methods will enhance the convenience of the conference participants. Usual methods for preregistration include submitting the registration form through the mail, by fax, or online.

Six to 11 Months Before the Conference

Six months before the conference, the planning committee should begin recruiting exhibitors, negotiate and sign contracts for other services, and compile all documents required for fulfillment of continuing education units (CEUs) and continuing medical education (CME) units.

Recruit Exhibitors and Sponsors   Many groups have a stake in the success of a conference. Obviously, the conference planners, sponsoring organization, and conferees hope that the symposium is a success. Businesses that sell their products to the target audience may wish to use the conference as a tool for marketing those products. Conference planners can take advantage of this desire by charging companies to display their products at the conference. This is an excellent way to keep the cost of attending the conference down while also meeting the needs of the businesses that support the profession. Businesses are typically invited to support the conference in one of two ways:

Advance Online Registration Form

Annual Meeting & Clinical Symposia
National Athletic Trainers' Association
2952 Stemmons Freeway Dallas, TX 75247
214.637.6282

Please complete this form in full and press the SUBMIT button at the bottom of this form. Use the tab key to maneuver between the fields. Do not use the enter key.

This form can only be used with a credit card.

Mailing Info: Registration packet will be mailed after May 1 to this address.

Last Name: * [   ] First Name: * [   ] Member Number: [   ]

Address: * [   ]

[   ]

[   ]

City, State, Zip * [   ]

Work Phone: [   ] Home Phone: [   ]

Spouse (if attending): [   ]

Child(ren) & Age(s) (if attending): [   ]

Emergency Contact Name & Relationship: [   ]

Emergency Contact Phone: [   ]

 * Required

Badge Info: Name badges will be prepared from this information.

Nickname for Badge: [   ]

Credentials (Limit 3): [   ]

Institution: [   ] City, State: [   ]

▶ **Figure 2.10** An example of the first page of a web-based conference preregistration form.

Courtesy of the National Athletic Trainers' Association.

- **Sponsor.** Sponsors are businesses that provide either a sum of money or a gift in kind that is used to support one or more aspects of a conference. For example, conference planners may solicit funds from various businesses related to sports medicine to support the costs associated with an individual speaker. Planners may solicit other sponsors to pay for a meal function or other social event. Sponsors should receive public recognition at the conference and an expression of gratitude for their contribution.

- **Exhibitor.** Exhibitors are companies that are invited, for a fee, to display their merchandise at the conference. Exhibitors are commonly assigned to a booth (the larger or more prominently placed the booth, the higher the fee) in an exhibit hall near, but not infringing on, the rooms where the sessions will be held. If exhibitors will be invited to participate, breaks should be built into the conference schedule to allow and encourage the conferees to visit the exhibit hall.

Contract for Miscellaneous Services   Even the simplest conference has many expenses, each of which must be planned for. Each item of substantial cost should be agreed to in advance in the form of a signed contract. Most vendors that supply the conference will have their own contracts. Conference planners should review contracts carefully for acceptable terms. Most conferences require the following services:

- Audiovisual equipment
- Pipe and drape (the curtains used to create exhibit booths and demarcate other spaces)
- Transportation
- Security
- Printing
- Mailing and marketing
- Meeting room space
- Hotel sleeping rooms
- Food functions

Many of the items listed can be negotiated based on the size of the conference. For example, late checkouts can be requested for course participants when the meeting might end on a day after the typical 11:00 a.m. checkout time. Also, as noted earlier, audiovisual equipment, catering, and room space are all negotiable.

Continuing Education Units   The BOC (www.bocatc.org) establishes criteria for continuing education for athletic trainers to maintain certification status. Organizations and individuals that offer continuing education courses have the opportunity to become **approved providers** of continuing education for athletic trainers through the BOC. Becoming an approved provider requires the completion of an application process that demonstrates compliance with the standards set forth; this is an effort to ensure that a level of quality is in place for course offerings. Applicants are asked to provide examples of course agendas, cancellation policies (a policy a provider would have in place for participants of courses that get cancelled; such a policy is needed in order to receive recognition as an approved provider by BOC), and other relevant components of continuing education management.

Being an approved provider also entails responsibilities for each course offering. Much of the preparation occurs months before the course is delivered. Templates for certificates of attendance and completion need to be developed. Course evaluations will need to be developed and issued for all participants. A roster with the name, contact information, and certification number of participants needs to be maintained for potential auditing purposes. The BOC website is very thorough and explains all of the details of the requirements for approved providers.

Three to Five Months Before the Conference

The final planning activities to be completed include conference marketing and the preparation of learning materials. Conference planners usually accomplish these tasks a few months before the beginning of the conference.

Market the Conference A conference will fail if people do not attend. The marketing process is one of the elements that will inform potential conferees and encourage them to attend. In many ways, a conference brochure is like a person's resume: A good first impression is attractive to the consumer, whereas a poorly designed and cheap-looking advertisement for a course may lead to the perception of a lack of quality offerings. For this reason, saving money on the marketing aspect of the conference should be considered very carefully. Even the best speakers can't make up for lost revenue as a result of an insufficient number of participants. A variety of methods can be used to market a conference. Some require detailed access to a database of names and addresses of the target audience. Conferences marketed to health care professionals are generally more successful if the conferees can earn required continuing education credits by attending. Marketing should begin several months before the conference because most professionals plan their travel schedules far in advance. Methods for marketing a conference include the following:

- **Direct mail.** Either the postal service or e-mail can be an effective way of reaching potential conference attendees. Professional organizations to which the members of the target audience belong often sell mailing lists.

- **Web-based advertising.** If the conference will be advertised online, the website that presents the advertisement must be one that substantial numbers of the target audience visit frequently. A mass e-mail message containing a link to the online advertisement is a useful strategy.

- **Print advertising.** Advertisements placed in professional and trade publications that are commonly read by members of the target audience can be effective. Some journals and newsletters will list the conference in a free calendar of events section, but such publications may charge a fee for regular advertising space. If the conference targets a local audience, the local newspaper may be a good choice for informing prospective conferees. A press release sent to the local newspaper describing the conference may or may not result in a story, but planners always have the option of buying space for an advertisement.

Prepare Learning Materials A practice common to most conferences is providing attendees with a packet of learning materials. These materials vary in content and scope. Some are simply reprints of the speakers' PowerPoint notes. Others include abstracts of each presentation. A book containing the abstract or outline of each speaker's presentation is known as a **proceedings**. Conference participants very much appreciate proceedings that are complete. Pages omitted or left blank because speakers have not turned in prepared outlines detract from proceedings. Though the task can be somewhat cumbersome, conference planners must provide frequent reminders of deadlines to speakers so that participants will have access to handouts in a timely manner.

Conference planners should consider at least three strategies when preparing learning materials:

- **Hard-copy proceedings.** The most common method of providing conferees with learning materials is to distribute a hard-copy proceedings. Depending on its scope and quality, the proceedings may be included in the registration fee or sold to conferees for an additional charge. Large conferences sometimes contract with publishing companies to provide this service.

- **Online proceedings.** Another method for distributing conference proceedings is to place the abstracts or outlines online and allow attendees to download and print parts that they find useful. This method offers considerable cost savings but is less convenient for attendees.

Conference organizers who wish to become approved providers of athletic training continuing education programs should visit the Board of Certification website at www.bocatc.org and click on the "Approved Providers" tab.

■ **CD or DVD.** An increasingly popular method of disseminating conference proceedings is to place the presentation outlines and documents on a CD or DVD that can be distributed at the beginning of the conference. This method allows participants to follow the presentations on a laptop or notebook computer without requiring Internet access at the conference. It also allows speakers to provide outlines and accompanying documents without concerns for size limitations. If a conference chooses to distribute print materials, there can be a large cost associated with producing and copying those materials. The cost of producing CDs or DVDs for a large number of participants is not significant, and the time required to make the number needed will depend on whether they are made by hand or prepared by a business service.

Conferences as Fund-Raising Events

Conference planning requires careful thought, and it helps to have experience to ensure a profitable, high-quality program. A combination of experience, careful planning, and some luck ultimately determines the success or failure of a conference. One method of minimizing risk and attempting to raise funds for organizations such as student athletic training clubs is through the offering of a continuing education course. All of the key elements in operating a successful course that have been previously described in detail apply to managing a successful fund-raising event of this kind. There are a few areas, however, that can assist in the reduction of overhead costs that will have an impact on potential revenue generation.

Typically, these types of events are targeted toward more local participants, possibly clinical instructors (CIs) of a program and clinicians in the geographical region. Thus e-mail distributions and physically dropping off brochures are options that can significantly cut down on costs. Courses can be given in just a day so that hotel stays are not required. Meeting space can be "borrowed" at minimal to no cost through use of one of the school's classrooms or meeting rooms, or possibly at a local clinic or hospital facility that has larger conference rooms for meeting purposes. Audiovisual equipment can also be borrowed from the school or local facilities.

Perhaps two of the largest costs to consider are provision of food and the speaker's honorarium and travel expenses. When the plan is to host a continuing education course as a fund-raiser, it is possible to seek sponsorships from local and other businesses that the program regularly supports through annual purchases of athletic training supplies. Often these businesses are happy to provide funding to support continental breakfasts or snacks and beverages. In some cases, the business may also offer to sponsor the speaker. Having one speaker who possesses enough expertise to provide all of the content for a course is much easier and less expensive than having multiple speakers. In some cases, speakers will exhibit altruistic levels of generosity and waive any honorarium to support the fund-raising effort, although conference planners should not expect a speaker to waive travel costs such as gas, airfare, airport parking, or meals associated with travel. Speakers who support a fund-raising conference by waiving their honorarium may or may not wish this acknowledged, and meeting facilitators and moderators should be cognizant of their preference. Whether or not the speaker waives the honorarium, giving a gift that serves as a keepsake of the meeting, one related to the location or the host group, is a kind gesture. Gifts may be items that remind speakers of the city or the university they visited to assist with the fund-raiser, and such gifts may have more lasting meaning than an honorarium.

PROGRAM EVALUATION

Athletic trainers are regularly called on to assess various aspects of a sports medicine program. How is Bill's knee rehabilitation coming along? Is he on schedule? Was the drug education seminar we hosted last week effective? Will the behavior of the athletes change as a result? Questions like these help determine the quality of the program. Unfortunately, even the most thorough and well-conceived strategic and operational plans don't always produce the desired

Sports medicine program evaluation is a critical, but often ignored, part of the athletic trainer's managerial responsibilities. Program evaluations can be either formative or summative. Evaluations typically use goals, objectives, criteria, and outcomes, based on patient charts and other data sources.

> ### ■ Types of Evidence to Support Sports Medicine Program Effectiveness
>
> - Patient files
> - Injury summaries and statistics
> - Treatment summaries and statistics
> - Client testimonials
> - Athletic training student graduation and certification statistics
> - Critical incident reports
> - Staff accomplishments
> - Client surveys
> - Alumni surveys
> - Surveys of employers of alumni

results. To maximize the value of a sports medicine program, athletic trainers must engage in **program evaluation** regularly.

Worthen and Sanders (1973) have defined *evaluation* as "the determination of the worth of a thing. It includes obtaining information for use in judging the worth of a program, product, procedure, or objective, or the potential utility of alternative approaches designed to attain specified objectives" (p. 19). The athletic trainer should answer two underlying and related questions when evaluating a sports medicine program: What would the likely effects be if the sports medicine program ceased to exist? How are those who have access to the program better off than those who do not have access to the program? Each of these questions is crucial; the answers will ultimately help the organization determine if it is committing an appropriate amount of human and financial resources to sports medicine. Answers to these questions, and indeed to questions about every area of the program evaluation, should be supported by documented evidence.

Evidence of sports medicine program quality can and should be derived from several sources. Patient files, injury and treatment summary statistics, and client testimonials are examples of useful data. Educational programs should evaluate student graduation and certification rates. Surveys of satisfaction among clients and alumni can provide valuable evidence of perceived program quality because they allow respondents to reflect for a time before providing feedback. None of this evidence is sufficient in isolation. Considered together, however, it can help provide an overall assessment of the effectiveness of the sports medicine program. Although the athletic trainer will certainly have to render judgments based on professional experience, others who judge the program will need tangible proof that the sports medicine program is accomplishing its mission.

Chart Auditing

Patient chart auditing is one of the most common methods for evaluating the effectiveness of a sports medicine program. The patient chart should contain a detailed history of the patient's problems, treatment goals, specific interventions, and reactions to those interventions (see chapter 6). As such, it is an excellent data source from which to draw conclusions regarding the effectiveness of the sports health care provided by the program. Although many chart-auditing techniques exist, internal and external techniques are most common.

Members of the sports medicine staff typically perform an **internal chart audit** procedure, which serves as an important component of a Total Quality Management process for the sports medicine program (see chapter 1). Chart auditing is an internal check to ensure that certain quality standards are being upheld in the treatment of injured patients. The procedure might examine a number of factors. For example, the director of a sports medicine clinic might be concerned that a large number of anterior cruciate ligament (ACL) patients are having a portion of their reimbursement requests denied because they are exceeding the allowable number of visits. One way to find out why this is happening is to pull the charts of all ACL patients for the preceding year and look for common elements. Was there a common surgeon? Were one or two clinicians seeing most of the patients who had their insurance claims denied? Were the patients mostly older industrial workers or younger physically active people? After staff members have identified a pattern, they can develop and implement a plan to address the causes of the problem.

Computerized patient databases make internal chart audits fairly painless. Searching for every patient with an ACL injury, for example, and discovering common elements between patients are simple tasks with a computer. When records are not computerized, the process must be performed by hand, which can be extremely time-consuming.

Internal chart auditing should be performed in a peer review format; in other words, clinicians should not review their own charts. It is more objective and ultimately more beneficial to have a peer review another provider's chart with a fresh set of eyes. The provision of constructive feedback by a peer reveals strengths and weaknesses in overall delivery of care and serves as a thorough assessment of outcomes in relation to interventions.

A second kind of chart-auditing process is known as an **external chart audit**. External chart auditing is used by accreditation agencies to ensure that a sports medicine program is upholding commonly held standards of practice in patient care (see the earlier section "Accreditation" and discussion of external evaluators in the section "Summative Versus Formative Evaluation"). Third-party reimbursement agencies also use external chart audits to determine the appropriateness of claims for reimbursement. One of the most common instances of external chart auditing occurs when practitioners bill Medicare for the services they provide to qualifying patients. Either a **carrier** or an **intermediary** evaluates these claims, which must be extensively documented to qualify for reimbursement (Esposto 1993). When an intermediary or carrier evaluates a Medicare claim, it looks for a record of the patient's progress and a rationale for reimbursement. The chart must contain information sufficient to document that the services were directly related to a treatment plan established by the physician or other health care provider. The chart must also document that the services provided were reasonable and necessary. The Medicare guidelines for determining what is reasonable and necessary include the following:

■ The treatment must be accepted as standard for the effective remediation of the patient's condition.

■ The patient's condition must be such that only the services of the particular health care provider could be used to provide the care.

■ There must be a reasonable expectation that the patient's condition will improve in a specific period.

■ The treatment plan must be reasonable with respect to the amount, duration, and frequency of treatment.

Another way to perform external chart auditing is to hire experienced consultants who will offer expert reviews in a preferable manner to the client. The fee paid to the consultant is often based on the number of hours of work required. Though this may seem like an unnecessary expense, the use of an experienced reviewer adds value to the audit. Furthermore, using external consultants for chart audits as part of an ongoing plan, as opposed to implementing an external review only after problems or concerns have been identified, will likely improve quality control. In particular, external consultants can help an organization plan for upcoming accreditation reviews.

Summative Versus Formative Evaluation

Athletic trainers may be called on to perform two types of program evaluations: **summative** and **formative evaluations** (Fitz-Gibbon and Morris 1987). Summative evaluations typically describe the effectiveness or accomplishments of a program, whereas formative assessments are used for program improvement purposes. The summative evaluation includes

■ a summary statement of program effectiveness,

■ a description of the program,

■ a statement of documented achievement of program goals,

- unanticipated outcomes of the program, and
- comparisons with other similar sports medicine programs.

The formative evaluation includes

- identification of potential problems in the sports medicine program,
- discussion of areas that need strengthening,
- recognition of program strengths, and
- ongoing assessment of program objectives.

Good program evaluation is expensive in terms of both overt and covert costs. Ideally, athletic trainers should use rigorous experimental research designs incorporating control or nontreatment groups for every program evaluation. This method is the best way to determine whether a sports medicine program is having the intended effect. Unfortunately, only athletic trainers with the appropriate graduate school training will have the research and statistical skills necessary to carry out such experimental designs. In addition, athletic trainers often find it impossible to carry out evaluation projects of this scope and complexity because they take too much time away from their other duties. The athletic trainer should strive to include as much comparative information as possible in the program evaluation to help other stakeholders appreciate the quality of the program compared with other programs of its type.

One way in which athletic trainers can provide evidence of quality in comparison to sports medicine programs at similar institutions is to use other athletic trainers as **external evaluators**. This is similar to using external reviewers for chart auditing. For example, athletic trainers trained in program evaluation are employed to judge the quality of athletic training education programs for schools requesting accreditation. External evaluators can also be useful for reducing bias. Athletic trainers will find it difficult, or even impossible, to be objective about their own programs. Asking expert third parties, who have little to lose or gain, to assess the program helps lend credibility to the evaluation results (Joint Committee on Standards for Educational Evaluation 1981). For the purposes of internal reviews, scientific reporting is not necessary. In fact, to the contrary, the more practical the information and the greater the potential for immediate application, the more favorably a report will be received.

Before the external evaluator arrives, the institution must commit itself to allowing reasonable access to the people and information the evaluator will need to make accurate judgments and generate useful suggestions for improvement. A competent external evaluator will want to have access to all the evidence. In addition, a good external evaluator will interview the athletic trainers, team physicians, athletic administrators, coaches, athletic training students, athletes, and other physically active patients to gain a broad-based perspective of the quality of the sports medicine program. After the site visit, the evaluator should prepare a report that lists perceived strengths and weaknesses of the sports medicine program and specific steps that the institution could take to improve the program. It is helpful to provide external reviewers with as much information as possible in advance of a site visit. Such information should include, but not necessarily be limited to, all department and organizational policy and procedure manuals, the website URL, and especially the goals that the organization is looking to achieve with the aid of the external review.

Goals, Objectives, and Criteria

Program evaluation should be based on an analysis of the goals and objectives of the athletic training program. Evaluation of goals and objectives should use measurable criteria established in advance of the evaluation. **Goals**, general statements of program intent, are derived from the mission statement. Two or more objectives support each goal. **Objectives** are more specific than goals and identify how the program intends to achieve a particular goal. **Criteria** are highly specific, and typically quantifiable, statements that provide the yardstick for determining whether a particular objective has been accomplished. Examples of a goal and supporting objectives and criteria from the Memorial Hospital case at the beginning of the chapter might include the following:

Goal: The Memorial Hospital Sports Medicine Outreach Program shall provide easy access to sports medicine services for high school student-athletes.

Objective #1: High school student-athletes will have access to Outreach Program staff within 24 hours of the onset of injury.

Criterion for objective #1: 80% of those high school student-athletes responding to the Outreach Program annual patient satisfaction survey will indicate that they were seen within 24 hours of the onset of their injuries.

Objective #2: High school student-athletes will incur minimal travel in accessing the services of the Outreach Program staff.

Criterion for objective #2: 90% of those high school student-athletes responding to the Outreach Program annual patient satisfaction survey will indicate that they traveled less than 5 miles from their homes to be seen by an Outreach Program staff member.

Frequency of Program Evaluation

How often should a sports medicine program be evaluated? Although there is no universal answer, some guidelines apply regardless of the setting in which the sports medicine clinic is housed:

- **Collect and collate evaluation evidence continuously.** If data are collected only immediately preceding the evaluation, sufficient time may not be available to complete the task. Gathering the evidence is the most time-consuming aspect of program evaluation.

- **Perform a mini-evaluation every year.** This approach has two advantages: The athletic trainer will have to compile evidence of program effectiveness for a reasonable time frame, and the evaluation will identify program weaknesses that require immediate attention.

- **Conduct a complete evaluation of the sports medicine program every three to five years.** This schedule will allow the athletic trainer to examine strategic issues such as mission congruence and program goals and objectives, which shouldn't change often.

Program Self-Study

Part of the mission statement for the Memorial Hospital Sports Medicine Outreach Program specified that evaluation would occur on an ongoing basis to ensure quality care for the high school student-athletes being served. One of the ways Janet could evaluate the effectiveness of the program would be to design and implement a self-study process every three to five years (see figure 2.11). The self-study should critically examine all the major elements of the program. It should result in a report to the primary stakeholders of the sports medicine program (Morris and Fitz-Gibbon 1978). Reports from external evaluators and condensed transcripts of documentary evidence should be included as appendixes.

Outcomes

One of the major thrusts related to program evaluation that has developed since the late 1980s is objective measurement of patients' functional abilities using **outcomes assessment**. Outcomes assessment is a type of evaluation process designed to provide objective, measurable evidence that the care provided by the athletic trainer was effective in improving the patient's functional ability. Outcomes assessment is likely to play an increasingly important role in health care in general and for athletic trainers specifically. As Denegar and Hertel (2002) asked, "What do certified athletic trainers do that makes a difference in the health care of the physically active?" As the dollars available for health care continue to shrink at the same

SPORTS MEDICINE OUTREACH PROGRAM SELF-STUDY

Instructions

The self-study for the sports medicine program shall consist of four areas: general considerations, patients, staff, and program. The athletic trainer in charge of the program shall answer the questions below and prepare a report with supporting evidence to be submitted to the Director of Rehabilitation Services and the Vice President for Patient Services. In addition, the Director of Rehabilitation Services, in consultation with the athletic trainer, shall select an appropriate external evaluator. The external evaluator's report shall be included in the self-study as an appendix.

General considerations

1. What is the mission of the program? Is the mission statement consistent with the mission of Memorial Hospital? Is the mission statement consistent with national standards for the delivery of sports medicine services?

2. Does the program work well in the context of the Department of Rehabilitation Services? How does the program take advantage of available resources? Do the program's staff members work well together? Do they work well with the rest of the hospital staff?

3. Who provides leadership for the program? Are the program leaders effective?

4. What are the priorities of the program? Are they appropriate? Do they mesh well with the priorities of Memorial Hospital? Do the priorities of individual staff members mesh well with the priorities of the sports medicine program?

Patients

1. Do patients achieve the short- and long-term goals established at the beginning of their treatment programs? Do patients have easy and quick access to evaluation and treatment services? Do the students of the Ashton County high schools use the program? If not, why not? Are the program's patient loads consistent with national averages?

2. Does the program help reduce the incidence of injury in the Ashton County high schools? If not, what factors account for this? In what ways can the program be improved so as to reduce the incidence of injury?

3. Are the students of the Ashton County high schools better educated with respect to healthy lifestyles than students elsewhere? What efforts have been made to educate students regarding healthy lifestyles? What additional efforts should be/could be made in this area?

Staff

1. How effective are staff members as providers of sports medicine services? Are some staff members ineffective? What can be done to resolve the problem?

2. Do staff members possess the standard credentials for delivery of sports medicine services? Do they engage in programs of continuing education?

3. Are staff members considered experts in their fields? Can they boast of professional accomplishments consistent with experts of regional or national reputation?

4. Are staff members performing in a manner consistent with their position descriptions and codes of professional conduct?

5. Is the size of the staff appropriate for the tasks it must accomplish? Could the same job be done with the same quality with fewer staff members?

Program

1. Is each component of the sports medicine program effective? Which components are the strongest? Which are the weakest? How could the weak components be strengthened?

2. Is each component of the sports medicine program necessary? If not, should some components be eliminated? Are there additional components that should be added to the program? Who would they serve? What is the desired effect of any new component?

3. Is the sports medicine program cost effective? Does the income it generates support its budget? Is it efficient? How could it become more efficient?

▶ **Figure 2.11** Self-study form for a hospital-based sports medicine clinic.

time athletic trainers are actively seeking access to third-party reimbursement, quality assurance processes and utilization reviews will become critical factors in determining who will be paid and who will not (Stewart 1993). Health care professions that cannot demonstrate that their interventions are effective and medically necessary will find themselves without access to third-party reimbursement in the increasingly competitive managed care market. In addition, organizations that cannot document that their interventions are cost-effective will be bypassed in favor of those that can.

The focus on outcomes assessment is particularly important for athletic trainers employed in clinics and hospitals. These organizations remain financially sound only if they receive reimbursements for their services, either through government programs like Medicare and Medicaid or through private insurers. As the private insurance market continues to make the transition from a traditional fee-for-service model to a managed care model, it will be more important than ever for these organizations to be able to document that they improve their patients' function in an efficient and cost-effective manner. Hospitals and clinics that cannot produce documentary evidence to demonstrate the effectiveness of their patients' functional outcomes will have a difficult time getting the contracts from managed care organizations that will, to an increasing degree, be their lifelines.

Spending for medical research is reaching all-time high levels, yet challenges remain with regard to translating basic science research into clinical applications (Moses et al. 2005). For the profession of athletic training to advance and subsequently justify the undisputed benefit of the certified athletic trainer, it will be necessary to avoid a glaring disconnect between the increasing body of knowledge produced by athletic training researchers and clinical practice (Hertel 2005). It is also vital that published data be compiled in such a way that the average athletic trainer in a clinical setting could locate and comprehend essentials of research findings. For example, it has been estimated that in today's world, the average health care provider would need to read 19 journal articles per day every day of the year to remain abreast of the changes in health care (Hootman 2004). Others have stated that it takes an average of 17 years to translate research findings into clinical practice (Fineout-Overholt et al. 2005). The use of critically appraised topics (CATs) has been helpful in condensing research information from peer-reviewed studies (Law 2002a). A CAT is basically a summary, in a couple of pages, on a focused clinical question, with the information divided into categories such as clinical question being addressed, date of completion of the CAT, treatment approaches, comparative interventions, and the outcomes obtained.

Outcomes assessment is important for athletic trainers who work in professional, collegiate, and high school settings. Although systematic assessment of outcomes has not traditionally occurred in these settings, the increasing pressure that most athletic trainers are under from cost-conscious administrators makes it important to be able to document that athletic trainers provide an excellent service in an economical fashion. Outcomes data could potentially serve a useful purpose in justifying new staff or in defending against an athletic director who wants to contract all sports medicine services to an outside agency. Streator and Buckley (2000) suggest that outcomes studies in these settings should help answer the following questions:

- Does the involvement of an athletic trainer in the athletic program result in decreased incidence of injury?
- Does the involvement of an athletic trainer in the athletic program result in reduced insurance claims?
- What are the cost savings associated with employing athletic trainers in the athletic program?

Additionally, results of outcomes assessments may assist with identifying the medical coverage required for each setting and support the need for full-time athletic trainers and an improved ratio of athletic trainers to athletes. Currently, in many high schools fortunate enough to have a full-time athletic trainer on staff, the athletic trainer is responsible for the

■ Example of a CAT

Effects of combining OKC and CKC exercises on quad strength and knee laxity in athletes recovering from ACL reconstruction

Clinical Bottom Lines: 1. In athletes who have undergone Anterior Cruciate Ligament (ACL) reconstruction, a combination of open kinetic chain and closed kinetic chain resulted in greater improvement of quadriceps strength than closed chain exercises alone. 2. A combination of opened kinetic chain and closed kinetic chain exercises did not improve knee laxity statistically versus closed kinetic chain exercises alone in this population.

Citation: Mikkelsen, C., Werner, S., and Eriksson, E. Closed kinetic chain alone compared to combined open and closed kinetic chain exercises for quadriceps strengthening after anterior cruciate ligament reconstruction with respect to return to sports: A prospective matched follow-up study. *Knee Surgery, Sports Traumatology, Arthroscopy.* 2000; 8: 337-342.

Clinical Question: In athletes who have undergone ACL reconstruction, is a combination of open kinetic chain (OKC) exercise and closed kinetic chain (CKC) exercise more effective than closed kinetic chain exercise alone in improving quadriceps strength and knee laxity?

The Study: The purpose of the randomized (RCT) controlled trial was to look at the rehabilitation of ACL reconstruction using a combination of OKC and CKC exercises versus the same program using only closed kinetic chain exercises. Subjects received treatment from the same therapist that took the measurements. The study used both a pretest and a posttest. The RCT was not blinded. Reliability procedures were not established.

The Study Patients: The study consisted of 44 athletes, 34 males and 10 females, aged 18-40 years who were recovering from ACL reconstruction using a bone patellar tendon bone graft at the same hospital.

Experimental Groups: All subjects were randomly assigned to one of two groups. One group performed a combination of open kinetic chain and closed kinetic chain exercises (n=22). The other group performed closed kinetic chain exercises alone (n=22). Therapy lasted six months. The participants were very similar to that in my clinical question.

The Evidence: The outcome measures were quadriceps torque, measured by a Kin-Com dynamometer, and knee laxity, measured by KT 1000 arthrometer. The study showed statistical evidence that there was a measurable difference in quadriceps torque (p < 0.01) but no difference in knee laxity by those who performed a combination of open chain and closed chain compared to closed chain exercises.

Comments: 1. The study is limited as it only shows short-term effects of open kinetic chain exercises on the ACL reconstruction. Also, the researchers used equipment that not all therapists may have to measure outcomes. 2. Further studies should be done to show the long-term effects of ACL reconstruction on knee laxity. 3. The study provided statistical evidence that a combination of OKC and CKC exercises increased quadriceps torque compared to CKC exercises alone.

Appraised by: Riley Phelps
Date Appraised: August 7, 2008

Reprinted, by permission, from University of Nevada, Las Vegas. Available: http://pt.unlv.edu/ebpt/index.html.

supervision of hundreds of athletes. In these situations, the lone athletic trainer must prioritize work assignments so as to be where the risk of injury is greatest, thus neglecting coverage and care for many other student-athletes.

In the college and university setting, positive outcomes can be used for recruiting purposes; school officials, administrators, and coaches can provide parents of incoming student-athletes with information about the provision of care to their children.

Many methods are used to conduct outcomes assessments. The three most common models, however, are patient chart documentation, randomized clinical trials, and patient surveys. Each has strengths and weaknesses (see table 2.1). All three are important sources of outcomes data. The usefulness of each of these methods, however, depends on the degree to which standard research protocols that reduce the likelihood of yielding spurious conclusions are employed. Outcomes studies that fail to employ control groups, to randomize patient selection and therapeutic methods, or to blind the researchers and the subjects may yield suspect results. Note also that many factors beyond the control of the athletic trainer can affect the outcome of a patient's care, including factors related to initial clinical findings and patient characteristics (Streator and Buckley 2000; see figure 2.12).

TABLE 2.1 Strengths and Weaknesses of Different Outcomes Assessment Models

Model	Strengths	Weaknesses
Patient chart documentation	1. Provides outcomes for specific patients 2. Required for Medicare reimbursement	1. Labor intensive 2. Dependent on charting skills of practitioner 3. Does not systematically control for situational variables
Randomized clinical trials	1. Uses rigid controls to reduce confounding factors 2. Controls variance 3. Useful for examining very specific problems	1. Requires the use of a control group 2. Poor focus on broad or multiple issues 3. Time intensive
Patient surveys	1. Easy to administer 2. Useful for examining a broad range of issues 3. Useful for assessing patient satisfaction	1. Instruments must be subjected to a validation process 2. Lack of patient specificity 3. Self-reported data are often unreliable

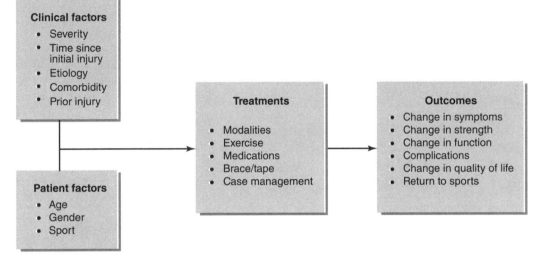

▶ **Figure 2.12** Factors affecting clinical outcomes.

Reprinted by permission from S. Streator and W.E. Buckley, 2000, "Clinical outcomes in sports medicine," *Athletic Therapy Today* 5(5): 60.

One of the most visible ways in which outcomes assessment has been performed in athletic training has been the NATA Reimbursement Advisory Group's three-year outcomes study. The study used an instrument called the Athletic Training Outcomes Assessment (ATOA) to link specific treatments with outcomes and to assess athletic training procedures for efficacy and efficiency (Keirns, Knudsen, and Webster, in Konin 1997). The ATOA considers a number of factors, including type of injury, body part, type of treatment, affective variables, comorbidities, and patient outcome expectations (see figure 2.13). Bear in mind that this outcomes study has many of the weaknesses of other outcomes studies that use self-reported patient surveys, including the lack of a control or comparison group (Albohm and Wilkerson 1999). Campbell (1999) reports that data from the three-year study yielded the following results:

1. Athletic training methods produce excellent overall outcomes, with the best results in functional outcomes and physical outcomes.

2. Athletic training techniques are effective in treating injuries at all body locations, especially in the lower extremities and spine.

3. Industrial patients treated with work-hardening techniques by athletic trainers had excellent outcomes.

4. The total number of treatments provided is a positive factor in determining positive outcomes.

ATHLETIC TRAINING OUTCOMES ASSESSMENT©

TO BE COMPLETED AT INITIAL ENCOUNTER

Site-Athletic Trainer Code _____   Patient Name_____   Age _____   Sex _____

(for site use only)

Site Type _____

1. Sports Medicine Clinic
2. Clinic—High School/College
3. High School Training Room
4. College/University Training Room
5. Professional Training Room
6. Industrial Setting

Referring Source _____

1. Self
2. Coach/Supervisor
3. Insurer
4. Primary Care Physician/Generalist
5. Orthopedic Physician/Specialist

Payer _____

1. Medicaid
2. Medicare
3. Managed Care
4. Workers' Compensation
5. CHAMPUS (government/military)
6. Private Insurance
7. Institution
8. Patient

TO BE COMPLETED BY ATHLETIC TRAINER AT INITIAL EVALUATION

Duration Between Injury/Surgery and Beginning of Athletic Training Treatments _____ days
(Put 0 if treatments begin on the same day as the injury/surgery.)

Location of Injury/Surgery _____
(Give only the <u>one</u> most primary location. If another injury, identify as a comorbid factor.)

1. toe(s)	4. lower leg	7. hip	10. abdomen	13. cervical	16. arm	19. wrist
2. foot	5. knee	8. pelvis	11. lumbar	14. head	17. elbow	20. hand
3. ankle	6. thigh	9. groin	12. thorax	15. shoulder	18. forearm	21. finger(s)

Type of Injury _____
(Give only the <u>one</u> most primary injury. If another injury, identify as a comorbid factor.)

1. joint dysfunction	4. sprain; grade I	7. skin/wound infection	10. fracture
2. joint degeneration	5. sprain; grade II	8. bursitis	11. avulsion
3. joint hypomobility	6. sprain; grade III	9. musculotendinous injury	12. neurologic disease

TO BE COMPLETED BY PATIENT AT INTAKE AND DISCHARGE

Patient—Your responses to this questionnaire will help your athletic trainer and this clinic determine rehabilitation outcomes for specific medical conditions in response to specific treatments. This will help us optimize our treatment services to you and other patients. Your responses will be kept confidential and will not affect your care in any way. Thanks for your assistance.

AT INTAKE   **AT DISCHARGE**

AT INTAKE						AT DISCHARGE				
CRITICAL PROBLEM	SEVERE PROBLEM	MODERATE PROBLEM	MINOR PROBLEM	NO PROBLEM		CRITICAL PROBLEM	SEVERE PROBLEM	MODERATE PROBLEM	MINOR PROBLEM	NO PROBLEM

Instructions—Please rate your current capacities specific to the injury for which you will receive, or have received, treatments. Please answer all questions as best you can, even if some of the questions seem somewhat irrelevant to you. Circle the appropriate response according to the (0 1 2 3 4) scale; 0 - critical problem, 1 - severe problem, 2 - moderate problem, 3 - minor problem, 4 - no problem.

0 1 2 3 4	**Work Activities**—lifting/lowering, holding/handling, carrying, pushing/pulling, bending over, squatting/stooping, kneeling, crawling, reaching, turning/pivoting, gripping/pinching, fingering	0 1 2 3 4
0 1 2 3 4	**Sports/Recreation/Wellness Activities**—running, jumping, throwing, catching, kicking, swinging, withstanding impacts, weightlifting, specific sport/recreation/wellness activities	0 1 2 3 4
0 1 2 3 4	**Movement**—getting into desired positions, range of motion, speed of motion, bilateral differences (e.g., limping), need for support device	0 1 2 3 4

▶ **Figure 2.13** Excerpt from Athletic Training Outcomes Assessment.

Adapted from JAMES A.F. STONER, MANAGEMENT, 2nd Edition, ©1982, pp. 268, 271. Prentice Hall, Englewood Cliffs, New Jersey.

5. Patients have a high degree of satisfaction with athletic trainers and their services.

6. Athletic training outcomes are consistent across site types, referring sources, and payer groups.

7. As the number of days increased between an injury and the onset of treatment provided by a certified athletic trainer, the patients' favorable perceptions of their outcomes decreased.

Another important outcomes study that has helped demonstrate the efficacy and efficiency of the care provided by athletic trainers was conducted by an independent outcomes research company, Focus on Therapeutic Outcomes, Inc. (FOTO). The FOTO study, conducted in 1999, compared patient responses to care provided by athletic trainers with that provided by physical therapists in the same clinical setting. The study showed that the outcomes associated with the care provided by athletic trainers, including various measures of value and patient satisfaction, were similar to those associated with care provided by physical therapists. Although the FOTO study provides a good starting point for the systematic study of athletic training outcomes, it has received criticism because it did not assess measurable patient function outcomes valued by the insurance industry. Future studies should be structured so as to analyze improvements in patient function, which will better enable the insurance industry and other important external markets to assess the cost-effectiveness of athletic training care.

Evidence-Based Practice

Over the last couple of decades, there has been an increased effort internationally to support assessment techniques and interventions as they relate to all aspects of medicine. The term **evidence-based medicine** has evolved as an approach to improving practice efficacy. Among other variations of this term are "evidence-based practice" and "evidence-based health care." Sackett and colleagues (1996), considered one of the forefathers of evidence-based medicine, coined the phrase and defined it as "the conscientious, explicit, and judicious use of current best evidence in making decisions about the care of individual patients." When incorporating the evidence into clinical practice, one should use a systematic approach toward reviewing peer research data so that unbiased clinical decision making can occur (Belanger 2002). Steves and Hootman (2004) noted the following reasons for the importance of evidence-based medicine for athletic training:

1. Improvement of care for the patients

2. Promotion of critical thinking

3. Ongoing and continued evaluation of treatment methods

4. Allows for athletic training to further contribute alongside health professions in peer-reviewed published evidence

5. Improved potential for third-party reimbursement

6. Overall enhanced reputation for the profession

The authors have furthermore identified five components of evidence-based medical practice for athletic trainers to adhere to:

1. Define a critically relevant question

2. Search for the best evidence

3. Appraise the quality of the evidence

4. Apply the evidence to clinical practice

5. Evaluate the outcomes of the applied evidence

Watson (in Law 2002) described the **relative value** of a particular intervention as it relates to the overall cost of providing the service. With reference to five types of economic value (cost–consequence analysis, cost-minimization analysis, cost-effectiveness analysis, cost–utility analysis, and cost–benefit analysis), part of the perceived success of an intervention relates to how the intervention compares in outcomes results to other comparable treatments when the cost per delivery of the intervention is factored in. For example, if two interventions yielded the same result for a patient but one was less costly than the other, the lower-cost intervention would be better to use for the overall population since this could translate into a significantly larger savings of dollars spent for health care. Pharmaceuticals is an area in which this is clearly seen. Many brand-name drugs also have a "generic" equivalent that is approved to provide similar outcomes at a much lower cost to the consumer.

Since evidence-based medicine approaches to clinical care are a relatively new concept in organized health care, many current practitioners were not formally educated about the process and have been forced to learn the importance of the evidence, as well as how to identify and utilize evidence, as part of their professional growth. There is growing support for teaching evidence-based medicine concepts as a standard part of today's medical and health care curriculum in an effort to promote this style of clinical practice as a learned normative method (Burns and Foley 2005; Cliska 2005). The BOC considers the application of evidence-based medicine in the practice of athletic training a professional responsibility. Similarly, the educational competencies as outlined by NATA include using evidence-based medicine as a foundation for the delivery of care for all entry-level athletic trainers.

One outcome that has been sparingly introduced into clinical practice as a result of evidence-based medicine is the use of **clinical practice guidelines**, or **CPGs**. Clinical practice guidelines have been defined by Nicholson (in Law 2002) as "systematically developed statements that assist practitioner and patient decision about appropriate health care for specific clinical circumstances." Perhaps one of the more well-known CPGs is the one related to the assessment process for an acute ankle injury:

The Ottawa Ankle Rules (OAR)

X-rays are only required if pain exists in the malleolar zone and any one of the following:

- Bone tenderness along the distal 6 cm of the posterior edge of the tibia or tip of the medial malleolus, or
- Bone tenderness along the distal 6 cm of the posterior edge of the fibula or tip of the lateral malleolus, or
- An inability to bear weight both immediately and in the emergency department for four steps.

Challenges With Implementing Evidence-Based Medicine

Despite the need for the profession of athletic training to join all other medical and allied health providers in the implementation of sound, evidence-based practice, not all have embraced the concept in its entirety. The two most common reasons are that (1) a large percentage of athletic trainers are not practicing in a setting that requires oversight of outcomes as they relate to using evidence-based techniques (i.e., reimbursement) and (2) the concept of evidence-based medicine has been formally taught in entry-level athletic training education programs for only the past couple of years. More specifically, the following barriers to successful integration of evidence-based practice in clinical settings have been identified (Haynes and Haynes 1998):

- Amount and complexity of available research
- Difficulties in developing evidence-based clinical policies
- Limited access to evidence for some clinicians
- Ineffective continuing education programs
- Challenges with patient compliance

Information relating to the professionally described role of evidence-based medicine for athletic trainers can be found in the following two documents:

National Athletic Trainers' Association. 2011. *Athletic training educational competencies*. 5th ed. Dallas: Author.

Board of Certification. 2010. *Role delineation study/Practice analysis*. 6th ed. Omaha: Author.

Maher and colleagues (2004) have also described barriers to evidence-based practice specifically in the physical therapy profession, identifying the following reasons behind the barriers:

1. Publication bias, with authors submitting for publication only those studies that have yielded positive outcomes

2. Indexing of journals, as many practicing clinicians do not have access to subscriptions for databases, and many databases do not include trials performed earlier

3. Difficulty of obtaining access to the full text of some published articles

4. Language barriers, as some studies are not published in English

5. Limited number of systematic reviews that assist with assessment of internal validity of the published research

6. Difficulty in translating published studies into clinical practice

7. Difficulty in drawing conclusions from the evidence when conflicting reports are available

8. Difficulties of influencing the integration of the evidence into a patient's own health care decision-making process

It is clear that much more needs to be done for a complete cultural shift toward universal acceptance of evidence-based medicine to occur. Collaborative efforts toward removing the perceived and real barriers to implementing evidence-based medicine will allow for further advancement of quality health care services based on sound evidence. Furthermore, all scientists, educators, and clinicians will need to come closer to a consensus for rating systems that are used to both evaluate and report the evidence. One important concept that has plagued the profession of athletic training as well as medicine as a whole is the fact that in some cases, positive patient outcomes can be achieved despite the lack of peer-reviewed scientific studies that explain why. A lack of studies to support an assessment or intervention does not in and of itself mean that the approach does not work.

> The following two websites serve as resources for evidence-based medicine databases:
> Center for Evidence-based Physiotherapy, www.pedro.org.au/, and Centre for Reviews and Dissemination at York University, www.york.ac.uk/inst/crd.

APPLICATIONS TO ATHLETIC TRAINING: THEORY INTO PRACTICE

The following three case studies will help you apply this chapter's concepts to real-life situations. The questions at the end of the case studies have many possible correct solutions. These studies may be used as homework or exam questions or to stimulate class discussion.

■ Case Study 1

The chairperson of the Department of Sport and Exercise Sciences met Susan Quigly, the college's athletic trainer, in the hallway. After exchanging the news of the day, the chairperson said, "By the way, I've been working on the NCAA self-study, and one of the sections deals with drug education programs and policies. I know we are just a small college that doesn't have many problems with drugs, but I can't send this thing over to the president without addressing the issue, especially in light of the emphasis the NCAA places on it. Would you be willing to organize a program so that we can at least meet the NCAA guidelines?"

"What would you want such a program to include?" asked Susan. "This could potentially be a huge project."

"You're the expert," replied the chairperson. "Let me know what you come up with."

Susan had strong opinions on the use and abuse of alcohol and other drugs. Several of her family members had suffered the negative effects of drug and alcohol use. She had plenty of examples of how alcohol had affected her students. She decided that if she was going to take on this program, she wasn't going to allow any half measures. She knew that for a problem as complex as drug and alcohol use among college students, she would have to develop a comprehensive program to be successful.

(continued) ▶

(continued)

After checking with several other athletic trainers who had developed programs for their schools, Susan began writing a proposal for the program. She decided to include the following elements:

- A standards-setting workshop led by a trained facilitator to help the coaches and team captains develop their own rules and sanctions for alcohol and other drug use
- A policy statement that would address the college's concern about the drug and alcohol issue with procedures to provide an action plan to deal with the problem
- A series of educational seminars and workshops for the student-athletes that would form the bulk of the drug and alcohol education program
- A research study to find out the extent of the problem on campus and determine the effectiveness of the program

The entire program would cost approximately $3,000 for the first 18 months. Because the department wouldn't allocate any funds for the project, Susan wrote a grant proposal to a local community foundation that covered the cost. Susan was pleased and confident. After six months of planning, the program was finally ready to go.

QUESTIONS FOR ANALYSIS

1. Based on what you know of Susan's planning effort, how successful is the drug and alcohol education program likely to be? How would you have planned this program?

2. Who are the inside interests in this case? Who are the outside interests? How is this program likely to affect them? How should they be involved in planning it?

3. How much support do you think Susan will be able to develop for the program? What strategies should she use to develop support?

4. How should Susan evaluate the effectiveness of the program? What elements should she include in the evaluation plan?

5. How should Susan write the policy that she wants to see adopted? Develop an example of a process and a procedure that might support such a policy.

6. If you were in Susan's position, would you have handled anything differently? What alternative actions would you have taken?

■ Case Study 2

Dan Wu was halfway through his first year as the chairperson of the Department of Athletic Training Studies at a midsized university. The department he led offered an accredited undergraduate major in athletic training. The department was housed in the College of Allied Health and had graduated an average of 10 students per year for the past eight years. Two full-time faculty members and three adjunct members who had release time from the athletic department staffed the department.

Dan received a memo from the dean of the College of Allied Health informing him that it was his department's turn for a departmental review. In keeping with the new policy of allowing greater administrative freedom to department chairpersons, Dan would be allowed to collect and present the evidence that he thought the provost and the dean's council should use to judge the effectiveness of the department. The dean told Dan that he would have five months to submit his report.

A few days later, Dan was having lunch in the faculty cafeteria when the dean walked over. "Dan," the dean said, "you should know that the dean's council has been given instructions to reduce our budget by 10% next year. After discussing the problem, we all agreed that the only way to do it without weakening all the programs is to eliminate

one of them. I wanted you to know that, unofficially, your department is one that is being considered in the cutback. No decision will be made until after the departmental reviews come in."

QUESTIONS FOR ANALYSIS

1. What evidence should Dan present when preparing the report for the departmental review? What plan for collecting the evidence would you develop if you were in Dan's position?

2. Which aspects of the evidence should Dan highlight, considering the uncertain future of his department? How could he best feature this evidence for maximum effect?

3. Would an external evaluator be useful in this situation? What qualities of the external evaluator would lend credibility to the report?

4. Besides the departmental self-study, what other steps could Dan take to safeguard the future of the department? What are the likely effects of these actions? Could any of these actions have negative consequences?

Case Study 3

Chris Kyle is beginning his senior year as an athletic training student at a small college. His class includes eight students who want to attend the upcoming NATA Annual Meeting & Clinical Symposia in June. Though it is just a few hours' drive away, they will likely need to raise money to offset the costs of conference registration, gas, hotel accommodations, and food.

The athletic training student club discussed the various methods of fund-raising, and most of the students expressed concerns over the amount of time they would need to spend on fund-raising efforts while they maintain an intense curricular load and clinical education requirements. They decided that the much relied upon approaches of selling candy, holding car washes, having bake sales, and others of the like would never provide the level of funding they would need to reach their goal of having everyone attend the national meeting.

Chris expressed his concerns to his club advisor during the first week of classes in September. His advisor mentioned that in recent conversations, some of the athletic training program's CIs inquired about obtaining CEUs within the next few months since the end of the three-year reporting period was December 31 of this year, just four months away. Chris' advisor told Chris that he would help the club put together a CEU course. He also told Chris that if the course was profitable, he would allow all of the proceeds to be used toward the students' trip.

QUESTIONS FOR ANALYSIS

1. If Chris were to encourage the club to participate in the planning of a fund-raising CEU program, what priorities would the students need to consider to determine whether or not the effort would be profitable?

2. With essentially a little less than four months for planning, what challenges would the students face in determining the logistics of the course?

3. What criteria should the students use in identifying topics or a course content theme? How will they determine who will give the presentations?

4. How should the students assign responsibility among themselves to ensure that all aspects of course preparation are taken care of?

5. Are there any specific incentives that could be implemented to encourage participants to register early?

6. Given the current economic challenges that all businesses are facing, what steps could the students take to secure sponsorship for the program?

SUMMARY

Program management encompasses the summative process that athletic trainers must consider when overseeing an organization or activity. All programs and organizations should begin by establishing a vision statement that serves as a succinct description of what the program should eventually become. A mission statement is also an important planning tool that can convey the goals and philosophies of a program and further identify, for example, the particular services to be offered, the primary market for those services, and the technology to be used in delivery of the services. All developing programs should include a strategic planning process in an effort to foresee elements of implementation. Strategic planning processes should include some form of self-analysis, such as a WOTS UP or SWOT analysis. Strengths, weaknesses, opportunities, and threats can be thoroughly assessed through internally and externally derived data collected from stakeholders to better align a program for success. These findings may also help formulate program policy and procedures that will assist in operational tasks.

Facility planning may be required for organizations envisioning any form of small- or large-scale type of business or event, and many considerations need to be taken into account to ascertain the necessities. When meetings are involved, a large majority of the time is spent during the planning phases. Typically, the larger the size of the meeting or conference, the greater the amount of time that should be reserved for planning. An established time line should be followed to ensure optimal success. Small-sized departmental meetings also require planning, with agendas thought through in advance and disseminated to meeting attendees prior to any discussion. Ongoing evaluations of conferences should be performed in an effort to assess the outcomes of the delivery of an event. Regular smaller-sized meetings should also undergo a periodic review so that meetings can remain efficient, timely, and productive.

KEY CONCEPTS AND REVIEW

1. Understand and develop vision and mission statements for a sports medicine program.

Change is a pervasive aspect of organizational life that affects sports medicine programs. The development of vision and mission statements can help a sports medicine program create a philosophical infrastructure that will allow it to adapt appropriately to change. A vision statement should identify the service provider, the service to be provided, the recipients of the service, and the expected quality of the service. The mission statement is a broad, enduring statement of purpose that defines the scope of operations of the sports medicine program. The mission statement should direct the athletic trainer toward accomplishing specific tasks, motivate and inspire, and guide the development of goals and objectives.

2. Understand the principles underlying sports medicine strategic planning.

Planning is a set of activities that the athletic trainer should engage in to bring about a desired future state for the sports medicine program. Strategic plans are broadly written guides for developing specific program goals and objectives. The development of a strategic plan involves identifying the needs of both outside and inside interests; gathering information that identifies the historical and present status of the program; and analyzing the strengths and weaknesses of, the threats to, and the opportunities for the sports medicine program.

3. Develop and link sports medicine policies, processes, and procedures.

Operational plans are explicit steps that guide the actions of athletic trainers so that they can accomplish specific tasks. A policy is an operational plan for expressing the organization's intended behavior relative to a specific program subfunction. Policies require the approval of persons in legal authority, such as boards of trustees or owners. Processes are a collection of incremental and mutually dependent steps designed to direct the most important tasks of the sports medicine program. Procedures provide athletic trainers with specific direction for various processes.

4. Communicate and develop ownership in a sports medicine program among inside and outside stakeholders.

Planning will be ineffective unless the athletic trainer can elicit support for the plan by identifying and influencing allies, opponents, bedfellows, and adversaries. The agreement–trust matrix can be a useful tool in this process. Athletic trainers should employ specific strategies with each of these groups to gain support for their programs and ideas.

5. Understand the principles of effective meeting and conference planning and management.

Most people view meetings as a necessary evil, but if properly organized they can be productive engines of decision making. Meetings are generally most effective if athletic trainers organize in advance, divide the meeting into parts, control their own behavior, avoid new business and reports whenever possible, and have a future-oriented perspective. Conference planning is a specialized activity that some athletic trainer-administrators will have as part of their responsibilities. Planning an effective conference involves appointing a coordinator and a steering committee, establishing a theme and developing a program with the right speakers to accomplish the conference goals, establishing realistic time lines and budgets, selecting a site, developing a plan for registration, marketing the conference, planning for meals and entertainment, recruiting exhibitors and sponsors, preparing learning materials, and contracting for a variety of miscellaneous services.

6. Understand the principles of effective sports medicine program evaluation.

Athletic trainers should evaluate the effectiveness of their sports medicine programs to ensure that the programs will continue improving and to document program quality. Formative program evaluation identifies strengths and weaknesses and provides alternatives for improvement. Summative evaluation judges the quality of the program. Program evaluation is most valid when it uses the scientific method to compare program clients with persons who do not have access to the program. This process is often difficult, expensive, and impractical. As much comparative data as possible should be used to evaluate the program. The use of an external auditor, along with chart auditing and outcomes studies, can facilitate unbiased assessments. A periodic self-study process that involves collecting evidence of program quality and answering questions crucial to program development is recommended.

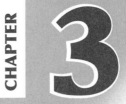
Human Resource Management

OBJECTIVES

After reading this chapter, you should be able to do the following:

1. Understand the different forms of organizational culture that can exist in a sports medicine program.

2. Formally define the relationships of the persons working in a sports medicine program by developing an organizational chart.

3. Understand the components of staff selection.

4. Develop a position description and a position vacancy notice.

5. Understand the recruitment and hiring process, especially as affected by discrimination and bias based on race, gender, disability, religion, or national origin.

6. Understand the differences among the three major supervisory models.

7. Understand the purposes, methods, and standards for evaluating athletic trainer performance.

► David Lewis had just completed his 10th year as the head athletic trainer at a major NCAA (National Collegiate Athletic Association) Division I university. David liked his job, and the feedback he received from most of the coaches and athletic administrators was positive. In short, David was content.

David was concerned, however, about one aspect of the job: Problems had developed with Judy Armstrong, one of his assistants. Although the coaches and athletes she worked with thought that she was doing a good job, Judy seemed to have difficulty working with the other athletic trainers on the staff. They perceived her as argumentative, inflexible, and arrogant. David decided on a face-to-face meeting to confront the problem.

David was not prepared for Judy's assessment of her problems with the rest of the staff. "David," she began, "I'm not the problem around here—you are! I'm no different in most respects from any of the other staff athletic trainers except that I'm not willing to keep my mouth shut and put up with all the garbage that goes on around here. For instance, none of us knows where our job responsibilities begin and end. Oh sure, we know what sports we're supposed to work with, but beyond that, who is responsible for the duties that overlap from team to team? Where is it spelled out? There are eight assistant athletic trainers here at the university, not counting graduate assistants. We are constantly stepping on each other's toes because we don't know what our own jobs are, let alone what the other person's is. And another thing. Where do I stand relative to the other athletic trainers? I've been here three years and my performance has never been evaluated! I might be able to put up with the lousy hours and the miserable pay if I just got some positive reinforcement for the good things I do from time to time. Think about it, Dave. The average employment length for assistant athletic trainers since you came is about two years. Why do you think everybody leaves so fast if this is such a great place? Don't pin this on me, because I'm not the problem!"

Although the meeting with Judy had put David in an angry and defensive mood, he sensed a kernel of truth in her arguments. He was not a strong personnel administrator, and he knew it. In fact, he hated most of the administrative duties that his position required of him. The assistant athletic trainer turnover problem had nagged him for years. Suddenly, the contentment that David had with his job vanished. He was frustrated.

By working faithfully 8 hours a day, you may eventually get to be a boss and work 12 hours a day.

—ROBERT FROST

The problems with personnel administration that led to David and Judy's confrontation are typical of many sports medicine programs. Athletic trainers are professionals who are, in general, oriented toward providing clinical services. Most have never had any training in how to manage human resources. Some athletic trainers excel at this aspect of administration without any formal understanding of human resource systems, but they are the exceptions. The most complicated tools the athletic trainer will ever work with are people. Without a system for managing those assets, a sports medicine program is unlikely to accomplish its mission. If this sounds like a familiar occurrence, you may recall the Peter Principle from chapter 1. This chapter focuses on the human resource function of a sports medicine program and the skills athletic trainers need to be successful in this area.

FACTORS RELATED TO THE SPORTS MEDICINE ORGANIZATION

The nature of the organization in which athletic trainers work has a powerful effect on many factors related to their employment. Three of the most important are the organization's culture, structure, and informal elements.

Organizational Culture

The first decision the athletic trainer in charge of a staff makes, consciously or unconsciously, is what kind of organizational culture the program will have. **Organizational culture** includes the basic values, behavioral norms, assumptions, and beliefs present in an organization (Owens 1987). The organizational culture of a sports medicine program largely defines what it means to be an athletic trainer in that setting. It influences the levels of commitment and loyalty of the athletic trainers working in the program.

Bennis and Nanus (1985) have described three general categories of organizational cultures (which they refer to as social architecture) that the athletic trainer should consider as part of sports medicine human resource management: collegial, personalistic, and formalistic.

1. Collegial culture. The sports medicine program with a **collegial culture** is one in which the emphasis is on consensus, teamwork, and participation in most decisions by all members of the staff, who tend to view each other as peers. The head of the department allows and encourages everyone to offer input so that the decision-making process is consensual. Although this type of organizational culture appears ideal, it is inappropriate in some settings. For example, when quick decisions are required, the consensus-oriented style of the collegial culture is inappropriate because formal authority is spread among the members of the staff. If the staff is small, the collegial culture is probably both appropriate and useful. For a larger-sized staff, this style may make it more challenging to reach a consensus of opinion.

2. Personalistic culture. The sports medicine program that Dave "leads" has a **personalistic culture**. This sort of program places little emphasis on policy and procedure. Each member of the staff makes her own decisions. Teamwork and group consensus are not high priorities. Although program leaders might be available for advice and counsel, the staff athletic trainers' problems are perceived to be *their* problems, not the program's. The personalistic organizational culture is a form of controlled anarchy. This type of culture is seen with smaller staff sizes, or in some cases with somewhat larger-sized staffs who operate independently out of multiple athletic training room facilities.

3. Formalistic culture. The sports medicine program with a clear chain of command and well-defined lines of authority operates in a **formalistic culture**. The formalistic culture is typical of bureaucratic programs that heavily emphasize policy, procedure, and rules. This kind of organizational culture discourages risk taking and deviation from the established source of authority. Although this arrangement might seem undesirable for a sports medicine program, the formalistic style offers certain advantages. First, decisions can be made more rapidly because various members of the staff have formal authority. Second, established policies and procedures can provide direction to staff athletic trainers and continuity in quality of service for clients. Finally, programs with large staffs might benefit from a formalistic culture because it divides and defines responsibilities and thereby enhances internal organization.

All work cultures that require individuals to work as a team to achieve overall success must rely on several common elements. While establishing cohesion among people in the work setting might involve numerous components, Lencioni (2002) has identified five areas of critical importance—dysfunctions—that he feels must be addressed in order for a team to reach its goals.

Sports medicine programs typically exist in organizations that exhibit one of three kinds of organizational culture: collegial, personalistic, and formalistic. Each is typified by certain values, beliefs, assumptions, and behavior norms.

1. Absence of trust. Trust is lacking when members of a team are not willing to acknowledge to one another that they are imperfect. Mutual trust underlies team success. Lencioni suggests that teams with trusting members are more likely to be cognizant of and admit to their strengths and weaknesses, seek assistance when needed, and accept feedback and criticism about their areas and roles; they have learned how to be more focused on important issues.

2. Fear of conflict. Teams that fear conflict will not make the best decisions. Teams that do not have a fear of conflict tend to have lively and interesting meetings, solve real problems quickly, minimize politics, and move forward by extracting and exploiting the ideas of all team members.

3. Lack of commitment. Teams with members who lack commitment to the organization tend to create an environment characterized by ambiguity about directions and priorities and to breed a lack of confidence and fear of failure. They tend to revisit discussions again and again without coming up with meaningful solutions. In contrast, a committed team aligns itself around common objectives, develops an ability to learn from mistakes, takes advantages of opportunities before competitors do, and moves forward or changes direction when necessary without hesitation or guilt.

4. Avoidance of accountability. Avoiding accountability creates resentment among team members who possess different performance standards, which likely leads to mediocrity. Key deliverables and deadlines are missed unless other team members pick up someone else's burden, likely leading to further team resentment. With accountability, all performers, especially those with a poor track record, will feel pressure to improve. Accountable members of a team will raise the standards for expectations and reduce the amount of time necessary for corrective action related to performance management.

5. Inattention to results. The fifth dysfunction of a team is inattention to results. When team members do not pay attention to results, the result is failure to grow and stagnation. This is a common fault of many organizations in which leadership has been in existence for a relatively lengthy period of time and is comfortable and set in its ways of operating. A person or operation that remains still while competitors and even colleagues improve has been "run over by the train." Attention to results leads to a greater likelihood of retaining achievement-oriented employees and minimizing individualist behaviors, as well as yielding unselfish employees who will at times put the team's goals and interests above their own.

Organizational Structures

Every sports medicine organization has a structure. The **organizational structure** of the sports medicine program plays an important role in how well staff members accomplish the program's mission. Each athletic trainer in the program has a different job to perform. Although duties may overlap and one athletic trainer may have duties similar to another's, each is responsible for distinct duties. The exception, of course, is the sports medicine program staffed by only one athletic trainer, a situation that is not uncommon at most high schools and some small colleges. Organizational structure need not be a concern for athletic trainers in these environments.

When designing the organizational structure of a sports medicine program, athletic trainers must consider the desired span of control. **Span of control** refers to the number of subordinates who report to a given supervisor. Although management researchers disagree on the precise formula for establishing a span of control, most agree that supervision of employees, including athletic trainers, is easier and more effective if supervisors are directly involved with three to six subordinates (Ouchi and Dowling 1974). Organizational structures are typically depicted in organizational charts.

The **organizational chart** is a graphic illustration that shows the formal relationships among the various athletic trainers and other health care workers in a sports medicine program. Organizational charts are useful because they show staff members their roles in relation to the

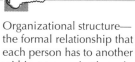

Organizational structure—the formal relationship that each person has to another within an organization—is best described by one of three types of organizational charts: function oriented, service oriented, or matrix.

overall program. In the opening case, Judy would probably have better understood the role David expected her to play if he had taken the time to develop an organizational chart for the university's sports medicine program. This task is especially important for newly hired athletic trainers because they lack a historical perspective of "how things are done around here."

Although a graphical depiction of the organizational structure of a sports medicine program can take many forms, most are charted according to function or service or in a matrix form.

Function-Oriented Organizational Chart

The section "Function-Oriented Organizational Chart": "Advantages and Disadvantages of a Functional Structure." Adapted from JAMES A.F. STONER, MANAGEMENT, 2nd Edition, © 1982, pp. 268, 271. Prentice Hall, Englewood Cliffs, New Jersey.

The organizational chart based on function is probably the most common in sports medicine settings. A functional organizational structure makes supervision easier because supervisors specialize along lines of expertise (see figure 3.1). Functional organizational structures are especially well suited to sports medicine clinics or universities with large staffs, because they facilitate allocation of staff members to projects for which they have special skills and knowledge.

Functional organizational structures also have several disadvantages. It can be difficult to make rapid decisions in these structures because requests often have to make their way up the chain of command. Functional organizational structures can also make it difficult to establish accountability for particular areas of responsibility. Consider the structure depicted in figure 3.1. If athletic training students are consistently failing the Board of Certification (BOC) examination, who should be held accountable? Is the athletic trainer in charge of clinical education at fault, or is the recruiting and placement coordinator guilty of bringing poor students into the program? Finally, the functional approach to organizing a sports medicine program can isolate staff members because it places little emphasis on sharing ideas or teamwork to accomplish program goals. From a team perspective, groups, committees, and especially departments within an organization that work in a function-oriented fashion tend to become possessive at times and to view compromise and collaboration as a weakness or as losing something. Groups that approach issues with this type of mentality are said to be functioning in a silo manner, without a positive interest toward interdisciplinary teamwork.

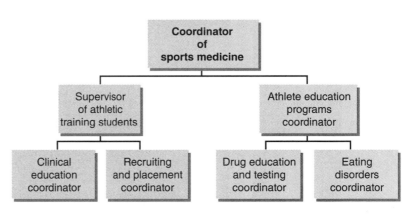

▶ **Figure 3.1** Sports medicine organizational chart: division by function.

■ Advantages and Disadvantages of a Functional Structure

Advantages
- Suited to a stable environment
- Fosters development of expertise
- Allows specialization
- Requires minimal internal coordination
- Requires fewer interpersonal skills

Disadvantages
- Slow response time in large programs
- Can lead to bottlenecks because of sequential task performance
- Less innovative; narrow perspective
- Might create conflicts over program priorities and staff responsibilities
- Little emphasis on sharing ideas and teamwork
- May lead to a silo effect

Service-Oriented Organizational Chart

The section "Service-Oriented Organizational Chart": "Advantages and Disadvantages of Service-Oriented Organizational Structures." Adapted from JAMES A.F. STONER, MANAGEMENT, 2nd Edition, © 1982, p. 274. Prentice Hall, Englewood Cliffs, New Jersey.

Another way to define the structure of a sports medicine program is to organize the staff according to the services they provide. Figure 3.2 provides an example from a large university that operates a sports medicine clinic in addition to the traditional sports medicine services provided by athletic department athletic trainers. With the exception of the box for the coordinator's position, the boxes in this chart represent athletic trainers who have responsibilities to certain client groups. This type of organizational chart is especially appropriate for programs that serve a diverse clientele.

Like its function-oriented counterpart, the service-oriented organizational chart has both advantages and disadvantages. One of the advantages of this system is that it facilitates coordination of services to any one client group because of the relatively strict division of responsibility. Accountability is easier to obtain because athletic trainers work with well-defined client groups. Finally, the chief decision maker can usually act more quickly and easily because intermediate supervisors have more authority to make their own decisions.

Among the disadvantages of this system are problems balancing power and authority. When service groups are tightly defined, athletic trainers working with a particular client group might tend to place the interests of that unit over the mission of the total program. Power struggles between members of the various program units may result. Another disadvantage with the service-oriented organizational structure is that it sometimes inflates personnel costs. Strictly delimiting service groups means that the expertise of an athletic trainer working in one unit is often unavailable to an athletic trainer working in another. Consequently, additional athletic trainers are required to balance the expertise between units. Supervisory expenses go up proportionally.

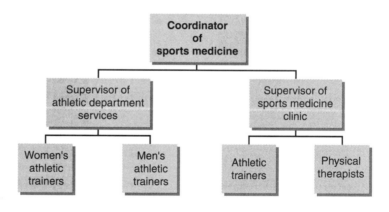

▶ **Figure 3.2** Sports medicine organizational chart: division by service.

Advantages and Disadvantages of Service-Oriented Organizational Structures

Advantages
- Suited to fast change
- Allows for high service visibility
- Allows full-time concentration on tasks
- Clearly defines responsibilities
- Permits parallel processing of multiple tasks

Disadvantages
- Fosters politics in resource allocation
- Inhibits coordination of activities
- Restricts problem solving to task needs
- Permits in-depth competencies to decline
- Creates conflicts between tasks and priorities
- Can inflate personnel costs

Matrix Organization Chart

Many athletic trainers will be tempted to structure their sports medicine programs in terms of function or service. Unfortunately, most traditional sports medicine programs do not match these models. Athletic trainers should consider an alternative to function or service paradigms: the matrix structure. The **matrix structure** combines the strongest features of the service and function models (Kolodny 1979).

In matrix structures, athletic trainers and other members of the sports medicine team report to two or more "bosses," depending on the project they are working on. The organizational chart for a matrix organization has both horizontal and vertical elements. If David accepts Judy's advice and develops an organizational chart for the university's sports medicine program, he might design a structure similar to the one in figure 3.3. The vertical elements show the chain of command in the program. The horizontal elements depict project teams that take advantage of the athletic trainers' specialization in certain areas. Not everyone has to be placed on a project team. Some athletic trainers will lack expertise in some areas. Others will be new to the organization and might need time to become acclimated. In educational settings like David's, some of the athletic trainers might have release time to teach sports medicine courses, making it difficult to assign them to project teams.

The advantages of the matrix system as a model for deploying athletic trainers include the ability to efficiently use the staff's expertise. In addition, the matrix structure reduces coordination problems and enhances economic efficiency by assigning only the necessary number of athletic trainers to any given project.

The matrix model also has disadvantages. Athletic trainers need a high level of interpersonal communication skill to work effectively with various coworkers on different tasks. For example, in the opening case study, Judy found that, like most athletic trainers, she needed to accomplish a number of tasks with other staff members. Because her interpersonal skills were not highly developed, she was unable to get along with her fellow athletic trainers. Another disadvantage of the matrix system is that athletic trainers can become frustrated and morale can suffer when people are switched between projects or when one project ends and another begins. Because many projects have a finite life span, this is a common problem.

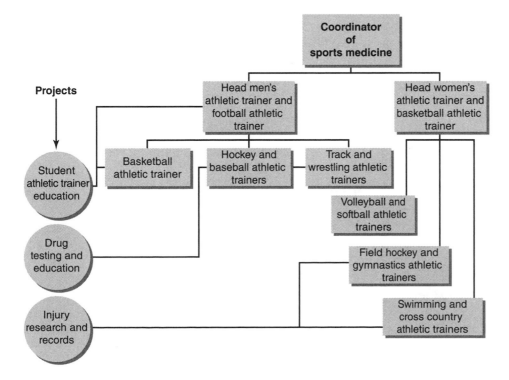

▶ **Figure 3.3** A matrix organization structure.

Advantages and Disadvantages of the Matrix Organizational Structure

Advantages
- Gives flexibility to the organization
- Stimulates interdisciplinary cooperation
- Involves, motivates, and challenges people
- Develops athletic trainers' skills
- Frees program coordinator for planning

Disadvantages
- Can create a feeling of anarchy
- Encourages power struggles
- Might lead to more discussion than action
- Requires high level of interpersonal skill
- Can be time-consuming to implement

Informal Organizations

Organizational structures, with their accompanying charts, are a useful starting point in helping athletic trainers and those with whom they work understand their roles in a sports medicine unit. Unfortunately, these devices rarely tell the whole story about how a sports medicine unit really functions. The formal organization, as defined by the officially approved organizational chart, is usually accompanied by the informal organization. Although the formal organization represents the theoretical relationships among the various members of the sports medicine unit, the informal organization represents the relationships as they exist and change from day to day. Whether athletic trainers are managers or employees, only those who understand both the formal and informal organizations will succeed in any given setting.

Why do athletic trainers and others join informal organization groups? They do so for many reasons, but Drafke (1994) believes that these are the most common:

- **Social contact.** The informal organization allows people to join small groups and form relationships, thus filling an important human need. People develop friendships at work. The informal organization allows this to occur.

- **Satisfaction of needs.** The relationships developed at work can provide for many of the psychological needs that most people have. The informal organization often bolsters self-esteem because it allows people to exercise power and assume leadership in a small group even when they have no formal authority to do so.

- **Power.** Many people join groups in the informal organization because they sense that they will enhance their power by doing so. A group is often able to influence the outcome of a decision, whereas an individual might not be.

- **Peer pressure.** Athletic trainers frequently join a group in the informal organization because of peer pressure to do so. A person who doesn't ally himself with a group might be shunned.

- **Problem solving.** Most people in the informal organization look to their peers as the first source in obtaining advice on how to solve work-related problems. This method is frequently less intimidating than seeking the advice of one's superior on the formal organizational chart.

- **Goal congruency.** Informal organization groups often form because of shared beliefs or goals. These goals might or might not be limited to work-related functions. Athletic trainers might choose to join a group based on common interests with other members of the group.

- **Understanding.** Often an individual joins a group in the informal organization because the group members encounter similar kinds of problems at work. Athletic trainers are more likely to ally themselves with other groups of athletic trainers because of this shared experience and desire for understanding.

Relationships between people in an organization often have nothing to do with the formal organizational structure. People form relationships in organizations for at least 11 reasons: social contact, satisfaction of needs, power, peer pressure, problem solving, goal congruency, shared understanding, information and communication, knowledge and expertise, formal organizational support, and physical proximity.

- **Information and communication.** The informal organization is potentially a tremendous information source. Athletic trainers often choose which groups to join based on how much information the group is privy to. Athletic trainers who share information about organizational issues—whether officially sanctioned or not—will find others flocking to their group to hear the latest news. Knowing when to pass on unofficial information and when not to is an important survival skill.

- **Knowledge.** The person who occupies the manager's role in the formal organization does not always have the most knowledge on a given subject. Athletic trainers will frequently seek out others in the informal organization for answers to their questions rather than going directly to their supervisors.

- **Formal organization support.** The power structure of the informal organization commonly functions to keep the department or institution going when the formal organization is flawed or temporarily incomplete. The strategy of taking action now and apologizing later, as opposed to asking permission, is common in both health care and athletic organizations. This strategy often works because the informal organization influences day-to-day operations more than the formal organization does.

- **Physical proximity.** Many people join groups in the informal organization because they work with the group members every day. Indeed, it is difficult to join a group when contact is infrequent.

STAFF SELECTION

The basis for human resource management in sports medicine is **staff selection**. Although the term *staff selection* might imply only identifying and hiring new athletic trainers, it has a much broader meaning in law. The Equal Employment Opportunity Commission's *Uniform Guidelines on Employee Selection Procedures* (1978) defines *staff selection* as any procedure used as a basis for any employment decision. Athletic trainer hiring, promotion, demotion, retention, and performance evaluation are all considered selection activities by law (see figure 3.4). To comply with the *Uniform Guidelines,* athletic trainers must be sure their employment practices do not adversely affect any group protected under the law. The only exception to these rules occurs when an organization can prove that it discriminates because of "business necessity." The following sections provide practical suggestions for athletic trainers with staff selection responsibilities.

Staff selection is commonly assumed to include just that—selection of employees. Staff selection is actually a much broader construct and includes any procedure used to make employment decisions.

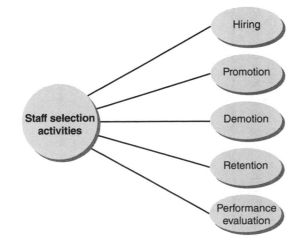

▶ **Figure 3.4** Staff selection activities in sports medicine.

To access the complete text of the *Uniform Guidelines on Employee Selection Procedures,* visit www.uniformguidelines.com.

Position Description

A formal document that contains information about the required qualifications for, and the work content, accountability, and scope of, a job is known as a **position description**. The position description is an important communication link between the athletic trainer and the supervisor that creates a common understanding of the role the athletic trainer should play in the program. Although many supervisors assume that their staffs agree with them about the duties for which they are responsible, Myers (1985) concluded that less than 50% of the employees he surveyed agreed with their supervisors on the standards and responsibilities of their jobs. When position descriptions are poorly written or are absent altogether, athletic trainers are unlikely to be able to meet the undefined expectations of their supervisors. Unfortunately, many athletic trainers do not have position descriptions (Ray 1991a) (see figure 3.5). In addition, many athletic trainers' position descriptions are poorly written, couched in trait-oriented language, or lacking in weights for various job descriptors.

The athletic trainer's position description should be divided into two sections: the job specification and the job description (see figure 3.6). The **job specification** describes the qualifications an athletic trainer should have to fill the role (Haddad 1985). An element that helps clarify the job specification is the **person specification**. The person specification translates the job specification into meaningful qualities that the person must have to be successful in the role. It also helps operationalize and define what those qualities must be for this particular job. The **job description** lists the responsibilities for which the athletic trainer will be held accountable (U.S. Small Business Administration 1980b). Each responsibility should be assigned a weight so that the athletic trainer understands which duties are considered the most important (Fowler and Bushardt 1986).

The weights assigned to various responsibilities can be determined in a variety of ways. One method is to determine what percentage of the athletic trainer's time will be devoted to a particular responsibility. This method would place more weight on "taping ankles" or "wound care" than on "performing CPR." An alternative would be to assign weights according

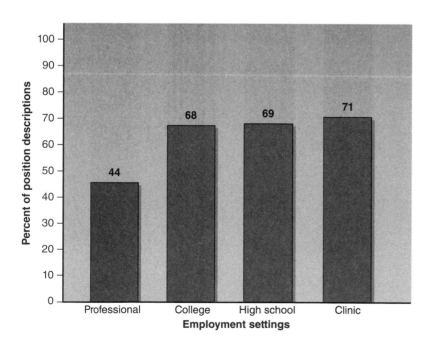

▶ **Figure 3.5** Position description frequency among athletic trainers.
Data from Ray 1991.

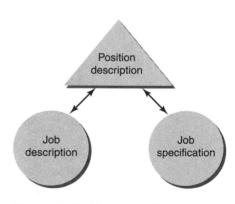

▶ **Figure 3.6** Position description components.

to how critical the job responsibility is. Using this method, "performing CPR" would clearly be weighted more heavily than "taping ankles" or "wound care." No matter which method is used, the weights must reflect the values of the organization. The casual observer should be able to see a clear representation of the organization's mission in the weighting of job responsibilities. Another important element in successful weighting of job responsibilities is a realistic assignment of weights. If every job responsibility is weighted as a 5 on a 1 to 5 scale of importance, the position description will not help the athletic trainer understand what is most important and what is less critical. It is also a good idea to clarify what minimal versus preferred qualifications are for the position. This is helpful for informing potential applicants of what is minimally required while simultaneously suggesting that the organization might be looking for individuals with more educational background, clinical experience, or research skill sets depending on additional considerations related to the position being advertised.

Athletic trainers who write position descriptions struggle with several important questions. Should the items be specific or general? Should the document describe what ought to be or what is? Although no definitive answers to these questions would meet the needs of every situation, general guidelines do exist. Being as specific as possible when delineating the duties and responsibilities of the athletic trainer is generally useful. Explicit descriptions are important because they provide clear direction for the athletic trainer. To avoid allowing employees to perform only minimal job responsibilities, Sikula (1976) suggests adding general phrasing near the end, such as "and any other duties related to the performance of this job as assigned by the Coordinator of Sports Medicine."

The question whether the job description should be normative or descriptive is not easy to answer. Ideally, the athletic trainer should have some input into her position description. She probably knows the most about the job and its responsibilities (Aldrich 1985). Unfortunately, when incumbents write their own job descriptions, they tend to be narrowly focused and to ignore tasks the incumbent does not enjoy, no matter how important they are to accomplishing the mission of the sports medicine program. For this reason, the program head should perform a final check on all position descriptions. The combination of input from the supervisor and the subordinate into the position description will more likely result in a balance between the needs of the employee and those of the sports medicine program. Position descriptions for new athletic trainers should be written as normatively as possible so that the new employee can begin to adapt to the new work setting. In any case, the position description should reflect only the characteristics of the job, not ambiguous personal characteristics like loyalty, initiative, and trust.

Finally, no matter which approach is used, the position description should be reviewed and modified as needed, at least once a year, to reflect changes in the athletic trainer's qualifications or the work environment (Bruce 1986). For an example of what Judy's position description might look like, see figure 3.7.

Recruitment and Hiring

Attracting and retaining qualified, competent staff members is crucial to the overall success of a sports medicine program. **Recruitment** of athletic trainers and other allied health care professionals should be viewed from two perspectives: the long-range need for human resources within the sports medicine program (see figure 3.8) and the immediate staffing needs.

The long-term staffing plan depends, to a significant degree, on the strategic plan of the sports medicine program. How is our client base likely to change? How will the accomplishment of our goals and objectives affect our need for staffing? The long-range recruiting plan should consider a number of factors, including the likelihood of promotion or transfer of present staff members, upcoming retirement plans, and the projected availability of athletic trainers and other allied health care workers in the labor pool. All these factors are important.

POSITION DESCRIPTION

Job title: Assistant Athletic Trainer

Date: July 1, 2012

Department: Intercollegiate Athletics

Status: Salaried Nonfaculty

Incumbent: Judy Armstrong

Supervisor: Linda Black, Head Women's Athletic Trainer

Written by: David Lewis, Coordinator of Sports Medicine, and Judy Armstrong

Approved by: James Wilson, Director of Intercollegiate Athletics

JOB SPECIFICATION

Factor	Job Specification	Person Specification
Education	Requires minimum of bachelor's degree	Must have a bachelor's degree
Certification	Requires credentials consistent with Ohio law and recognized national standards	Must be BOC certified, hold a valid Ohio license, and be certified in CPR
Working conditions	Requires travel over weekends and holidays, and exposure to all kinds of weather	Must have flexible schedule and be in good physical condition
Physical demands	Requires lifting of injured athletes, manual dexterity, and administration of CPR	Must be able to lift heavy weights and have functional use of all four extremities

JOB DESCRIPTION

Job Responsibilities	Relative Importance (1 = low 5 = high)
Coordinates and delivers athletic training services to members of the field hockey and gymnastics teams including, but not limited to, coordination of physical exams, evaluation and treatment of injuries at practices and games, design and supervision of rehabilitation programs, counseling within the limits of expertise, and prepractice/game taping	5
Refers injured athletes to appropriate physicians according to guidelines in the Standard Operating Procedures	5
Submits injured athlete status reports to coaches by 11:00 A.M. of the day following the injury	4
Maintains computerized injury/treatment database according to guidelines in the Standard Operating Procedures	3
Coordinates NCAA Injury Surveillance program by conducting in-service training for student athletic trainers, collecting and checking the accuracy of individual and weekly injury report forms, and mailing completed forms to the NCAA by Monday of each week	3
Prepares annual injury and treatment report for all sports by June 1	3
Exhibits behaviors in strict compliance with the NATA Code of Professional Practice	5
Performs other duties not specifically stated herein but deemed essential to the operation of the sports medicine program as assigned by the Coordinator of Sports Medicine or the Head Women's Athletic Trainer	Varies

▶ **Figure 3.7**   Sample position description.

For example, if the program structure will support an additional athletic trainer but the pool of qualified applicants is inadequate, the human resources plan for the sports medicine unit might need to be revised. Each of these factors should be evaluated annually so that future staffing needs can be met.

The other perspective in the recruitment process is the immediate need for staffing the sports medicine program. Immediate staffing needs typically arise because of five changes in the makeup of the present staff: radical program changes, termination (for either personal or professional reasons), retirement, noncompliance, and death. Each of these can result in the immediate need to fill a vacant position (see figure 3.9).

Neither long-term nor immediate staffing needs of the sports medicine unit can be fulfilled unless those needs are successfully integrated into the overall institutional or departmental staffing plan. Athletic trainers are often frustrated when their staffing requests are denied or put on hold. Too often, the athletic trainer-manager responds to this negative outcome by saying, "Athletic training always gets shortchanged around here. Our needs are always considered last priority." Frequently, the reason for these decisions is not that athletic training and its needs are low priorities, but that athletic trainer-managers have not carefully cultivated institutional decision makers, who face pressure from many competing interests. The athletic trainer-manager must communicate the staffing needs of the sports medicine program to institutional decision makers so that they will receive frequent reminders about how important those needs are to the operation of the program.

Many institutions that employ athletic trainers have specific procedures in place for recruiting and hiring all personnel. In these institutions, the athletic trainer in charge of staffing the sports medicine program has little choice but to become well informed about the policies and procedures and to adhere to them scrupulously. Most institutional recruitment and hiring policies and procedures are designed to prevent blatant forms of discrimination based on race and gender. In many cases, the athletic trainer will be required to document every step of the recruitment and hiring process to ensure that all qualified applicants have equal opportunity in the process. McCarthy (1983) has suggested that employers ask the following questions of their recruitment and hiring practices to determine if they could be discriminatory:

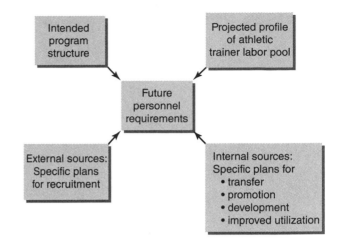

▶ **Figure 3.8** Long-range recruiting considerations.

CASTETTER, WILLIAM B., PERSONNEL FUNCTION IN EDUCATIONAL ADMINISTRATION, 4th Edition, 1986, by permission of Pearson Education, Inc., Upper Saddle River, NJ.

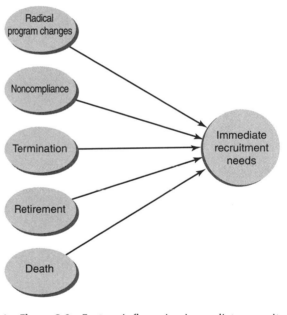

▶ **Figure 3.9** Factors influencing immediate recruitment needs.

- Are hiring restrictions based on sex, national origin, age, or religion or bona fide occupational qualifications?
- Are the prerequisites listed in the job specifications valid indicators of success as an athletic trainer?
- Is there a legitimate necessity for policies and procedures that adversely affect any given class of employee?
- Are the questions asked in the hiring interview directly related to the prospective employee's ability to perform the job responsibilities?
- Have reasonable accommodations been made to enable people with disabilities or persons of various religious beliefs to perform the job?
- What precautions have been taken to ensure that present recruitment and hiring policies and procedures do not perpetuate past discriminatory practices?

Validity and Reliability in Hiring

Besides ensuring that racial and gender bias are systematically purged from the hiring process, the athletic trainer in charge of staffing must consistently use hiring criteria that are predictive of success in the position. **Validity** in staff selection criteria is important for several reasons. First, the use of valid hiring criteria is more likely to produce an athletic training staff that functions well in its role. Second, using valid hiring criteria enhances efficiency in the staff selection process because productive employees are less likely to leave the organization, which would create gaps that must be filled. Finally, valid hiring criteria can help demonstrate that the hiring process was fair and free from bias.

Establishing validity in hiring criteria is a difficult process that often takes years to accomplish. A significant amount of trial and error might be involved in validating the process. In general, athletic training managers ought to scrutinize every established criterion for a particular position and ask themselves two questions:

- Could a person who did not meet this criterion be reasonably expected to succeed in this position?
- How likely is it that a person who meets this criterion will succeed in this position?

If the answer to the first question is yes, the criterion is not valid and should be discarded. The answer to the second question is a bit trickier. The athletic trainer-manager must predict a probability value based on his knowledge of the position and his experience. If the answer to the second question is "quite likely," then the criterion is probably valid. If, on the other hand, the athletic trainer-manager cannot predict how successful candidates would be even if they met the criterion, the criterion is probably not valid. We use the modifier "probably" because the only way a manager can definitively assess the validity of employment criteria is by collecting data over time and determining the relationship between various employment criteria and success or failure in the position.

Reliability in staff selection is the degree to which employment standards and practices are applied with consistency to all candidates. As with validity, reliable procedures are important to ensure that bias is reduced to a minimum. Reliable procedures also help produce the same information when applied to different candidates. For example, suppose that all candidates for an athletic training position with a large urban police or fire department were required to submit to a drug-screening procedure. If the procedure resulted in an unacceptably high rate of false positive or false negative results, it would be an unreliable staff selection criterion because its use provides different information for candidates with similar characteristics. Ensuring that all candidates go through an identical screening process, including the questions asked during the interview, will enhance reliability.

Hiring practices vary greatly from organization to organization. Some sports medicine programs employ an informal process, whereas others adhere to rigid procedures. Most will use a system that resembles the following 10-step process.

Step 1: Request for Position

Athletic administrators, general managers, principals, and clinic administrators will not consider filling a vacancy or adding a new position unless the athletic trainer makes a specific request. Some organizations require that the athletic trainer complete a specific form as part of the request process. Others require a position description. Obviously, administrators will generally screen requests for additional personnel more cautiously than they will requests for position replace-

---

■ Common Steps for Recruiting and Hiring Sports Medicine Personnel

1. Request for position
2. Position request approval
3. Position vacancy notice
4. Application collection
5. Telephone interviews
6. Reference checks
7. On-site interview
8. Recommendation and approval for hiring
9. Offer of contract
10. Hiring

ments. Such requests should be detailed enough to document need, based on both present and forecasted program conditions. The athletic trainer-manager could use many potential sources of information to justify the position. Outcomes data, patient load, revenue statements, and student–faculty ratios are just a few examples of the kinds of justification most administrators will require before they approve a position.

Step 2: Position Request Approval

After the athletic trainer in charge has submitted the request to the appropriate administrative officer, the request will probably be approved, denied, or held up pending further study. Athletic trainers should try to anticipate the data that administrators will need to make a decision.

Step 3: Position Vacancy Notice

Once the request for position is approved, the athletic trainer might be required to advertise the position vacancy to satisfy collective bargaining agreements and state and federal guidelines. Position vacancies should be posted both internally, so that present sports medicine staff who wish to apply for a position may do so, and externally. Position vacancy notices may be posted externally in any of the following locations:

- Local newspapers
- National Athletic Trainers' Association Placement Vacancy Notice Service, www.nata. org (click on "Career Center")
- *NCAA News*
- *Chronicle of Higher Education*
- Publications of the American Alliance for Health, Physical Education, Recreation and Dance
- Publications of the American Physical Therapy Association
- Publications of the American College of Sports Medicine

Finally, many athletic trainers find it useful to send a copy of the position vacancy notice to program directors of accredited athletic training education programs, alumni mailing lists, or other forms of e-mail distribution lists composed of athletic trainers.

The position vacancy notice should not be a carbon copy of the position description but should include a summary of the major responsibilities, a list of prerequisite qualifications, and a brief description of the major attributes of the institution or organization. In addition, the position vacancy notice should have the name, address, and telephone number of the person responsible for coordinating the hiring effort for the sports medicine program along with a list of required application documents. Typical application documents include a resume or curriculum vitae, letter of application, letters of reference, and transcripts. Many institutions require notice of nondiscrimination near the bottom of all position vacancy notices (see figure 3.10).

Although creating the position vacancy notice is an important step in the hiring process, athletic trainers who wish to attract the best candidates to their programs must rely on their networking skills to do so. For example, assume that David Lewis in the opening case has a position vacancy in his program. He has been in the business for many years and has been prudent in getting to know many athletic trainers around the country. He is familiar with two or three highly qualified athletic trainers who he knows would be a good match for the position in his program. If he wants to attract them to this position, he will have to take an active role in informing them about the position and encouraging them to apply. He should send them a copy of the position vacancy notice, but he should also speak with them personally to express his interest in attracting them to his institution. Athletic trainer-managers responsible for staff selection should maintain a file on people who they think would be excellent candidates for future positions in their organizations. When openings occur, they should contact these people directly and encourage them to apply.

POSITION VACANCY
Ohio Technological University
Assistant Athletic Trainer

OTU is seeking applications for the position of assistant athletic trainer in the Department of Intercollegiate Athletics. Primary responsibilities include the delivery of athletic training services for the field hockey and gymnastics teams, although occasional work with other teams will be required. This position also includes responsibility for coordinating the sports medicine program's injury research and records program, including maintenance of the computer database and coordination of athletic training students involved in NCAA injury surveillance data collection.

Minimum qualifications include a bachelor's degree, BOC certification, an Ohio athletic training license, and current American Red Cross CPR certification.

Salary is negotiable and will be commensurate with experience. This position is a 10-month, renewable-term, salaried nonfaculty contract.

Ohio Technological University has an enrollment of 25,000 students and is located in an urban center of over 250,000. OTU offers 41 undergraduate majors and 15 graduate degree programs. The university is a member of the NCAA Division I and offers eight sports for men and eight for women. OTU is an equal opportunity, affirmative action employer. Women and members of minority groups are encouraged to apply.

Interested persons should send a letter of application, resume, three letters of reference, and undergraduate transcript by June 1 to

David Lewis
Coordinator of Sports Medicine
Ohio Technological University
Urban Center, OH 40000
(217) 555-5555

▶ **Figure 3.10** Sample position vacancy notice.

A word of caution regarding this technique is appropriate. Athletic trainers who actively recruit from the ranks of other sports medicine programs run the risk of being accused of stealing another organization's employees. This situation can lead to bad feelings and damaged institutional relationships. Although avoiding this unpleasant side effect of network-based employee recruiting can be difficult, the best approach is generally to work with the candidate to develop a strategy to minimize the consequences and preserve the relationship. In most cases candidates will not want their employers to know that they are considering another position until they are reasonably certain that they will in fact be hired by the new organization.

Nowhere is network-based recruiting more important than in the effort to identify, recruit, screen, and hire members of minority groups. Athletic trainers who wish to enhance the racial and cultural diversity in their programs face a difficult challenge because the number of ethnic minority certified athletic trainers is relatively small. To encourage members of minority groups to apply for their positions, athletic trainers will probably have to employ at least four strategies. First, they should mail the position vacancy notice to the athletic trainers at all historically black colleges and universities. Second, they should mail the position vacancy notice to the program directors at universities that offer accredited athletic training education programs. Third, they should send the position vacancy notice, along with a personal letter, to certified athletic trainers who identify themselves as members of a minority group. Finally, the athletic trainer will probably need to make direct contact with minority athletic trainers she is familiar with and personally invite them to apply for the position. Even with the use of all four strategies, recruiting minorities to a program may take a long time.

Step 4: Application Collection

The next step in the process is to receive and screen applications for the position. A common practice is to appoint a committee of interested persons with a legitimate stake in hiring the athletic trainer to screen applications. The operation of search committees varies widely. Some operate on consensus, whereas others follow strict parliamentary procedure and vote on the suitability of various candidates for the position. In some cases, the committee suggests a name to a director, dean, or other high-ranking administrator who is charged with making the final decision.

In any case, incoming applications should be sorted into three groups: unqualified applicants, qualified applicants with complete application files, and apparently qualified applicants with incomplete application files. As the application deadline approaches, the committee should send a letter to apparently qualified applicants with incomplete files requesting an immediate response if they wish to remain under consideration for the position. The committee should keep on file a copy of all correspondence with applicants as evidence of good-faith hiring practices on the part of the institution or organization.

What process should the committee use to assess a candidate's credentials? No foolproof method exists, but athletic trainers should be aware of certain "red flags" as they evaluate the materials submitted as part of the application package.

Application Letter   Athletic trainers should ask themselves the following questions as they read an application letter (see figure 3.11 for a sample letter).

- Is the letter personalized? An application letter addressed "To Whom It May Concern" indicates a gross lack of preparation on the part of the candidate.

- Is the letter well written? The application letter demonstrates the writing skills of the potential employee. A candidate whose application letter is poorly written and full of grammatical errors is likely to write poorly after he or she is hired.

- Does the letter briefly describe the candidate's experiences and qualities without duplicating the contents of the resume?

- Does the letter describe why the candidate thinks he or she is qualified for the particular position? Letters that do not contain this information are often form letters that candidates routinely include with all job application packets.

- Has the letter been proofread? One common error is not changing the name of the school, the employer, or a person in the letter when a candidate is preparing multiple letters that contain somewhat similar information.

Resume   Athletic trainers should ask themselves the following questions as they read an applicant's resume (see figure 3.12 for a sample resume).

- Is the resume professionally prepared? A poorly formatted resume often shows that the applicant has poor organizational skills.

- Does the resume contain all the usual categories of information? Common categories include personal information, educational background, professional experience, honors and awards, and references. Other categories that might be appropriate include publications, presentations, grants, and volunteer and community service.

- Does the resume reflect a continuous time line from the date the candidate entered school until the present? Gaps in the record are not necessarily bad, but they should be investigated if the candidate is chosen for a telephone interview.

- Does the candidate's experience reflect the kind of position for which she is applying? If the candidate has never worked in a setting similar to the one she is applying for a job in, it will be difficult to predict how well she is likely to perform based on experience.

- Do the previous professional experiences listed on the resume reflect stability? A resume filled with many jobs of short duration raises questions about the employability of the candidate.

A list of minority athletic trainers is available from the NATA Ethnic Diversity Advisory Committee. The EDAC sponsors a discussion list—LEDAT. To subscribe, contact LEDAT-subscribe@ yahoogroups.com. You can also participate in think tank discussion groups on a variety of employment-related topics; visit www.nata. org and click on "Think Tanks" under the "Social Media" section.

February 5, 2012

David Lewis, ATC
Coordinator of Sports Medicine
Ohio Technological University
Urban Center, OH 40000

Dear Mr. Lewis:

The purpose of this letter is to request that I be considered as a candidate for the assistant athletic trainer position at Ohio Technological University. I have been a high school athletic trainer for the past five years and am very interested in furthering my career at the university level. I am particularly interested in the position at OTU because it would allow me to build on the skills I have developed since finishing my master's degree. On a personal note, I am also interested in this position because it would allow me to move back to a region of the country where my parents and most of my family reside.

As you can see from my resume, two of the sports with which I have experience are gymnastics and field hockey. I have enjoyed working with these sports at the high school level, and I am anxious and excited to have the chance to work with college-level gymnasts and field hockey players. I have asked the coaches of the teams I have worked with in my present position to write to you in support of my application. I am confident that they will be able to help you gain a better sense of my athletic training skills in these two sports. I believe that my experiences as a college-level gymnast would also help qualify me for your position.

Thank you very much for considering my application. Enclosed you will find a resume and a list of references. I would be grateful for the opportunity to interview with you and your staff at any time you think would be appropriate. If you have any questions regarding my background or application, please do not hesitate to contact me.

Sincerely yours,

Amy Hays

Amy Hays, MS, ATC

▶ **Figure 3.11** Sample application letter.

- Are the references listed on the resume well-known, reputable members of the profession? References with whom the athletic trainer is personally acquainted are more likely to provide an honest appraisal of the candidate's qualities—both good and bad. Do the references include individuals who served in supervisory roles for the candidate? How long has a reference known the candidate and in what capacity?
- Does the resume reflect the candidate's experiences without exaggeration? Many candidates attempt to make their experiences sound more glamorous than they really were. For example, if a candidate indicates that he was an assistant athletic trainer at a Division I university and you deduce that this took place while he was a junior in college, he has probably inflated his experience as an athletic training student at that university.
- For an entry-level athletic trainer, does the resume reflect a skill set beyond the basic expectations for all entry-level athletic trainers?

Amy Hays, MS, ATC
1234 South Armstrong St.
Way-Out-West, CA 90000
999-555-2000
amyhays@network.com

Professional Goals

I would like to use the experience I have gained as a certified athletic trainer in the high school setting in a more competitive and athletically challenging environment. I would especially like to secure a position in a Division I university.

Educational Background

2011	Master of Science in Athletic Training, Big State University
2009	Bachelor of Science, Regional University (Major—Athletic Training Minor—Biology)
2007	Associate of Arts, Wiley County Junior College

Professional Experience

2009–Present   **Way-Out-West High School**   I serve as the head athletic trainer in a high school comprising 2000 students and 20 sports, including

Boys' Sports	Girls' Sports
Football	*Field hockey*
Cross country	*Cross country*
Soccer	*Soccer*
Basketball	*Basketball*
Swimming	*Swimming*
Gymnastics	*Gymnastics*
Volleyball	*Volleyball*
Track	*Track*
Baseball	*Softball*
Tennis	*Tennis*

In addition, I coordinate the school's drug and alcohol prevention program. My responsibilities also include maintenance of injury and treatment records.

2007–Present   **Western County Triathlon**   I serve as the medical director for this event, which draws over 1,000 participants from all over the state.

2007–Present   **Summertown Gymnastics Club**   I teach gymnastics at this club during the summer.

Certifications

2009–Present	Certified Athletic Trainer, National Athletic Trainers' Association Board of Certification
2008–Present	Certified Basic Life Support Instructor, American Red Cross

Memberships

2007–Present	National Athletic Trainers' Association
2009–Present	Far West Athletic Trainers' Association
2009–Present	California Athletic Trainers' Association

(continued) ▶

▶ **Figure 3.12**   Sample resume.

Honors and Awards

2009   Athletic Training Scholarship, Big State University
2006   Most Valuable Gymnast, Regional University

Publications

Hays, A. (2007). Scaphoid non-union in a gymnast: A case study. *California Sports Medicine,* 2(3):14–16.

References

These people have given their permission to be contacted for additional background on my experiences and qualifications:

Ms. Renee Bigelow
Athletic Director and Gymnastics Coach
Way-Out-West High School
1245 Western Dr.
Way-Out-West, CA 90000
999-555-8903

Ms. Lillie Thompson
Field Hockey Coach
Way-Out-West High School
1245 Western Dr.
Way-Out-West, CA 90000
999-555-8903

Dr. Martin Dykstra, ATC
Program Director
Graduate Athletic Training Program
Big State University
Bigville, OH 40001
444-555-1111

▶ **Figure 3.12** Sample resume. *(continued)*

Letters of Reference   An athletic trainer should ask herself the following questions when reading the letters of reference:

- How long has the reference known the candidate and in what capacity? A referring individual who has known the candidate for a longer period of time in a capacity related to the position being sought is able to provide more substantive information. Having known the candidate for a short period of time can make it difficult to provide information. Also, someone who is a classmate, acquaintance, family member, government official, or religious or spiritual leader may not be able to provide an accurate assessment of a candidate's ability to perform athletic training–related tasks.

- Does the writer recommend the candidate for the position? Some people are honest enough to indicate that in their opinion a candidate is not well suited for a particular position, although this type of comment is rare.

- Does the writer balance the candidate's strengths and weaknesses? Every candidate has both, and the useful letter of reference will mention them.

- Does the information in the letter confirm what appears on the resume? Inconsistencies should be verified through a telephone call to the person who wrote the letter of reference.

- Is the letter of reference excessively short or vague in its assertions? People who don't really want to recommend a candidate will often write a very short letter confirming the candidate's employment or educational status and little else. Another common technique is to use language that is so bland and nondescriptive that it becomes difficult to determine whether the writer actually recommends the candidate or not.

- Does the letter include references to actual job performance? A strong letter of reference will focus on the quality of the candidate's performance. Weak letters often focus on personality traits that, while valuable and desirable, might not reflect on the quality of the candidate's work.

- Does the letter address the referring individual's perception that the candidate will be successful in the position being sought? Candidates may be better suited for certain positions than for others. Candidates should choose individuals as references based on the position they are applying for and should select people who can provide the most accurate assessment in relation to the particular job.

Step 5: Telephone Interviews

After the qualified applicants have been identified, members of the search committee should interview especially promising candidates by telephone. Telephone interviews in advance of on-site interviews are useful for weeding out unsuitable applicants and providing additional information not readily communicated in application letters or resumes. Telephone interviewers should be friendly and informative, but they should avoid making statements that the candidate might interpret as promises or oral contracts that might be binding on the institution. Questions asked in the telephone interview should elicit additional information unavailable in the application documents. Interviewers should ask each candidate the same questions in the same order to ensure reliability. Questions should always focus on candidates' job-related behavior, not on personal characteristics (Drake 1982). Table 3.1 presents some examples of legal and illegal questions that athletic trainers should be aware of when conducting interviews (Falcone 1997; Fry 1993).

TABLE 3.1 Examples of Legal and Illegal Interview Questions

Illegal question	Legal question
Are you a U.S. citizen?	Could you, after employment, submit verification of your legal right to work in the United States?
Do your religious beliefs allow you to work on Sundays?	Weekend and holiday work is a condition of this position. Is that acceptable to you?
Are you married? Do you have children?	Weekend and overtime work is a condition of this position. Is that acceptable to you?
Do you have any illnesses or disabilities?	Can you perform the essential job functions of this position with or without accommodation?
Did you serve in the military? What kind of discharge did you receive?	Did you serve in the military? Were any of the jobs you performed similar to those in this position?
Where did you learn to speak Spanish?	Do you speak any languages other than English that would be useful in this position?

Step 6: Reference Checks

After further narrowing the applicant pool through telephone interviewing, the search committee should begin checking references. This aspect of the recruitment and hiring process is important because it allows the potential employer to validate the information supplied by the candidate. Some application materials need not be checked. Notarized transcripts, diplomas, and certificates are usually, but not always, valid. Expiration dates and signatures should be checked.

The most valuable information source is usually the applicant's previous employers or, for entry-level applicants, internship supervisors. An applicant's performance in similar employment settings is the best predictor of how the person will perform the new job. Notes from all conversations should be kept in the applicant's file for future reference by other members of the search committee.

Step 7: On-Site Interview

On-site interviews are costly and time-consuming. Only those applicants who are obviously well qualified for the job should be interviewed on-site. Candidates about whom the search committee has serious reservations should not be interviewed. The on-site interview is important for both the candidate and the organization. The interview allows the candidate to become familiar with the work setting, and it allows the search committee to see the candidate in the work setting.

The on-site visit can be organized in many ways. Most visits should include a number of interviews with institutional stakeholders such as coaches, athletes and other physically active patients, athletic administrators, owners, team physicians, and other athletic trainers. Time should be set aside for the candidate to ask questions about the job. Candidates should have an opportunity to tour the facilities and inspect their potential worksites. The visit should typically be one or two days in length, depending on the level of responsibility of the position and the number of people who need to be involved in the interview process. If David Lewis, the athletic trainer in the opening case, was conducting an on-site interview for a candidate in the Ohio Technological University sports medicine program, the visit might be structured like the one in figure 3.13.

The people with whom the candidate will work closely should have the largest amount of interview time with him. Interviews with people the candidate will have limited contact with or those with only a tangential interest can be more limited in time and scope. Candidates interviewing for faculty positions should have time allocated for meeting with students enrolled in the program. This interaction can be beneficial for both the candidate and the students.

Bringing a candidate to campus for an on-site interview means it is believed that the individual possesses the minimal qualifications for the position based on the documents reviewed to date and the preliminary interview process. During the on-site visit, a part of the process should be used to confirm the candidate's ability to fill the role based on further inquiry and discussion. In addition, and perhaps most importantly at this point in time, the idea is to determine the "fit" of the candidate. As with any team, simply having the best players at every position does not necessarily guarantee a winning season unless the chemistry is right and the teamwork is effective. Determining whether or not a candidate is a good fit for an organization may be difficult to do objectively. Feedback from all of the stakeholders that have taken part in the interview process is helpful; and feelings, perceptions, and other indicators may be relied on to make such a decision.

An important aspect of the on-site interview that many managers fail to recognize is the need to sell the job to the candidate. Too often, we assume that the mere offer of a job will be enough to induce a candidate to accept. This is frequently not the case. A significant part of the interview process should be devoted to highlighting the benefits of the job, the organization, and the community.

Reliability in the on-site interview is just as important as in the telephone interview. Irrespective of how the interview is organized, a structured process will enhance the reliability of the selection procedure. In a structured interview, the interviewers, preferably the same

Itinerary for the visit of

John Olmstead
Candidate for the position of head men's athletic trainer

Monday, June 11

10:00 A.M.	Arrive at Urban Center Airport, met by David Lewis.
10:30 A.M.	Meet with Linda Black, head women's athletic trainer, Fieldhouse athletic training room.
11:45 A.M.	Lunch with Athletic Training Students Club representatives Jim Gleason and Elaine Williams.
1:30 P.M.	Meet with James Wilson, director of intercollegiate athletics, central administration building.
2:45 P.M.	Meet with Dr. Reid Chesterfield, team physician, Student Health Service.
3:30 P.M.	Meet with Greg Campbell, head football coach, Memorial Stadium.
4:15 P.M.	Meet with Lucy Sneller, director of human resources, central administration building.
5:00 P.M.	Check into Campus Inn.
6:30 P.M.	Dinner with David Lewis, coordinator of sports medicine, and Rick Ellis, assistant athletic trainer, Campus Inn Grill.

Tuesday, June 12

7:30 A.M.	Breakfast with Tom Hernandez, head men's basketball coach, University Club.
8:30 A.M.	Meet with members of the search committee, Fieldhouse conference room.
11:00 A.M.	Fly home. Jim Gleason will accompany you to the airport.
11:00 A.M.	Search committee meeting, Fieldhouse conference room.

▶ **Figure 3.13** Sample on-site interview itinerary.

people, ask each candidate the same questions in the same order. This process helps improve the chances that the search committee members will have the information they need to make distinctions between the candidates.

It is also helpful to schedule time for rest periods or breaks for the candidate, as well as social time when the employers and candidate can interact in a less formal environment. This can occur during casual dinners after a formal interview has taken place. If candidates are asked to give a presentation of any kind as part of the interview process, providing time for setup can be very helpful to the candidate, especially if audiovisual or other technological aids do not always operate as expected.

Step 8: Recommendation and Approval for Hiring

After the candidates have been interviewed on-site, the search committee must make a recommendation for hiring to the person in the organization with formal authority to approve it. Supporting documentation, including the candidate's resume, transcripts, letters of recommendation, and interview notes, should accompany the recommendation for hiring so that the decision maker has the necessary information to make a final choice. Search committee members should be sure they make a final recommendation for hiring based solely on the qualifications of the candidate and not on personal characteristics unrelated to the job, such as race, marital status, national origin, or creed.

Step 9: Offer of Contract

After the search committee has selected the most outstanding candidate, whoever is authorized to negotiate a contract with the candidate should call and orally extend an offer of employment. If the parties can agree on terms of employment over the telephone, the authorized institutional representative should prepare a formal employment contract consistent with institutional rules, collective bargaining agreements, and state and federal laws. The contract should include the starting date for the job, length of employment, salary and benefits, position title, and job responsibilities as specified in the position description. In addition, the contract should include a clause stating that the athletic trainer agrees to abide by the terms and conditions delineated in the institution's employee handbook. Two copies of the signed contract should be sent to the athletic trainer with instructions to sign and return one of the copies by a given date, usually within 10 to 14 days. Less formal ways of handling the offer of contract are certainly available, but the less formal the process, the greater the chances for misunderstanding and trouble later.

Step 10: Hiring

After a candidate has signed a written employment contract, the institution should send a letter to the other applicants thanking them for their interest in the position and informing them that the position has been filled. In some cases, it is considered gracious to personally call any candidates who were interviewed on-site and not offered the job to inform them of the hiring. Too many institutions, unfortunately, ignore this important courtesy. Another step that some institutions take at the end of the hiring process is to distribute a press release to the media announcing the addition of the new athletic trainer to the sports medicine staff. This valuable public relations tool for the sports medicine program makes the new athletic trainer's induction into a relatively unfamiliar work setting more comfortable. Providing the newly hired athletic trainer with an orientation manual can be very helpful during the preparation and transition process. Information on topics such as any training that needs to be completed, policies and procedures for computer access and usage, and other daily functions necessary to perform the job should be included.

Finding Your Job

Everything up to this point in this section has been written from the perspective of the athletic trainer-administrator who is looking for just the right person to join her staff. Because many readers of this text are either undergraduate or graduate athletic training students who aren't yet in a position to be doing the hiring, it seems fitting to include a few tips for helping you find your first job. Although the preceding material will help you understand the recruiting and hiring process from an employer's point of view, you should consider many additional facets of employment when looking for a job.

Identifying Job Openings

If you are a student just getting ready to graduate and enter the workforce, one of the questions you have undoubtedly asked is, "Where can I find a job as an athletic trainer?" Athletic training positions are advertised in many places. The career center at your university may have a database of recently posted positions. Similarly, your professors probably receive many letters every month advertising athletic training positions in all kinds of settings. The classified "help wanted" section of your local newspaper is usually not a rich source of athletic training positions, but you may find local schools, hospitals, or companies advertising there from time to time. Other ways to identify potential athletic training jobs include the following:

■ **Networking.** Your ability to develop and stay in touch with the many contacts you have made while in school might be the best job search strategy you can employ. The supervisors and teachers you have had in various classes, clinical experiences, internships, and health-related summer jobs will know about jobs as they become available from time to time. Make sure that all these people have a current copy of your resume, and keep in touch with them so that they will know that you are looking for a job. Dunne (2002) recommends that you let everyone in your life—including family, friends, advisors, and mentors—know that you are job hunting. You might be surprised by the way you find out about your first job! Professional networking begins in the undergraduate classroom: Someday your classmates will be practicing certified athletic trainers whom you will have built relationships with. It is beneficial to maintain friendships throughout school and beyond, despite minor episodes or incidents that might irritate you during a brief moment in time. Burning bridges can ultimately serve no benefit for future networking purposes.

■ **Cold calling.** This technique can be especially effective if your job search is restricted to a limited geographic area. For example, if you have to find a job in a certain city, you should compile a list of all the agencies, clinics, hospitals, schools, universities, and professional sports organizations that are likely to employ athletic trainers in that city. Send all these a letter indicating your interest in working for them as an athletic trainer (even if you aren't sure if they have any openings—they may save your letter for a future opening). Include a resume with your letter. Follow up with a phone call to see whether the organization received your materials and inquire about any openings. This task is time-consuming. If the geographic area that you are searching is large, this method can take a long time, but it is a valuable tool because you will be saturating a particular market with your name and While cold calling can be effective in identifying position openings that otherwise would not be easy to find, it is important not to overdo contact with any single employer. This may be perceived as nagging.

■ **Web-based databases.** Athletic trainers can take advantage of many web-based job search services. Some are specific to athletic trainers, whereas others are broadly structured for all kinds of health care professionals. The NATA (www.nata.org) provides one of the most important web-based services, but there are many others. Besides searching specific athletic training–related databases, you can use an Internet search engine like Google or Yahoo with search terms such as "athletic trainer" and "job" or "position" to develop a long list of potential positions in nearly every employment setting. Web-based search engines that are more specific to health care jobs, and especially athletic training jobs, will yield results on positions more suitable for an athletic trainer. In addition, universities, colleges, and school districts have human resource pages where they post position vacancies.

> The following websites are useful sources of potential athletic training positions:
> www.nata.org
> www.aahperd.org/careers/
> http://acsm.healthjobsplus.com/
> http://ncaamarket.ncaa.org/search.cfm

■ **Conventions, conferences, and job fairs.** National and regional conventions, conferences, and job fairs are a common and convenient place for employers to recruit athletic trainers. The annual conventions of the NATA, the American Alliance for Health, Physical Education, Recreation and Dance, and the American College of Sports Medicine all host job fairs that provide employers and job seekers a venue to meet, interact, and interview. If you plan to look for a job at one of these conventions, bring plenty of copies of your resume and show up prepared to interview.

Choosing Where to Apply

Once potential opportunities have caught your interest, you will need to decide which ones are worth pursuing. This can be a time-consuming process that involves learning about each position. Whether it is an athletic training job or a graduate assistantship you are seeking, the process of inquiry will be similar. To objectively evaluate each opportunity, you can use a matrix such as the one in figure 3.14 to assess the individual components of each position and also perform a comparative summary analysis. Items for consideration in the vertical column of the matrix can be added or deleted based on criteria you feel are important to evaluate. Some things to consider when weighing the relative merits of an employment offer include the potential for job growth, benefits, salary, environment for communication and collegiality, job security, and job flexibility (Konin, in Konin 1997).

	GRADUATE SCHOOLS						
Cost of tuition							
Size of school							
Location of school							
Distance from home							
Safety of area							
Reputation of school							
Postprofessional accredited status							
Length of degree							
Financial assistance							
Facilities & resources							
Cost of living							
Prerequisite attainment							
Volunteer hours							
GRE scores							
No. of faculty							
Faculty qualifications							
Curricular design							
Clinical sites							
Board passing rate							
Total rating							

▶ **Figure 3.14** Guide to choosing a graduate school. Using the chart, rate the categories for each graduate school. Use a scale of 0 to 10, with 10 representing the best situation for you.

Making Contact

After you have compiled a list of potential employers, the next step is to make sure that they become aware of your interest, background, credentials, and skills. A well-prepared resume and cover letter are the most common ways to accomplish this, but you can and should use other methods to help you stand out from the crowd. Depending on how your cover letter and resume were delivered, it is usually a good idea to follow up with either an e-mail message or a phone call to make sure that the potential employer received them. For some jobs this will be your first conversation with the employer, and making a good impression is important. Yate (2002) suggests that this contact experience should have four goals:

- Get the employer's attention
- Generate interest in your application
- Create a desire in the employer to know more about you
- Encourage the employer to take action on your application

Here are a few ways that will help you accomplish those goals:

- Express your enthusiasm for the opportunity to work in the organization.
- Fill the employer in on any additional experiences you may have had since sending in your materials. Keep in mind that if you are an entry-level athletic trainer, you possess all of the same skills every recently certified entry-level athletic trainer has based on learned competencies and proficiencies. Thus, additional experiences can help separate you from others.
- Remind the employer of the special skills or experiences that help you stand out from the crowd, but do this in a manner that doesn't exaggerate your experiences.
- Ask the employer if he has any preliminary questions that he would like to ask you.
- Identify your time line for availability as it relates to a start date and your overall flexibility for work scheduling.
- Thank the employer for his time.
- Stay in touch with all potential employers in this way until the position is filled or you have accepted another job.

Resume Writing

In many cases, one's first chance to make an impression on a potential employer takes the form of a resume. It is very helpful to seek advice from others regarding the development, formatting, and updating of a resume that may be attractive from the viewpoint of an employer. However, be prepared to receive as many opinions on how to prepare a resume as the number of people you seek advice from. While there is no one perfect method or style of resume writing, you can follow some general guidelines on how to present an appealing document.

All resumes follow a format that is designed to subdivide the background information for an individual and present it in chronological (or reverse chronological) order. The following subcategories are suggested for inclusion for an athletic training graduate or relatively new certified athletic trainer:

- **Personal contact information:** This should include formal and preferred name, current mailing address, e-mail, and phone numbers.
- **Goals:** It is helpful to list a single focused professional goal. This may be a relatively short-term goal, such as the type of setting you want to work in, or it may be slightly more long-term, for example what you want to accomplish within the next three to five years as an athletic trainer.

■ **Educational experience:** List all of the educational programs you have attended or graduated from. Include name of the school, geographical location of the school (city, state), year of attendance or graduation, and major and minor areas of study.

■ **Employment experience:** List all places of employment. Be sure to include the name of the employer, your position and title, primary responsibilities, dates of employment, and location of employment setting (city, state).

■ **Honors and awards:** Identify any relevant honors, awards, and achievements that you have earned relative to your professional career, academic endeavors, or social contributions. If the name of an award is not self-explanatory, include a brief sentence that describes the achievement. Academic and professional awards should always be highlighted on a resume. There are other honors and awards you may or may not want to list, for example, Boy Scouts recognition or captain of high school athletic team. It may be a good idea to list such honors if in total they represent a pattern of leadership or accomplishment. Again, as one's professional career advances, honors like these may become less relevant to athletic training skills.

■ **Presentations and publications:** Include any professional presentations you have given (exclusive of formal classroom assignments) or work you have published; examples are a poster at a regional district athletic training meeting, a community sports safety presentation to coaches or parents, or an abstract published in a proceedings manual.

■ **Memberships and certifications:** List the organizations or associations that you are a member of. This may include student athletic training associations, NATA, academic honor societies, and community groups. List the years of your affiliation, and if the name of the organization is not self-explanatory, include a sentence that explains its purpose. Be sure to list any leadership or official positions you have held in any of these organizations.

■ **Additional information:** There may be items you think are important to list on your resume that do not seem to fit into a specific category. You may also not want to have one item under a subheading as it may look like a lesser accomplishment. If this is the case, you can create subcategory headings of your own or simply use the subheading "Miscellaneous." An example might include a nonpaid shadowing experience you completed that was beneficial to your career. This might also be a place where you can list any additional languages you speak or computer or other related skills you possess.

■ **References:** List the names and current contact information of individuals who have agreed to provide a recommendation for you. Include their names, titles and affiliations, employer, mailing address, e-mail address, and phone number.

As previously mentioned, there are numerous opinions regarding what to include or not include on a resume. The following are some considerations that should be left up to you:

■ **Personal information:** Some people list their age, health status, hobbies, family members, and even religious affiliation. Depending on the employment setting that you are seeking, this information may or may not be relevant.

■ **High school:** Where someone attended high school becomes less relevant the longer her career. In some cases, a high school attended is listed on a resume because it has some connection to the potential employer or employment setting.

■ **Nonathletic training work experience:** Since athletic training is a health care profession, work experiences as a waitress, clerk, retail manager, or other jobs may not be relevant toward demonstrating capability as an athletic trainer. However, in some cases, listing these experiences may demonstrate work ethic or skills such as leadership, supervision, accounting, interpersonal skills, or software management that are similar to those required of a successful athletic trainer. Most would agree, however, that listing these experiences is more helpful to a newly certified athletic trainer than to one who has been removed from entry-level education for years.

■ **Grade point average:** Individuals who have obtained an above-average grade point are encouraged to list this on the resume as part of their academic experience. Be sure to list not only the earned grade point average, but also the potential maximum, for example, 3.7/4.0. If you have earned honors or high honors, this should be listed. However, if you earned honors for just one or two semesters out of a possible eight, you might want to consider whether or not to include this information.

■ **Employment departure:** All employment experiences should be listed, regardless of their duration. With noticeably short stints of employment, it may be wise to list the reason for departure in an effort to proactively explain what might otherwise be viewed as a red flag. Acceptable reasons for departures may include family or home relocations, a return to school for further education, illness, or other life-changing circumstances.

■ **Order of events:** The decision about what order to list items in is a simple one. If you have held three jobs, you can list them in reverse chronological order, with the most recent one first, or in chronological order beginning with the first job. Regardless of which method you choose, the order should be the same for all subcategories of the resume.

■ **References available on request:** Some professionals recommend not including references with contact information on a resume but instead the phrase "References available on request." Though the issue is open to debate, it would appear that including information on references makes for a more thorough resume, allowing potential employers who choose to contact your references to do so without having to track you down. Furthermore, from a networking perspective, listing the names of your references may trigger a connection of some kind with the employer. This could prompt a quicker phone call to discuss your candidacy based on name recognition alone.

Cover Letter

A cover letter should always accompany a resume. The cover letter should be succinct, presenting an overview of your interest in and qualifications for the job. The cover letter typically includes the following:

■ Introductory paragraph stating formal intent to apply for the position

■ Body of letter highlighting your experiences in a single paragraph

■ Careful meshing of your abilities with employer's needs in a single paragraph

■ Summary paragraph informing recipient of how you can be contacted

Figure 3.15 shows an example of a cover letter.

Common Mistakes to Avoid

While there are numerous ways to write a resume and cover letter, there are also some common mistakes that employers see regularly. Unfortunately, these errors can create a negative impression of the applicant. Careful proofreading and attention to detail will help you avoid these mistakes.

■ **Inappropriate e-mail address.** Contact e-mail addresses that do not look professional, such as partydude@email.net, make a bad impression.

■ **Nonapplicable career goal.** Applicants sometimes forget that the career goal listed on the resume should be specific to each position they are applying for and should be modified accordingly. For example, the career goal "To serve as head athletic trainer in a secondary school setting" should be changed or deleted if the applicant has decided to send the resume with an application for a university position.

■ **Incorrect names.** Candidates applying for multiple positions often use the same basic cover letter. Unfortunately, failing to change the name and affiliation of the addressee is not uncommon. This is simply a matter of careless proofreading and makes an unfavorable impression, even though employers know that candidates do apply for multiple positions simultaneously in an effort to find the right job.

January 14, 2012
Mr. Marty Stamkos
Athletic Director
Light High School
Tampa, FL 33533

Dear Mr. Stamkos,

In response to your recent posting for an athletic trainer position at your high school, I would like to formally submit my application for consideration.

After carefully assessing the position description, I believe that my past experiences and current leadership capabilities would serve as a complementary fit at Light High School. As my resume reflects, my career experience as a certified athletic trainer has included four years in a secondary school setting, the past two as the head athletic trainer. In addition, I am CPR certified and will soon become a certified strength and conditioning specialist.

My leadership experience and interpersonal skills are strengths that will enable me to provide quality care and services to the student athletes. I am dependable and organized and also have a dedication to my work that others have commended me for regularly. I believe that all these characteristics would enable me to perform in an exemplary manner at your school. It is my continued career goal to be an athletic trainer in a secondary school setting, and your program appears to be exactly the type of setting I would like to work in.

Thank you for consideration of my application. I can be reached at anytime on my cell phone or by e-mail if you feel that I am a qualified candidate and are interested in setting up an interview.

Sincerely,

Wes Oates

Wes Oates, ATC

▶ **Figure 3.15** Sample cover letter.

■ **Misspellings.** Misspelling addressees' names or listing their credentials incorrectly is a common error that should be avoided with careful proofreading. Similarly, applicants not infrequently misspell names of individuals listed as references and provide inaccurate or outdated contact information, which causes difficulties for potential employers who may wish to contact references.

■ **Name dropping.** It may be appropriate to inform a potential employer that you learned of the opening through a particular individual. However, listing people's names can give the impression that you hope their professional reputation or stature will increase your chances of obtaining a position and is often not seen in a favorable light.

■ **Redundancy.** The cover letter should emphasize and highlight key components of a resume. More importantly, it complements and should serve as an opportunity to expand on the resume. Using the cover letter to merely repeat what is on the resume is not the best way to sell oneself to a potential employer.

■ **Exaggeration.** The cover letter serves to explain why you feel you are a good fit for a job. Even though the cover letter is crafted to portray your background and your interest in the job, you should be careful not to exaggerate your skills or accomplishments. Guard against overstating your merits especially if you are a recent graduate, as it will be assumed that you possess entry-level skills.

■ **Listing basic accomplishments.** In listing responsibilities and accomplishments in a job or clinical experience, do not include basic tasks that every athletic trainer performs. Employers will expect that you can carry out responsibilities such as taping ankles, cleaning the training room, and evaluating and treating injuries, and these should not be listed as skills or accomplishments.

■ **Aggressiveness.** It is helpful to note your availability for interviews. However, many consider it inappropriate to state that you will contact the employer soon after sending a resume. It is acceptable in some cases to follow up to ask about the status of a job inquiry. However, it is not necessarily as appropriate to state, for example, "If I do not hear from you within one week I will contact you to set up an interview."

Interviewing

Interviewing for a job can take several forms. Employers sometimes conduct preliminary interviews by telephone before arranging face-to-face interviews with the most promising candidates. As suggested earlier, some employers conduct interviews at conventions and job fairs, whereas others prefer to bring the applicant to the employment site. Whatever the interview technique or location, your first task as the interviewee is to prepare. Although you'll certainly need to be able to answer the employer's questions during the interview, you should also be able to summarize your experiences, qualifications, and skills in approximately 30 seconds. You should be able to articulate your professional philosophy. Be prepared to explain how you deal with difficult problems, using examples from your past. Find out as much as you can about the organization before the interview—the organization's website is a great place to start this part of your preparation. All this takes planning and practice. You should arrange for a videotaped mock interview so that you can practice and receive feedback. Many career counseling centers on college campuses offer this service.

The list of questions that one can be asked during an interview is endless. There are standard, expected questions such as "What are your strengths and weaknesses?" Other questions tend to be people's personal favorites and are unlikely to be anticipated during preparation for an interview. The following are examples of questions that a candidate for an athletic training position might be asked:

■ What would others say are your strengths and weakness?

■ Explain how you would be a team player. Perhaps provide an example of a previous AT-related experience.

■ How can you specifically make our organization better?

■ Why should we hire YOU?

■ What unique skills do you possess, and how will that make you a good AT?

■ Are you willing to work nights and/or weekends and travel when necessary?

■ What are your professional goals for five years from now? 10 years from now?

■ What are your thoughts on the current state of health care as it relates to athletic training services?

■ Currently we are struggling with reimbursement issues. What suggestions might you have to assist us with efforts to obtain fair remuneration for the services that we provide?

■ Recently, we had an AT student who was asked to perform a manual technique on a patient that the AT student was not terribly comfortable with performing. Normally, the AT performs the treatment, and the results provide the patient with two to three days of pain relief. On this particular day, the AT had a family illness and could not make it to work. It also happened to be the last treatment session for the patient given the fact that she was going to leave for a three-day drive to California where she lives in the winter. If you were the AT student in this situation, what would you do?

- What type of salary are you looking for?
- With respect to this position, what are the most important issues that will determine whether or not you would accept should we decide to offer a position to you?
- Are you familiar with CPTs? [If candidate answers no:] How would you plan to learn about them prior to beginning employment with us? [If candidate answers yes:] What code would you choose to use for a patient who has ABC health care as an insurance provider and participates in a hydrotherapy session for 45 minutes under your supervision?
- Why do you want to work with us?
- How do you handle stress? Please elaborate.
- How do your goals tie into the mission of our program and institution?
- What is the first thing you would like to do if hired here?
- How could we help you here with your professional goals and interests?

In addition to these professional and work-related questions, it is not uncommon for employers to ask a candidate what might be considered a unique type of question not related to athletic training simply in an effort to judge the candidate's innovativeness and creativity. These are also questions intended to elicit spontaneous answers:

- If you could be a piece of furniture, what would you be and why?
- If you could be any animal, what would you be and why?
- Tell me about the last good movie that you saw.

Lastly, employers try to hire positive-minded individuals who will be motivated to work and who do not thrive on negativity or pessimism. Be prepared to respond to questions that may be "traps." The intent of this type of question is to provoke a candidate to speak in a negative manner about a previous employer, colleague, or situation. Here are some examples:

- What did you not like about your last job? Why did you leave?
- Did you ever have any professors you didn't like? What did you not like about them?
- Tell me something that you do not like about yourself.
- Please describe your idea of a "bad" job.

First impressions are critical. Although the employer has seen your cover letter and resume, the interview is probably the first time he or she will meet you in person. Although employers should certainly be concerned about your knowledge, skills, and experience as important predictors of future job performance, they will also be developing an impression of how well you are likely to fit into the culture of the organization. They will determine in a relatively short time whether they like you—and whether the other employees with whom they work will like you. The following tips will help you develop a good first impression with prospective employers:

- **Dress professionally for the interview.** Any externals (clothes, grooming, excessive jewelry) that distract the employer from your conversation will create a poor impression.
- **Learn as much about the organization as you can before the interview.** Besides trying to learn the names of the people in the organization, attempt to discern in advance the culture of the place so that you can frame your answers in a way that will have as much effect as possible. Ideally, talk to people who work in the organization or know it well enough to give you advice.

■ **Be enthusiastic.** Express interest in the things the employer tells you about the organization. If you think that this is a place where you could be happy working, be sure to say so. Employers want happy, motivated employees. You'll have to demonstrate that you can be both.

■ **Be courteous.** Although it may seem obvious that an applicant should show courtesy, failing to say simple things like "please" and "thank you" has derailed the job prospects of many talented people. As someone being interviewed for a position in an organization, you are a guest in that place for a day. Your interviewers will remember your behavior long after they have forgotten your answers to specific interview questions.

Closing the Deal

An interview will create a first impression in the mind of the employer. You should take steps to build on that first impression after the interview ends. After the interview, repeat in modified form the steps you took to contact the employer before the interview. Here are a few things you can do to help the employer remember you after you have left:

■ **Send thank-you notes.** Send notes to every person with whom you spoke during your interview. The notes should be specific to the conversation you had with that person (for example, "I enjoyed learning about your days at Big Time University. My experiences there as an undergraduate were outstanding."). Be sure to thank the employer for taking time to interview you for the position. Encourage the employer to contact you if additional questions or concerns arise. You can send these notes by either mail or e-mail, but it is best to send them immediately after the interview.

■ **Postinterview references.** Although you probably had several people write to the employer on your behalf before the interview, you may want to have one of your most trusted and enthusiastic sponsors contact the employer after the interview ends—especially if the sponsor is personally acquainted with the employer.

■ **Keep in touch.** Stay in touch with the employer after the interview so that you can both keep current with the search and to demonstrate enthusiasm and eagerness for the position.

■ **Prepare for a job offer.** Soon after your interview you may be called and offered a job. An offer frequently includes all of the terms for employment, including the salary. To be prepared, you should have some idea of the terms of employment that would be acceptable to you. The NATA surveys athletic trainers annually and posts the results on their reported salaries; the information is categorized by the type of employment setting, gender, years of experience, and other categories of relevance (National Athletic Trainers' Association 2006b).

■ **Don't burn bridges.** Be sure to maintain amicable relations with the employer even in the face of rejection. You never know when another opportunity to work in that organization might arise. Your response to *not* being hired can be just as important to your reputation as an offer of employment. You might not be the right person for the job at this point in the organization's history, but that does not mean you won't be at some time in the future. If you receive a rejection letter, write back to thank the employer for considering you for the position and send your best wishes.

PERSONNEL DEPLOYMENT

The cost of employing people makes up the largest portion of the budget for most service-oriented enterprises, including those in which athletic trainers typically work. If an educational institution, health care facility, or business that employs athletic trainers is to operate effectively and efficiently, it must deploy the right number of staff at the right times and in the right places. Too often, employers hire athletic trainers and, without doing adequate planning for reasonable workloads that yield effective patient outcomes, expect them to manage every aspect of athlete or employee health care needs.

Factors Affecting Personnel Deployment Decisions

Nelson, Altman, and Mayo (2000) recommend that institutions consider the following five elements when planning staff deployment:

■ **Activities to be performed.** What jobs are critical to the successful operation of the sports medicine operation? When and where are these tasks performed? The answers to these questions should flow from the goals and objectives of the sports medicine program as outlined in chapter 2. Activities not related to the program's mission, goals, and objectives draw needed staff resources away from the things that matter most.

■ **Required abilities.** What level of professional competence is required for each of the identified tasks? Which professional credentials, licenses, or certifications are required by law or commonly accepted standards? When considering the kinds of abilities required for the activities performed in the program, organizations should think about more than technical athletic training skills. Equally important are things like communication skills, interpersonal skills, and organizational and management skills.

■ **Number of required staff.** How will the number, timing, and location of tasks, along with rules governing reasonable workloads, affect the number of personnel required to accomplish the mission? (See the discussion of the Fair Labor Standards Act later in this chapter.) Standards that help establish the necessary number of athletic trainers cover some employment settings in which athletic trainers work. For example, accredited athletic training education programs are required to maintain a ratio of students to clinical instructors no greater than 8:1. The NATA has established recommendations and guidelines for the number of athletic trainers needed to staff college and university sports medicine programs adequately (see the later section on appropriate medical coverage).

■ **The way in which the staff currently uses its time.** Are the athletic trainers currently in place using their time efficiently? Effectively? Are they working on the right kinds of tasks given their level of training and expertise? A number of methods exist to analyze staff activities. Using a combination of existing records, supervisor observations, and employee self-reports, it is possible to determine the kinds of activities that athletic trainers are involved with. Mayo and Goodrich (2002) recommend conducting both numeric and process analyses from time to time as a way of determining the appropriateness of staff activities (see the next section on workload analysis).

■ **Finding staff to accomplish the goals of the program.** Are resources available to hire additional athletic trainers if they are needed? Can athletic trainers be reassigned to achieve greater efficiency? Can other personnel assume some of the duties now assigned to athletic trainers? Too often the first impulse—especially in athletic training, in which understaffing has been a chronic problem for many years—is simply to hire more staff to accomplish the mission of the sports medicine program. The athletic trainer-administrator has the responsibility, however, to accomplish the mission at the least possible cost. Given that staff salaries and benefits make up most of the costs, additional hiring is not always the best action. The athletic trainer-administrator should consider other options such as task reallocation, task elimination, outsourcing for certain tasks, and use of part-time personnel for some aspects of the program.

Workload Analysis

The athletic trainer-administrator can use many methods to monitor the work being performed by his staff for the purpose of determining appropriate staffing levels. Mayo and Goodrich (2002) recommend two that seem appropriate for sports medicine settings: numeric analysis and process analysis.

- **Numeric analysis** is the process of determining a staff member's workload by calculating and comparing the amount of time a person spends on certain tasks with the outputs—the measurable results. An example of numeric analysis commonly employed in sports medicine clinics is the number of patients treated by each staff member per day, per week, per month, or per year. A similar example from athletic training education would be the number of credit hours taught by a faculty member per semester or per year. Calculations of this type are most useful if they are tracked over time so that increases or decreases in workloads can be observed. Where national standards exist, numeric analyses can also serve as helpful indicators for determining whether a particular staff member or a group of athletic trainers is working below, at, or above the standard.

- **Process analysis** is a technique for streamlining the number and complexity of steps needed to provide a service to a customer. Tasks that require the fewest number of steps—and whose steps are the simplest to perform—typically require fewer people to perform. Athletic trainer-administrators who want to staff their programs at the lowest reasonable level should brainstorm with their staffs to identify all the steps required to complete any given task. Two or more athletic trainers may be performing the same task using completely different steps. Analyzing those steps may produce a consensus on the most efficient way to perform the task.

A word of caution regarding process analysis is appropriate. Although this technique can be useful in sports medicine and other health care settings, risks are associated with its rigid implementation. Health care professionals may understand that a certain degree of conformity to organizational processes is necessary for efficiency, but they are likely to complain if they must sacrifice their professional autonomy and judgment. For example, if a school's head athletic trainer advocates a taping method that uses 6 fewer inches of tape per procedure and imposes this method on the other members of the staff, she should not be surprised if her staff meets the directive with limited enthusiasm. Although the procedure is technically more efficient, the cost savings are likely to be minimal. Athletic trainer-administrators must balance gains in efficiency with the staff's needs for professional autonomy.

Appropriate Medical Coverage

Although the staff deployment concepts outlined in the previous section apply to almost any business or industry, the NATA's *Recommendations and Guidelines for Appropriate Medical Coverage of Intercollegiate Athletics* provides the most specific staffing recommendations available to the athletic training profession in a college and university setting. As the title suggests, the guidelines provide colleges and universities with a system for determining the number of certified athletic trainers required to render adequate health care services to their student-athletes. The model on which the guidelines were established was developed from published injury data, national surveys of collegiate medical coverage, guidelines from a variety of sports medicine organizations, and other sources. Similar documents now exist that offer guidelines and suggestions for appropriate medical coverage in other settings.

The staffing recommendations in the guidelines are based on the concept of the health care unit (HCU). Each sport is assigned a base Health Care Index (HCI) of one to four units based on injury rates for time-loss and non-time-loss injury and the volume of treatments typically associated with injuries in that sport. A full workload for each certified athletic trainer is 12 HCUs. The HCI for a particular sport can be modified based on a number of factors, including squad size, inclusion of a nontraditional season, travel requirements, and administrative duties. Athletic trainer-administrators can calculate the number of certified athletic trainers required to provide appropriate medical coverage by applying the base HCI in table 3.2 to the formula shown in table 3.3.

To access the NATA's *Recommendations and Guidelines for Appropriate Medical Coverage of Intercollegiate Athletics,* visit www.nata.org and click on "Statements" and then on "Position Statements."

TABLE 3.2 Base Health Care Index by Sport

Sport	IR	TX/I	IR·TX/I	HCI
Baseball	19.3	11.5	222	1.7
Basketball—M	29.3	11.0	322	2.4
Basketball—W	32.4	16.3	528	4.0
Crew—M	7.2	12.9	93	0.7
Crew—W	22.0	13.0	286	2.2
Cross country—M	21.7	8.6	187	1.4
Cross country—W	23.7	9.4	223	1.7
Fencing—M	15.7	16.2	254	1.9
Fencing—W	24.1	12.6	304	2.3
Field hockey	34.8	10.8	376	2.8
Football	42.5	9.7	412	3.1
Golf—M	6.5	9.8	64	0.5
Golf—W	13.8	11.0	152	1.2
Gymnastics—M	29.0	16.8	487	3.7
Gymnastics—W†	48.1	27.9	1,342	4.0
Ice hockey—M	33.9	7.2	244	1.8
Ice hockey—W	12.3	10.7	132	1.0
Indoor track—M	31.9	11.4	364	2.8
Indoor track—W	32.3	11.8	381	2.9
Lacrosse—M	23.9	10.0	239	1.8
Lacrosse—W	27.9	11.8	329	2.5
Outdoor track—M	18.3	8.0	146	1.1
Outdoor track—W	21.1	7.1	150	1.1
Soccer—M	35.0	10.7	375	2.8
Soccer—W	42.3	11.2	474	3.6
Softball	28.1	10.7	301	2.3
Swimming and diving—M	12.8	7.6	97	0.7
Swimming and diving—W	15.5	9.5	147	1.1
Tennis—M	21.7	9.3	202	1.5
Tennis—W	24.5	10.7	262	2.0
Volleyball—M†	35.0	22.7	795	4.0
Volleyball—W	36.8	12.6	464	3.5
Water polo—M	12.0	18.3	220	1.7
Water polo—W	22.2	7.9	175	1.3
Wrestling	41.8	9.1	380	2.9

To determine the maximum risk (value of 4), the IR·TX/I recorded for each sport was divided by the highest IR·TX/I recorded for any one sport where sufficient representative data were available (e.g., women's basketball). Sports indicated by (†) had higher IR·TX/I, but this was based on limited data.

TABLE 3.3 Sample Worksheet—Adjustments to Base Health Care Index

A Sport	B Base HCI (from table 3.2)	C Days/season†	D Athletes/team	E Total athlete exposures (C·D)	F Exposure modifier (E/1,000)	G Adjusted HCI (B·F)	H % of year	I Adjusted HCI/year	J Travel (20 days = 1 HCU)	K Admin duties
Baseball	1.7	132	30	3,960	4.0	6.7	50%	3.3	1.5	
Basketball—M	2.4	132	15	1,980	2.0	4.8	50%	2.4	1.5	
Basketball—W	4.0	132	15	1,980	2.0	7.9	50%	4.0	1.5	
Cross country—M	1.4	144	10	1,440	1.4	2.0	50%	1.0		
Cross country—W	1.7	144	10	1,440	1.4	2.4	50%	1.2		
Field hockey	2.8	132	25	3,300	3.3	9.4	50%	4.7		
Football	3.1	120	100	12,000	12.0	37.5	50%	18.7	0.5	
Gymnastics—W	4.0	144	10	1,440	1.4	5.8	50%	2.9	0.5	
Lacrosse—M	1.8	132	30	3,960	4.0	7.2	50%	3.6	0.5	
Outdoor track—M	1.1	132	40	5,280	5.3	5.9	50%	2.9		
Outdoor track—W	1.1	132	40	5,280	5.3	6.0	50%	3.0		
Soccer—M	2.8	132	30	3,960	4.0	11.2	50%	5.6	1.0	
Soccer—W	3.6	132	30	3,960	4.0	14.2	50%	7.1	1.0	
Softball	2.3	132	25	3,300	3.3	7.5	50%	3.8	1.5	
Volleyball—W	3.5	132	15	1,980	2.0	7.0	50%	3.5	1.0	
Wrestling	2.9	132	30	3,960	4.0	11.4	50%	5.7	0.5	
Totals								**75.8**	**11.0**	
							Total health care units (add all units in columns I-K)		**87.0**	
							Total full-time ATCs (Total health care units/12)		**7.25**	

†Figures represent total number of allowable practice days for both in and out of season for NCAA Division I. Individual institutional values should be adjusted based on competitive level and the extent of both traditional and nontraditional season activities.

Reprinted, by permission, of National Athletic Trainers' Association.

STAFF SUPERVISION

The concept of management as defined in chapter 1 includes the notion that managers coordinate the activities of a group of people toward a common goal. They accomplish this partly through supervision. **Supervision** is a process whereby authority holders observe the work activities of an employee to improve the outcomes of the employee's work or the professional development of the employee. Supervision is different from summative evaluation. The purpose of summative evaluation is to place a value on the quality of an employee to determine appropriate employment actions, including retention, promotion, demotion, transfer, discharge, and compensation level. In the opening case, Judy was upset that David had never evaluated her performance during the three years she had worked for him. Judy lacked both summative evaluation and supervision. She didn't know whether she was meeting the expectations of the program. She became frustrated because David didn't appear to care about her, her work, or her professional development.

Supervision is one of the most difficult managerial functions for an athletic trainer to master for several reasons. First, unless the employees whom the athletic trainer supervises are perfect in every way, supervision requires some degree of confrontation. Second, almost every supervisory problem is unique in some way. Responding to the employment-related problems of athletic trainers requires creativity and emotional investment in the staff and their development. Finally, effective supervision requires the athletic trainer to consider the opinions and perspectives of others. Athletic trainer-supervisors should develop strategies to reduce the level of bias they bring to situations so that the needs of both the sports medicine program and its employees can be met. Athletic trainers can use many different supervisory models. Tanner and Tanner (1987) have described four: inspection, production, clinical, and developmental. This discussion combines the inspection and production models because their differences are minor.

It is not uncommon for athletic trainers in supervisory roles to find themselves in a position of supervisory neglect. Directors of athletic training clinical services and directors of athletic training education programs are not often directly supervised by other athletic trainers. Clinical athletic training directors may be supervised by an athletic director or a principal at a school, whereas those in academia may report to a department chair or dean with a nonathletic training background. It is imperative for athletic trainers in these circumstances to educate their supervisors on their role and function so that their supervision and summative evaluations are performed fairly and are reflective of their duties. Interestingly, while 46% of the NATA membership is composed of women, only 37% of women have supervisory positions and leadership roles (Perez et al. 2006).

> Athletic trainers may be required to supervise other employees to improve their work outcomes or professional development. The three kinds of supervisory models are inspection-production, clinical, and developmental.

Motivation

Before we look at the various supervisory models, it will be helpful to consider the role that supervisors play in motivating employees. Motivation of workers is generally considered an important supervisory function, yet it remains a poorly understood and applied management concept in most work settings. The supervisory models described in this section differ in many ways from each other, in part because of the different assumptions they make about the nature of motivation in the workplace. The inspection–production model, for example, has its roots in the scientific management movement of the early 1900s (see chapter 1, pp. 6-7). One of the most important assumptions underlying that theory is that financial reward is the sole motivation for people to work. We now know that motivation in the workplace is a complex phenomenon influenced by many factors besides the promise of financial gain.

Motivation is a complex concept. Answers to three basic questions are necessary to understand the part played by motivation in the supervisory roles that athletic training managers must assume (Steers and Porter 1987).

1. What energizes human behavior?

2. What directs or channels human behavior?

3. How can human behavior be maintained or sustained?

Each of these questions lies at the heart of the broader question, "How do I motivate the athletic trainers under my supervision to do the best job possible?" None of these questions has easy answers, and that is the primary reason this book does not have a table titled "How to Motivate Athletic Trainers." We have learned quite a bit about motivation, however, and it seems that the concept can be broken down into four basic components (see figure 3.16):

1. Needs or expectations of the employee

2. Employee behavior

3. Employee goals

4. Feedback from the supervisor or other sources

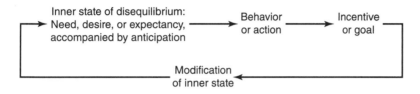

▶ **Figure 3.16** A basic model of motivation.

DUNNETTE, MARVIN D., KIRCHNER, WAYNEK, PSYCHOLOGY APPLIED TO INDUSTRY, 1st Edition, ©1965, p.125. Reprinted by permission of Pearson Education, Inc., Upper Saddle River, NJ.

Although this model does a good job of explaining workplace motivation at its simplest level, it is a poor predictor of employee behavior in actual job settings. At least four confounding factors complicate this model:

▪ **Motives can only be inferred, not seen.** Knowing why employees act the way they do at work is often difficult. Although their behavior might be observable, the motivation for that behavior is often not. For example, if Judy in the opening case puts in extra time in the athletic training room by volunteering to cover special events and other similar functions, we would know only that she is a hard worker. We wouldn't know what her motivation is for consistently volunteering. Perhaps she wants the extra money. Maybe she has a limited social life and meets her affiliation needs only through her work. Maybe she wants David's job and sees this as a way to demonstrate that she is capable and worthy of promotion.

▪ **Motives conflict with each other and are subject to change.** Most of us deal with conflicting motivations in many segments of our lives. These motives are usually not static; they change, as do the other situational variables in our lives. For example, Judy's behavior might be the result of conflicting motivations. If she has young children at home, the motivation to get ahead at work might conflict with her desire to fulfill her role as a parent. If she is the primary breadwinner, she might see the extra work as an opportunity to supplement the family income. As her children grow older, their needs (and hers) will change, resulting in a different set of motivating factors.

▪ **Individual differences exist with regard to motives**. If everyone responded to the presence of motivators in the same way, supervision would be easy. Unfortunately, what motivates one person is often insufficient to motivate another. Judy is motivated (by something) to work extra hours in the athletic training room. David might not be. He might be the last to arrive and the first to leave every day. He could receive extra pay by covering special events, but he chooses not to. The two athletic trainers have the same motivator (extra pay) but exhibit different behavior.

■ **Goal attainment modifies behavior in different ways.** Besides the fact that people are motivated by different things, they often respond differently to achievement of the same goals. Again, take the example of Judy and David. After David was appointed head athletic trainer, he coasted, rarely volunteering for extra work even if it meant extra pay. Assume that Judy would like to be head of the program one day. Will she also coast after she achieves that goal? Will she continue to volunteer for extra duties? Or will she work even harder in the hope that she might be promoted to a position on the athletic director's staff?

As you can see, although motivation seems to be a straightforward concept, its application is complex and difficult to predict. As you read the following sections, keep in mind the assumptions that each supervisory model makes about the nature of human behavior at work.

When you eventually attain a position in which you must supervise athletic trainers and other health care professionals, you will have to choose a supervisory style that meshes with your basic assumptions about what motivates people.

Inspection–Production Supervision

The primary characteristic of the **inspection–production** model of supervision is an emphasis on authoritative managerial efficiency. Athletic trainers who prefer this approach to supervision insist on strict observance of program policies and procedures. This model views the services provided by the sports medicine program as products and the athletic trainer employees as the raw materials used to develop those products. In the inspection–production model, supervising athletic trainers require all employees of a sports medicine program to develop a comprehensive list of goals for the year. Then they carefully check progress toward accomplishing those goals during the course of the year. The overriding emphasis of this model is on accomplishment of program goals and objectives and on attainment of the program mission.

The advantage of the inspection–production model is that it can be effective in helping a sports medicine program accomplish its goals. It sets well-defined limits on job-related behavior for all employees and consequently enhances common understanding of the athletic trainers' roles. This approach to supervision is usually associated with formalistic bureaucratic organizations that have many levels of supervisory management.

Using the inspection–production system of supervision in service-oriented enterprises, including sports medicine programs, has several disadvantages. This model was originally developed and implemented in industrial settings where inputs and outputs could be easily measured. Measurement of inputs and outputs in most sports medicine settings is difficult. Although some measures of program success or failure should be developed, interpretation of them will vary widely depending on the audience.

Another problem with this model is the nature of the work that athletic trainers do. Most athletic trainers perform a variety of jobs, and not all of them are easily observed or quantified. For example, if David Lewis wanted to be sure that Judy Armstrong was meeting the program standard for taping effectiveness and efficiency, he could simply observe her as she prepared a team for a practice or game. But how would David inspect the effectiveness and efficiency of Judy's counseling skills? Her rehabilitation skills?

Finally, the inspection–production method of supervision can cause professional employees such as athletic trainers to feel unappreciated and unfulfilled. Because the dominant ethos is program goal accomplishment and not professional development, athletic trainers will rarely appreciate what little developmental feedback they receive. They will tend to view such feedback in negative terms.

Clinical Supervision

Clinical supervision is the process, borrowed from education, of direct observation of an athletic trainer at work and the subsequent development of plans to remediate deficiencies in performance (Acheson and Gall 1987). The process requires the supervisor to observe a sample of the athletic trainer's performance, analyze the strengths and weaknesses of the performance, and collaboratively develop a structure for helping the athletic trainer overcome the weaknesses. This type of supervision can be particularly appropriate for student interns, although it is useful for professional staff as well. Among the many supervisory techniques that can be applied within the clinical supervision model, one of the most promising for athletic trainers is work sampling (Hagerty, Chang, and Spengler 1985). Work sampling identifies the type of work that athletic trainers do and the amount of time they spend doing it. Hence, it can be an effective tool for both clinical supervision and job analysis. Work sampling consists of logging the activities of athletic trainers at randomly selected times and analyzing the data to judge the nature and quality of the work that they are performing. Appropriate activities facilitate the goals and objectives of the sports medicine program. Inappropriate activities duplicate effort, lack a connection to the purposes of the program, fulfill purely personal or social wants, or allocate too much time to tasks that are not suited to the athletic trainer's qualifications.

Among the advantages of clinical supervision is its emphasis on collegial working relationships and cooperative planning. The clinical model of supervision promotes the professional status of the athletic trainer and involves the athletic trainer in as much of the supervisory process as possible. The role of the supervising athletic trainer is consultative rather than authoritative.

The primary disadvantage of the clinical system of supervision is that the supervising athletic trainer must devote large blocks of time to supervising individual employees. Because clinical supervision requires direct observation of an athletic trainer's performance and most supervising athletic trainers have significant responsibilities in the treatment of injured clients, finding the time to implement a truly clinical system of supervision is difficult. Another problem with clinical supervision is that accurate interpretation of observed supervision data requires training.

Developmental Supervision

Developmental supervision involves collaboration between a supervising athletic trainer and employees. The emphasis is on helping employees develop professionally while meeting the needs of the sports medicine program. The overriding theme of developmental supervision is participative management—employees discuss common problems and suggest and implement creative solutions. The system is intended to improve both the sports medicine program and its employees by increasing employee involvement in problem solving. It acknowledges the interdependence of the goals of the program and those of the athletic trainers.

The primary advantage of the developmental model is its emphasis on personal growth and its integration of athletic trainer and sports medicine program goals. The developmental system tends to build an organizational culture that emphasizes meeting the needs of athletic trainers to improve program quality. Athletic trainers working in organizations with this focus are generally happy and content with their professional development.

Unfortunately, well-developed, happy employees do not guarantee overall program success. Collegiality and collaboration are desirable only when they bring different perspectives and new ways of thinking to difficult problems. Heavy emphasis on collaboration can delay problem solving because of the need to preserve the collegial organizational climate.

Which supervisory model is best? Is one model more appropriate for a university setting? For a sports medicine clinic setting? These questions are difficult to answer, because the three supervisory models have never been empirically investigated in sports medicine settings. But we can intuitively draw a few tentative conclusions. First, most sports medicine programs should probably integrate elements of each model into their supervisory plans. When possible, programs should use collaborative problem solving because athletic trainers will have a greater sense of ownership in the resulting solutions. When questions arise about the effectiveness of an athletic trainer, direct observation of his work and suggestions for improvement by the supervising athletic trainer would probably be useful. At times, however, the supervisor will have to take other actions. If an employee has not responded well to attempts at collaborative problem solving or suggestions from the supervisor, the supervising athletic trainer may have no alternative but to impose a solution to correct the actions of the employee.

PERFORMANCE EVALUATION

Performance evaluation is the process of placing a value on the quality of an athletic trainer's work. Performance evaluation is important for at least two reasons. First, it can help a supervising athletic trainer make valid and reliable distinctions between athletic trainers who are performing at or above program expectations and those whose work is unsatisfactory. Second, a properly implemented system of performance evaluation helps the athletic trainers being evaluated identify areas of weakness and eliminate or reduce them.

Figures 3.17 (pp. 114-118) and 3.18 (pp. 119-120) provide examples of performance evaluation instruments based on the opening scenario. Remember, however, that any performance evaluation instrument not based on a specific athletic trainer's weighted job description and not designed for a particular purpose is useless. Performance evaluation is *not* the annual completion of a form. Performance evaluation is a process done throughout the entire year that involves mutually establishing goals, creating performance standards for accomplishing those goals, measuring the level of accomplishment, mutually understanding how well the athletic trainer met her goals, and mutually developing plans to remediate performance deficiencies and continue professional development. Measuring performance often requires the input of the athletic trainer being evaluated, the athletic trainer's peers, the supervisor, the clients, and the consulting physicians. Any performance evaluation instrument not built on these principles would be so riddled with caveats as to render it meaningless. In some circumstances, coaches are also asked to provide input regarding the performance of the athletic trainer. While their feedback is viewed by some as relevant, it is important to take into account that coaches are very biased in their expectations of an athletic trainer and not always objective in their judgment of how appropriately the athletic trainer is performing his role. At times, a coach's opinion on how well an athletic trainer performs may simply be an opinion about how compliant the athletic trainer is with the coach's requests.

> Performance evaluation is an underused and generally poorly performed human resource tool in athletic training. Performance evaluation systems and methods should meet established standards so that they are legal and fair, useful, accurate, and practical.

Ohio Technological University
Department of Intercollegiate Athletics

Annual Performance Evaluation Instrument

Employee being evaluated: Judy Armstrong   Evaluation: July 1, 2011–June 30, 2012

Supervisor conducting evaluation: David Lewis   Date of feedback conference: July 10, 2012

This information may be shared only with: Judy Armstrong, Linda Black, David Lewis, James Wilson

Data sources used in the performance evaluation: Supervisor's direct observations and feedback from team physicians and athletic trainer coworkers as provided on the "Ancillary Data Source" form.

Purpose:

The purposes of the annual performance evaluation include (1) assisting employees to identify strengths and weaknesses of their performance in job-related responsibilities so they can work with their supervisors to improve performance, and (2) collecting job-related performance information that may be used for the following staff selection activities: promotion, demotion, retention, dismissal, and compensation. Only job-related performance may be used as the basis for this evaluation.

▶ **Figure 3.17** Performance evaluation instrument based on the opening case.

Role-Specific Ratings:

Instructions to evaluator: Assess the performance of the employee for each specific job responsibility. Rate only those responsibilities included on this employee's position description. Provide performance quality ratings using a 1 to 5 scale. Provide performance frequency ratings using a 1 to 5 scale. Multiply performance quality ratings by performance frequency ratings by relative importance points (from position description) for overall performance ratings. Provide rationale for each rating.

Performance Quality Ratings

1–Job responsibility is performed at an unacceptable level of quality (significant improvement is expected).

2–Job responsibility is performed at a below-average level of quality (significant improvement is expected).

3–Job responsibility is performed at an average level of quality (most other employees perform at this level).

4–Job responsibility is performed at an above-average level of quality (some improvement is possible).

5–Job responsibility is performed at an outstanding level of quality (no improvement is possible).

Performance Frequency Ratings

1–Job responsibility is performed 0–20% of the time.

2–Job responsibility is performed 21–40% of the time.

3–Job responsibility is performed 41–60% of the time.

4–Job responsibility is performed 61–80% of the time.

5–Job responsibility is performed 81–100% of the time.

JOB RESPONSIBILITIES FOR JUDY ARMSTRONG

Responsibility	Performance Quality Rating	Performance Frequency Rating	Relative Importance Points	Total Possible	Total Achieved
Coordinates and delivers athletic training services to members of the field hockey and gymnastics teams including, but not limited to, coordination of physical exams, evaluation and treatment of injuries at practices and games, design and supervision of rehabilitation programs, counseling within the limits of expertise, and prepractice/game taping.	Rationale:	Rationale:	5	125	
Refers injured athletes to appropriate physicians according to the guidelines in the *Standard Operating Procedures*.	Rationale:	Rationale:	5	125	

(continued) ▶

▶ **Figure 3.17** Performance evaluation instrument based on the opening case. *(continued)*

JOB RESPONSIBILITIES FOR JUDY ARMSTRONG

Responsibility	Performance Quality Rating	Performance Frequency Rating	Relative Importance Points	Total Possible	Total Achieved
Submits injured athlete status reports to coaches by 11:00 a.m. of the day following the injury.	Rationale:	Rationale:	4	100	
Maintains computerized injury/treatment database according to the guidelines in the *Standard Operating Procedures*.	Rationale:	Rationale:	3	75	
Coordinates NCAA Injury Surveillance Program by conducting in-service training for athletic training students, collecting and checking the accuracy of individual and weekly injury report forms, and mailing completed forms to the NCAA by Monday of each week.	Rationale:	Rationale:	3	75	

▶ **Figure 3.17** Performance evaluation instrument based on the opening case. *(continued)*

JOB RESPONSIBILITIES FOR JUDY ARMSTRONG

Responsibility	Performance Quality Rating	Performance Frequency Rating	Relative Importance Points	Total Possible	Total Achieved
Prepares annual injury and treatment report for all sports by June 1.	Rationale:	Rationale:	3	75	
Exhibits behaviors in strict compliance with the NATA *Code of Professional Practice*.	Rationale:	Rationale:	5	125	
				700	

(continued) ▶

▶ **Figure 3.17** Performance evaluation instrument based on the opening case. *(continued)*

Working Conditions:

Instructions: Describe any unusual working conditions beyond the control of the employee that may have affected his or her ability to perform the assigned duties.

Critical Incidents:

Instructions: Describe any critical incidents that occurred during the evaluation period that are consistent with the strengths and weaknesses of the employee's job-related performance.

Performance Improvement Plan:

Instructions: List below the steps the employee should take in order to improve his/her job-related performance.

Employee Response:

Instructions: Describe below any points of agreement or disagreement with your supervisor's evaluation of your job-related performance.

▶ **Figure 3.17** Performance evaluation instrument based on the opening case. *(continued)*

Ohio Technological University
Department of Intercollegiate Athletics

Annual Performance Evaluation
Ancillary Data Source Instrument

Employee being evaluated: Judy Armstrong   Evaluation: July 1, 2011–June 30, 2012

Supervisor conducting evaluation: David Lewis

This information may be shared only with: Judy Armstrong, Linda Black, David Lewis, James Wilson

Purpose:

The purpose of this instrument is to help supervisors provide employees with valid and reliable feedback regarding their performance by allowing them to collect information from peers and coworkers. The information may also be used to make employee selection decisions regarding promotion, demotion, retention, dismissal, and compensation.

Instructions: Use the specific job responsibilities below from the employee's position description to guide your assessments. *Assess only the employee's performance on these responsibilities. Assess only those responsibilities that you directly observed.*

JOB RESPONSIBILITIES OF JUDY ARMSTRONG

Responsibility	Comments
Coordinates and delivers athletic training services to members of the field hockey and gymnastics teams including, but not limited to, coordination of physical exams, evaluation and treatment of injuries at practices and games, design and supervision of rehabilitation programs, counseling within the limits of expertise, and prepractice/ game taping.	
Refers injured athletes to appropriate physicians according to the guidelines in the *Standard Operating Procedures*.	

(continued) ▶

▶ **Figure 3.18** Performance evaluation ancillary data source form based on the opening case.

JOB RESPONSIBILITIES OF JUDY ARMSTRONG

Responsibility	Comments
Submits injured athlete status reports to coaches by 11:00 A.M. of the day following the injury.	
Maintains computerized injury/treatment database according to guidelines in the *Standardized Operating Procedures*.	
Coordinates NCAA Injury Surveillance program by conducting in-service training for student athletic trainers, collecting and checking the accuracy of individual and weekly injury report forms, and mailing completed forms to the NCAA by Monday of each week.	
Prepares annual injury and treatment report for all sports by June 1.	
Exhibits behaviors in strict compliance with the NATA *Code of Professional Practice*.	

Signature	Position	Date

▶ **Figure 3.18** Performance evaluation ancillary data source form based on the opening case. *(continued)*

Status of Performance Evaluation in Athletic Training

Printed resources for athletic trainers on performance evaluation are few, and most are outdated and advocate a trait-oriented approach (Parks 1977; Penman and Adams 1980). Trait-oriented evaluation systems place a value on athletic trainers' performance by assessing human qualities. For example, if David were to evaluate Judy's performance using a trait-oriented approach, he would likely label her "aggressive," "unfriendly," and "difficult to get along with." Unfortunately, none of these terms refer to the quality of her work. Although trait-oriented systems are the easiest to implement, they usually lack validity and reliability (Dobbins and Russell 1986; Huber, Podsakoff, and Todor 1986). For example, Cascio and Bernardin (1981) reported a survey of 47 administrators that identified 75 different definitions of *dependability*.

Unfortunately, in many settings, formal evaluation of the performance of athletic trainers does not occur annually (figure 3.19). For example, in Ray's 1991 study of performance evaluation in all athletic training settings, only 35% of athletic trainers employed in the professional athletics setting reported being evaluated on an annual basis. Of those who were evaluated regularly, most perceived their performance evaluations differently from their supervisors. For example, athletic trainers and their supervisors had different perceptions about whether *Competencies in Athletic Training* and *Standards of Practice for Athletic Training* was used as a basis for evaluating athletic trainer job performance. One of the most likely reasons for this discrepancy is that nonmedical supervisors who were not familiar with the athletic trainer's job responsibilities conducted a significant number of the evaluations. In addition, only about half of those supervisors had any formal training in how to conduct a performance evaluation or interpret the data derived from the evaluation (see figure 3.20).

Another reason athletic trainers and their supervisors have differing opinions on the nature of performance evaluation is that many athletic trainers, even if they are formally evaluated, never receive feedback regarding their performance from their supervisors (see figure 3.21). This lack of communication is an important reason for the lack of understanding between athletic trainers and their supervisors.

Performance Evaluation Methods

Practitioners of performance evaluation disagree about which methods are most effective for rating employee job performance (Reinhardt 1985). The performance evaluation methods used should be appropriate for the purposes and defined uses of the evaluation (Schneier, Beatty, and Baird 1986). No single method of performance evaluation matches every setting or meets the needs of every organization. Table 3.4 summarizes the strengths and weaknesses of the most common performance evaluation methods.

Seven performance evaluation methods are used most often: management by objectives, written essays, critical incident reports, graphic rating scales, forced-choice rating, ranking, and behaviorally anchored rating scales. Fowler and Bushardt (1986) developed a method called the task-oriented performance evaluation system (TOPES) that they alleged to be a simple, job-specific method of measuring performance-related behavior. Unfortunately, TOPES has

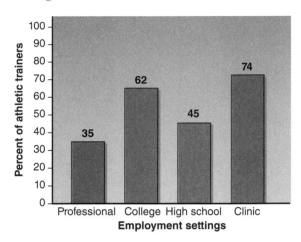

▶ **Figure 3.19** Incidence of athletic trainer performance evaluation by employment setting.
Data from Ray 1991.

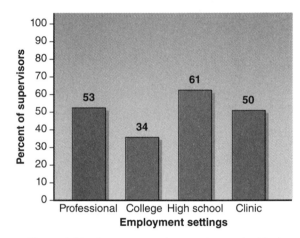

▶ **Figure 3.20** Percentage of supervisors of athletic trainers who have been formally trained in performance evaluation.
Data from Ray 1991.

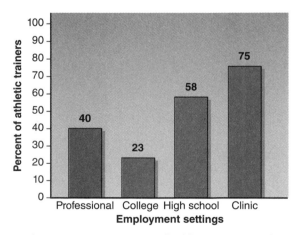

▶ **Figure 3.21** Percentage of athletic trainers who receive feedback regarding their performance from their supervisors.
Data from Ray 1991.

TABLE 3.4 **Strengths and Weaknesses of the Most Commonly Used Performance Evaluation Methods**

Method	Weaknesses	Strengths
Management by objectives	Tends to emphasize job characteristics that can be measured over those that cannot.	Employee is able to have input into the standards by which he or she is evaluated.
Written essay	Dependent on subjective data; validity dependent on writer's skill and judgment.	Evaluator can write a detailed profile of the employee's work.
Critical incident report	Can be subject to writer bias; often based on subjective data; negative incidents usually receive more notice than positive.	More detail regarding the employee's work can be provided.
Graphic rating scale	Scale elements often not valid or job related.	Simple to administer; low cost.
Forced-choice rating	Fails to provide specific feedback; not useful in human resource planning; does not relate job performance to selection criteria.	Simple to administer; low cost.
Ranking	Difficult to discriminate performance levels on multitask jobs; discourages cooperation among work group members.	Simplifies the task of allocating rewards.
Behaviorally anchored rating scales	Most useful for employees with identical job responsibilities; expensive and time-consuming to develop; difficult to update as job responsibilities change.	Evaluates behaviors rather than traits; specific to single job category.

not been field tested extensively or validated for different settings or uses. Work sampling, as described previously, can also be used as a form of performance evaluation. Keaveny and McGann (1980), in their research on the performance appraisal format and its influence on role clarity and evaluation criteria, determined that behaviorally anchored rating scales were superior to graphic rating scales in helping professionals understand the performance area being rated, the perceived performance level for each rating area, and the behavior changes that would be necessary to improve ratings for each performance area.

Performance Evaluation Standards

The Personnel Evaluation Standards (Joint Committee on Standards for Educational Evaluation 1988) has significantly influenced the practice of performance evaluation in a variety of settings. This publication provides widely accepted evaluation principles that educational professionals can use to improve their personnel evaluation systems. Many policy boards have adopted these standards as the official standards for judging performance evaluation systems. Although *The Personnel Evaluation Standards* was written for educational settings, the standards are rooted in valid and reliable evaluation principles and could be applied in noneducational settings. Athletic trainers employed in professional athletics, sports medicine clinics, and industry can benefit from the application of these standards because validity and reliability of performance evaluation are important in their job settings as well.

The Joint Committee on Standards for Educational Evaluation (1988) has identified 21 standards in four broad categories: propriety, utility, feasibility, and accuracy. A description of each standard along with an example of how it could be applied in an athletic training setting follows. Although the list seems long, keep in mind that performance evaluation is an important part of the athletic trainer-manager's responsibilities. Even small deviations from the ideal can result in damaging consequences for the employee, the supervisor, and the institution.

Performance evaluation systems for athletic trainers should be legal and fair, useful, practical, and accurate.

Propriety Standards

The following five **propriety standards** help ensure that performance evaluation is legal and fair.

■ **Service orientation.** Performance evaluation systems for athletic trainers should meet the needs of the persons they are intended to help, including athletic trainers, their clients, and their employing institutions. If the system neglects any of these groups, it should be reconfigured accordingly. Assume, for example, that David institutes a performance evaluation system in response to Judy's complaints. If David configures the system so that all that it consists of is a 15-minute feedback conference once a year, Judy's needs are unlikely to be met. The system would fail to serve those whom it was intended to help.

■ **Formal evaluation guidelines.** The procedures by which the athletic trainer's performance is evaluated should be recorded as written institutional policy and made available to athletic trainers so that they are aware of the process. The department handbook should include each step of David's new performance evaluation system so that Judy and her fellow athletic trainers are aware of and understand the system.

■ **Conflict of interest.** Evaluation procedures should eliminate conflicts of interest. For example, if Judy and her supervisor, Linda Black, were both candidates for the same job promotion, Linda would have a conflict of interest when evaluating Judy's performance. Formal evaluation procedures should specify how to avoid such conflicts.

■ **Access to personnel evaluation reports.** Only those who have a legitimate need to know should be allowed access to an athletic trainer's performance evaluation records. Each athletic trainer should know who has access to the information and under what circumstances they will have such access. Linda Black, David Lewis, and the athletic director might legitimately have access to Judy's performance evaluation, but nobody else should see it.

■ **Interactions with evaluees.** Athletic trainers should be treated with respect and dignity when being evaluated. When supervisors are judgmental, they are less likely to enhance trust in the performance evaluation system. They can promote trust by taking a counseling attitude (Dorfman, Stephan, and Loveland 1986). If David simply calls Judy into his office and assaults her with critical and threatening language during her feedback conference, the system is unlikely to achieve its goals.

Utility Standards

The following five **utility standards** ensure that an athletic trainer's performance evaluation is useful (Joint Committee on Standards for Educational Evaluation 1988).

■ **Constructive orientation.** If performance evaluation is to be useful, both athletic trainers and their supervisors must perceive that evaluation procedures result in improvements in professional development and accountability. If either perceives evaluation as a waste of time, the information obtained is unlikely to be useful. Performance evaluation should help athletic trainers improve their performance. David and Judy should together develop strategies designed to help Judy improve. If David does nothing but point out Judy's shortcomings, little will be accomplished.

■ **Defined uses.** Performance evaluation data should be used only for the purposes for which they were collected. Athletic trainers should be informed of these uses before data collection; the data might not be valid if used for other purposes. Athletic trainers are likely to lose trust in the system if the information is used for unstated purposes. For example, assume that David stated, in the written description of the system in the department handbook, that the purpose of the performance evaluation process was to "improve athletic trainer performance for the purpose of improving the quality of health care being provided to injured athletes." He would be violating the "defined uses" standard if he then used the information gathered during the process to decide whether to promote Judy when Linda Black resigned. David gathered the information for one purpose and used it for another.

■ **Evaluator credibility.** The people who evaluate an athletic trainer's performance should have institutional authority and should be knowledgeable about athletic training duties. In addition, they should be knowledgeable about the theory and practice of performance evaluation methods. Team physician and peer athletic trainer input can improve the credibility of evaluation because these people are often more knowledgeable about athletic training job responsibilities than coaches or athletic administrators are. If David works closely enough with Judy to understand her job responsibilities, and if he knows how to implement a valid and reliable performance evaluation system, he should have enough credibility to satisfy this standard.

■ **Functional reporting.** If performance evaluation is to be perceived as useful, athletic trainers should receive both formal and informal feedback on job performance. This feedback should be job related and timely, and it should contain specific suggestions for improving performance. If David evaluates Judy's performance in June but doesn't meet with her to discuss the results until October, the usefulness of the information decreases. Similarly, if David has no suggestions for helping Judy improve, she must try to figure this out on her own.

■ **Follow-up.** All recommendations from the performance evaluation should be implemented so that professional development can occur. An important component of the follow-up process involves forming a plan for professional improvement that focuses on identified weaknesses in an athletic trainer's performance. The athletic trainer and her supervisor should develop this plan jointly. To meet this standard, David must monitor whether or not Judy is improving her performance by implementing the plan that they developed together. If she isn't, and David does nothing about it, the system is a waste of time and money.

Feasibility Standards

The following three **feasibility standards** foster practicality in performance evaluation (Joint Committee on Standards for Educational Evaluation 1988).

■ **Practical procedures.** Performance evaluation procedures should intrude as little as possible into an athletic trainer's normal job-related activities. Athletic trainers will view evaluation procedures that require them to redirect significant amounts of energy and attention away from clients as impractical. If David developed a system that required Linda to follow Judy around for a week to monitor her work activities, he would probably learn a great deal about her performance, but the collection of information wouldn't be practical or efficient.

■ **Political viability.** All the users of the athletic trainer performance evaluation system should have input into its development so that they will accept and use it as intended. Evaluation systems designed without input from athletic trainers are unlikely to be effective for professional development—athletic trainers may view such systems as bureaucratic tools that interfere with their jobs. If David tried to impose a performance evaluation system on the members of the sports medicine staff without their input, they would probably resent it, and its usefulness would decrease significantly.

■ **Fiscal viability.** Institutions should recognize that effective athletic trainer performance evaluation systems require outlays of both time and money. Administrators who develop budgets should build the costs of evaluating performance into the overall institutional budget. A system that required Linda to follow Judy around for a week to observe her work would be expensive. Although Linda would learn quite a bit about Judy's performance, someone else would have to do Linda's work during this time, an arrangement that would be costly. This system would not be fiscally viable.

Accuracy Standards

The following eight standards are intended to improve the validity and reliability of a performance evaluation and thereby lend **accuracy** to the system (Joint Committee on Standards for Educational Evaluation 1988).

■ **Defined role.** Evaluation procedures for athletic trainers should use criteria that relate directly to the specific roles they are responsible for. This standard is especially important because of the variety of roles that athletic trainers often assume. If evaluation data are collected and interpreted without regard to role definition, they are likely to lack validity for evaluating job-related performance behaviors. Developing a weighted position description is an important first step in defining the athletic trainer's role. Judy's position description (see figure 3.7 on p. 84) is critical in helping both David and Judy understand the roles for which David will evaluate her. If David strayed from the roles described in her position description when evaluating her performance, he would be unfairly holding her to a standard that she could not have reasonably anticipated.

■ **Work environment.** The evaluator should record specific aspects of the athletic trainer's work environment during the performance evaluation process so that the final evaluation can take into account individual differences in working conditions. For example, if Judy was working with a new coach, that would be taken into consideration during her performance evaluation, because it is a factor beyond her control and might drastically alter the nature of her job.

■ **Documentation of procedures.** The evaluator should record the procedures followed during the evaluation process so that athletic trainers and other users of the information can compare actual with intended evaluation procedures. As David evaluates Judy's performance, he must be careful to record each step in the process. If David and Judy have a dispute that results from her performance evaluation, a third party should be able to examine the record to determine if there were any procedural flaws on David's part.

■ **Valid measurement.** Procedures developed or adopted for evaluating an athletic trainer's performance should measure the job-related behaviors they are intended to measure so that users can draw accurate conclusions about performance. Institutions should be able to defend the accuracy of the procedures. One potentially useful source of information regarding Judy's performance could come from the outcomes studies conducted in her department (see chapter 2). If David could link specific patient outcomes with the care that Judy provided, he would have objective data he could use to develop judgments regarding her effectiveness.

■ **Reliable measurement.** Institutions should ensure that methods used to evaluate performance are consistent across time and for different evaluators. Using multiple evaluators trained to follow specific evaluation procedures is a good way to build reliability into the evaluation system. David must be careful to apply the same evaluation techniques and methods when evaluating Judy's performance that he uses with every other member of the department. If he gathers information regarding Judy's performance from Linda Black, the team physician, and other members of the department, his assessment is more likely to be reliable.

■ **Systematic data control.** Information collected during performance evaluation should be recorded and stored so it can easily be retrieved in the future and so that future interpretations are similar to the conclusions drawn immediately after the athletic trainer's performance evaluation. If data are misplaced or lost, future evaluators might draw erroneous conclusions because they will lack a complete perspective. For example, the performance evaluation information that David develops for Judy this year must be stored in such a way that when he evaluates her next year he can use this year's information. The alternative is to hope he can remember the recommendations for improving Judy's performance when he evaluates her in the future.

■ **Bias control.** All possible biasing factors should be eliminated from athletic trainer performance evaluation so that accurate conclusions can be reached. Using multiple evaluators is an effective technique to help reduce bias. Evaluating only job-related behaviors also controls bias. Personal traits unrelated to the actual job performance expected of athletic trainers should not be part of the performance evaluation. Rigorous adherence to the other accuracy standards will help reduce performance evaluation bias. If Judy performs all the functions in her position description with a high degree of competence but David gives her low performance ratings because he simply doesn't like her, he is guilty of violating this standard. By using other evaluators, like Linda Black, as part of the process, he can reduce the possibility for bias.

■ **Monitoring evaluation systems.** Because the circumstances related to an athletic trainer's job might change over time, the systems used to evaluate performance should be modified as well. Institutional policies should require evaluation and modification of athletic trainer performance evaluation systems from time to time. David and the rest of the staff should meet periodically to decide whether the performance evaluation system is working well and to discuss how they might modify it.

FAIR LABOR STANDARDS ACT AND ATHLETIC TRAINING

Traditionally, the culture of athletic training has prescribed long hours at modest pay to meet the needs of injured athletes whose schedules rarely conform to the typical 40-hour workweek. Coaches, athletic directors, and athletes have come to expect that athletic trainers will stay in the athletic training room until they have attended to the last person, even if doing so requires 60 or 70 hours per week. Many in the profession who desire a higher quality of life are now challenging this culture, both in terms of a more reasonable workweek and a compensation package befitting the level of education required for practice in athletic training. One of the primary issues of concern to athletic trainers is whether they are exempt under the Fair Labor Standards Act (Hanak 2004).

Congress passed the Fair Labor Standards Act in 1938 and has since amended it several times. The act generally requires that employees be paid overtime (usually time and a half) or receive compensated time (1.5 times the hours worked in excess of 40) for work beyond 40 hours per week. The FLSA does not cover all employees. Executives, administrators, and professionals are generally exempt from the provisions of the law. All other employees are considered nonexempt. In 2004, the FLSA was changed again. It now stipulates that athletic trainers who work as employees fall within the learned profession exemption for overtime pay if they meet two criteria: They must be paid a minimum salary of $455 per week or $23,660 annually, and their primary duties must be work that requires advanced knowledge in the field of science or learning acquired through a prolonged course of specialized instruction (Newkirk 2004).

Athletic trainers in several states have challenged their exempt status and won the right to overtime by being reclassified as nonexempt. Athletic trainers in Kansas, with some exceptions, are considered nonexempt employees as the result of a case involving the athletic training staff at the University of Kansas. A similar situation exists in the state of Washington. High school athletic trainers in Texas, on the other hand, lost the right to be classified nonexempt in a 1999 case.

If athletic trainers are professionals, how can they be classified as nonexempt employees under the FLSA? The first point is that the word *professional* is used in different ways. Athletic trainers call themselves professionals because of their education, specialized knowledge, and practice standards. The FLSA, however, defines a professional as a person whose primary duties consist of either

■ the performance of a learned or educational profession entailing work which requires the exercise of discretion and judgment; or

■ the performance of work requiring invention, imagination, or talent in a recognized field of artistic endeavor (48A Am Jur 2d, Labor and Labor Relations § 3967, p. 813).

The two important elements in the preceding are "learned profession" and "exercise of discretion and judgment." A learned profession is one that requires an advanced kind of knowledge (usually beyond the high school level) in the field of science or education that the person obtained by prolonged and specialized instruction. Specific academic training as a prerequisite for entering a profession is usually required.

The Fair Labor Standards Act (FLSA) is a law intended to ensure that employees are justly compensated for work they do that exceeds the boundaries of the normal workweek. Athletic trainers might or might not be exempt from the provisions of the FLSA depending on how their jobs are structured.

The "exercise of discretion and judgment" element is much less well defined and is often problematic when the issue of whether or not athletic trainers should be classified as professionals (and therefore be exempt from the FLSA) is addressed. For example, in some states the provisions of a credentialing act require that physicians supervise athletic trainers. Some athletic trainers in the cases mentioned earlier have argued that because they do their work under the direction of a physician, they are not exercising discretion and judgment. In institutions without team physicians, athletic trainers might in fact exercise discretion and judgment, even though the work they perform is the same as that performed by nonexempt athletic trainers at a similar institution. Athletic trainers who teach at least 50% of the time are generally exempt and not entitled to overtime because teachers are considered professionals under the FLSA. Athletic trainers who spend more than 50% of their time in management or administrative roles might also be exempt.

APPLICATIONS TO ATHLETIC TRAINING: THEORY INTO PRACTICE

Use the following three case studies to help you apply the concepts in this chapter to real-life situations. The questions at the conclusion of the studies are open-ended, with many possible solutions.

Case Study 1

The new manager of the Wellness Center, a physician-owned sports medicine and rehabilitation clinic, instituted a policy requiring all supervisors to evaluate their employees and recommend salary increases. This new program was an attempt to implement a merit pay system at the center. In the past, all employees had received an across-the-board increase without regard to how they had performed during the past year.

Sandra Hotchkiss supervised the center's six certified athletic trainers. Upon receiving the memo mandating the new policy, Sandra decided that she would simply write a narrative describing each of the athletic trainers. She thought that such a narrative would be a useful guide for the new manager in awarding pay increases because it would provide in-depth analysis of the strengths and weaknesses of each athletic trainer. The following are examples of the evaluations she submitted.

Brian Robinson

Brian Robinson is one of the best athletic trainers employed by the center. He is thoughtful, works well with the patients, has a cheerful personality, and gets along great with the staff. Brian has received positive feedback from the athletic director at South High School, where he is assigned during the fall and spring. The athletes and parents seem to like him and there haven't been any problems that I am aware of, although I have only been out there a couple of times. My recommendation is that Brian be given a 3% salary increase.

Juan Diaz

Although I think Juan is basically a pretty good athletic trainer, he has had several problems over the past year. Juan

seemed to be in the middle of a couple of controversies at Martin Luther King High. I know King is an inner-city school and Juan has a lot of tough problems to overcome down there, but I just wish he could deal more effectively with them so we wouldn't have to spend time on them at the center. Juan hasn't been very effective in getting many referrals to the center from his high school. As I mentioned earlier, although I think Juan does a good job as an athletic trainer, I can't recommend anything higher than a 1% increase for him this year.

Sandra was surprised when three weeks later, on the day after the salary increases were announced, Juan stormed into her office and informed her that he was going to sue both her and the Wellness Center for discrimination based on negligent evaluation.

QUESTIONS FOR ANALYSIS

1. What were the strengths and weaknesses of the performance evaluation system that Sandra Hotchkiss initiated?

2. How could the center's new manager have approached the problem more constructively and effectively? How would this have affected Sandra? How would it have affected Brian, Juan, and the other athletic trainers?

3. Describe the performance evaluation system you would implement if you were in Sandra's position. What concerns, if any, would you express to the new manager regarding the new policy?

Case Study 2

John Freeman had just bought the local professional football franchise. He had made his fortune in the fast food restaurant business, starting with one small fried chicken restaurant and building it into a multimillion-dollar chain with restaurants all over the world. At his first meeting with the club's staff, John announced that he was bringing in a consultant to do a management audit of every department. He explained that sound management was the cornerstone of his success in business and in life. He expected each member of the staff to adopt that philosophy. Sound management, in his opinion, was the key to success in any business, and professional football was a business.

A few weeks later, Rick Condelato and the rest of the sports medicine staff spent the better part of two days answering questions and explaining the club's sports medicine operation to the management consultant. The consultant asked about policies and procedures. He examined the record-keeping system. He investigated the supply and equipment purchasing routines. He became familiar with how Rick selected student athletic trainers for summer training camp. As far as Rick could tell, the consultant left no stone unturned.

About a month later, the management consultant and John Freeman, the new owner, walked into the athletic training room and told Rick that they wanted to discuss the results of the recent management audit with him. "Rick," the consultant began, "for the most part, you are managing this part of the club's operations fairly effectively. You buy only what you need and you don't pay more than you have to. The procedures you have implemented are consistent with club policy, and they seem to be efficient and effective. But in talking with your assistants, the assistant coaches, and some of the players, I have determined that you don't do a very good job of utilizing your staff to its fullest potential. The information they provided leads me to believe that you don't delegate authority enough. You try to do too much by yourself. Take a look at the organizational chart I developed of your operation as it presently exists" (see figure 3.22).

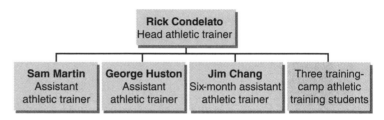

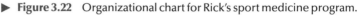

▶ **Figure 3.22** Organizational chart for Rick's sport medicine program.

"Rick," said John Freeman, "I want you to reorganize your staff so you can work more efficiently. From what everybody tells me, you're a good man and although I expect maximum effort, I don't want you to get burned out simply because you haven't organized your staff well enough. I expect to see your reorganization report on my desk by Monday of next week."

QUESTIONS FOR ANALYSIS

1. What is wrong with the current organizational structure in Rick's program? What problems are likely to arise based on the present structure?

2. How could Rick reorganize to reduce the amount of work he is responsible for and still accomplish everything that needs to be done?

3. If you were in Rick's position, what organizational structure would you devise to meet the mandate of the new club owner?

4. What strategies should Rick employ to make sure that his assistants develop ownership in the new organizational structure?

SUMMARY

Athletic trainers in supervisory roles will find themselves involved with human resource management. The proper management of human resources and personnel begins with establishing an organizational culture. No one culture fits all circumstances. However, setting a tone for how the operation will manage people is critical in order for personnel to understand working expectations. An organizational chart that reflects the hierarchy of positions, reporting structure, and roles and responsibilities helps to clarify the personnel structure. Having in place an organizational culture and chart can lead to an accurate development of position descriptions, which in turn facilitates the process of recruitment and hiring of employees that best fit the organization. There is much to consider when it comes to hiring, from the point of view of both the employer and the employee. Both parties should take ample time to consider all aspects of each employment opportunity, and particular attention should be

Case Study 3

Alicia Perkins is a senior athletic training student at a mid-sized university in New England. She is looking forward to taking her athletic training certification exam in April of this spring and getting a job as a certified athletic trainer in a secondary school setting. One of her clinical instructors informed her that a high school in the same district is planning to employ its first full-time certified athletic trainer for the upcoming school year. Alicia is very excited because the high school is located just 10 miles from where she currently lives.

Alicia was encouraged to send a resume to the school's athletic director now so that he can be made aware of her interest in the position. This is the first time Alicia has ever put together a resume for an athletic training position. She wants to be sure that her cover letter and resume are perfect, with no errors. She also wants to make sure that her resume is reflective of her experience to demonstrate that she is the best person for the job.

QUESTIONS FOR ANALYSIS

1. What challenges will Alicia have in preparing a cover letter and resume for a secondary school athletic training position prior to her achieving her certification?

2. Given that Alicia possesses many of the same skill sets as other entry-level athletic trainers, and arguably less experience than other athletic trainers who might apply for the same job at the secondary school, how can she promote herself as the best candidate for the position?

3. What are methods of networking that could benefit Alicia during the next few months prior to the formal posting of the position? Are there any behaviors or approaches Alicia should avoid so as not to come across as too persistent in her interest for the job?

4. What type of information can Alicia gather to prepare for an on-site interview to demonstrate her interest, qualifications, and fit for the job?

paid to the legal considerations of the hiring process and work environment to avoid any discriminatory procedures. Appropriate supervision contributes to more accurate employer performance assessment, a process that should include both formal and informal feedback in a timely and honest manner. Supervisory approaches can vary, taking into consideration both how one best manages as an individual and how one should accommodate to meet the needs of subordinates.

KEY CONCEPTS AND REVIEW

1. Understand the different forms of organizational culture that can exist in a sports medicine program.

Organizational culture includes the basic values, behavioral norms, assumptions, and beliefs of a sports medicine program. The type of organizational culture will have an effect on human resource management. The three major types of organizational cultures are collegial, personalistic, and formalistic.

2. Formally define the relationships of the persons working in a sports medicine program by developing an organizational chart.

An organizational chart best illustrates the relationships between the various members of a sports medicine program. Athletic trainers can describe these relationships in one of three ways: by function, by service, or in a matrix format.

3. Understand the components of staff selection.

Staff selection is a commonly misunderstood term. The *Uniform Guidelines on Employee Selection Procedures* describes staff selection as any procedure used as the basis for an employment decision. Hiring, promotion, demotion, performance evaluation, retention, and discharge are all examples of selection activities as defined by federal law.

4. Develop a position description and a position vacancy notice.

A position description is a formal document that describes the qualification requirements, work content, accountability, and scope of a person's job. The weighted position description is an important first step in helping athletic trainers understand the expectations of their employers. The position description generally comprises two sections: the job specification and the job description.

5. Understand the recruitment and hiring process, especially as affected by discrimination and bias based on race, gender, disability, religion, or national origin.

Recruitment and hiring are two of the most visible, expensive, and time-consuming aspects of the human resources function in sports medicine. Recruitment activities should be viewed in terms of long- and short-term needs. The prime directive in recruiting and hiring is that all qualified applicants should receive equal consideration. Athletic trainers and other sports medicine personnel must be hired based on their qualifications, not on race, gender, religion, or national origin. The recruitment and hiring process usually follows these 10 steps: request for position, position request approval, position vacancy notice, application collection, telephone interviews, reference checks, on-site interview, recommendation and approval for hiring, offer of contract, and hiring.

6. Understand the differences among the three major supervisory models.

The three major types of supervisory models are inspection-production, clinical, and developmental. The inspection–production model emphasizes authoritative managerial efficiency. Clinical supervision is the process, borrowed from education, of direct observation of an athletic trainer at work and the subsequent development of plans to remediate deficiencies in performance. The overriding theme of developmental supervision is participative management.

7. Understand the purposes, methods, and standards for evaluating athletic trainer performance.

Performance evaluation is the process of placing a value on the quality of an athletic trainer's work. In some settings, athletic trainers are not formally evaluated and lack position descriptions. Much of the performance evaluation literature intended for athletic trainers is based on a trait-oriented approach. Trait-oriented evaluation is usually biased and is rarely useful for improving performance. Athletic trainers should acquaint themselves with the 21 performance evaluation standards developed by the Joint Committee on Standards for Educational Evaluation. They are intended to guide the development of performance evaluation systems and to offer improvements in four major areas: propriety, accuracy, utility, and feasibility.

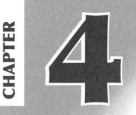

Financial Resource Management

Brief sections of this chapter were adapted, by permission, from R. Ray, 1991, "Training room efficiency," *Athletic Business* 15(1): 46-49; and from R. Ray, 1990, "An injury-free budget," *College Athletic Management* 2(1): 42-45.

OBJECTIVES

After reading this chapter, you should be able to do the following:

1. Understand the different kinds of budgeting processes and apply them to an athletic training setting.

2. Coordinate the purchasing of athletic training equipment, supplies, and services to maximize the use of program funds.

3. Manage the athletic training program's inventory of equipment and supplies.

► Stan Curtis was a certified athletic trainer for a large metropolitan school system in Grant, California. Stan's job was to provide athletic training services for school district athletes in a centralized athletic training facility. The facility was located in a municipal stadium, where the schools played football, soccer, baseball, and softball and ran track meets. In addition, Stan supervised the certified athletic trainers who worked in the district's six high schools. Every aspect of running the district's sports medicine program, from budgeting and purchasing to maintaining an inventory for each school, was Stan's responsibility.

One day in early June, Stan received a phone call from his boss, the director of cocurricular activities. "Stan, I'm not going to be able to approve those purchase orders you sent over the other day," she said. "The recent defeat of our tax referendum has really screwed up the district's finances. I don't think any of your athletic trainers are going to lose their jobs because they're all tenured and have been in the system for quite a while, but your supply budget is definitely going to feel the pinch. Not only are you going to have to reduce it by 30% immediately, but from now on you're going to have to justify every line item. I'm sorry about all this, Stan, but I've got my orders and there isn't anything I can do about it. I'll send those POs back to you today."

Stan was troubled. He didn't know how he was going to be able to cut 30% of his budget and still provide the same services at the same level of quality. In the past, the budgeting process had been simple. He had checked with the athletic trainers at the schools to find out what they would need for the upcoming year. If it sounded reasonable and the whole thing fit within the amount he had to work with, he ordered the supplies and that was that. He knew that his athletic trainers were going to be furious about this. Budgeting was about to become a whole new ball game.

We haven't got the money, so we've got to think!

—ERNEST RUTHERFORD

The common denominator in almost every management problem is money or the lack of it. Money is the engine that drives athletic enterprises, regardless of the level of competition. Sports medicine programs associated with athletic programs are subject to all the economic pressures that those programs experience, whether the setting is a high school, college, university, professional team, or hospital. For athletic trainers working in independent sports medicine clinics, the need for sound financial management practices is even more acute because economic downturns usually affect those operations more rapidly. The shallow resource pool typical of independent clinics compounds the effects of poor financial management. The amount of money an athletic trainer will have to operate a sports medicine program in an educational setting varies greatly depending on the level of competition engaged in by the institution's teams (Rankin 1992). The economics of the health care industry at any given time also affects how athletic trainers manage financial resources. Around the turn of the century, there was a movement away from traditional third-party reimbursement toward managed care models, resulting in a drastically altered financial landscape for most sports medicine clinics. Highly profitable publicly traded health care corporations were gobbling up small, independent clinics at a phenomenal rate (see figure 4.1). Most sports medicine clinics have had to expand their services to include nontraditional activities such as performance enhancement and nutritional counseling. Traditional rehabilitation is being transformed so that athletic trainers might see a patient only a few times, with the bulk of the rehabilitation consisting of liberal doses of advice and a program of home exercise. These changes have a significant effect on health care professionals—including athletic trainers—who operate, own, manage, and work in these environments.

The purpose of this chapter is to help athletic trainers become more astute stewards of their institution's financial resources by presenting the theory and application of various techniques for budgeting, purchasing, and inventory control. The chapter presents these three topics as distinct and separate processes, but in reality they are closely related to each other in a financial planning network (see figure 4.2). Although the ideas discussed in this chapter are applicable to almost any setting, athletic trainers should realize that certain types of sports medicine clinics, as small businesses, require more financial planning than this book can suggest. At a minimum, athletic trainers should consider six components of a financial analysis when operating sports medicine clinic: sales, costs, profits, revenue, return on investment (ROI), and growth earnings (Barnes, in Konin 1997). Athletic trainers who manage independently owned and operated sports medicine clinics should seek the counsel of experienced management consultants, attorneys, and accountants. In addition, the U.S. Small Business Administration publishes a management series that can help these athletic trainers become more familiar with the variety of issues facing owners of all types of small businesses.

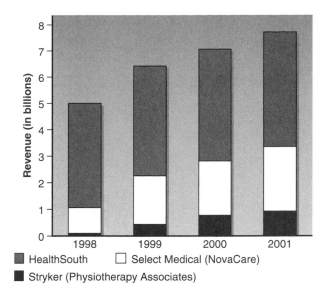

▶ **Figure 4.1** Revenues of three large private-sector employers of athletic trainers.

BUDGETING

Budgeting financial resources is a process that organizational leaders ask program heads to accomplish. Athletic trainers and others responsible for planning and delivering sports medicine services must develop skills in planning and implementing budgets so that needed services are delivered in an effective, timely manner and allocation of financial resources is consistent with the strategic plans of both the institution and the sports medicine program.

A **budget** is a plan for the coordination of resources and expenditures (Horine 1991). A budget also serves as a tool for estimating receipts and disbursements over a period of time (Mayo 1978). Beyond its practical uses as a restraint on resource waste and as a predictive tool for the financial health of a sports medicine program, a budget is a quantitative expression of the athletic trainer's management plan. As such, it is both a strategic plan for how the sports medicine unit will function over a given period and an operational plan for how it will accomplish its goals.

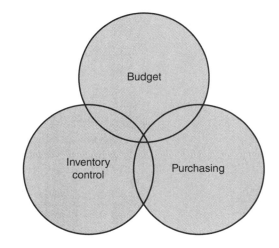

▶ **Figure 4.2** Interrelationships of financial activities of the sports medicine program.

Although many practitioners think of budgeting as a task that begins and ends in a narrow time frame during a particular part of the year, the wise athletic trainer views budgeting as a continuous process of prioritizing, planning, documenting, and evaluating the goals of the sports medicine unit and translating those goals into concrete plans for how to expend available resources. Because athletic seasons stretch over all 12 months and new programs of all types are added to the athletic trainer's responsibilities, the budgeting process requires constant attention to fund status and ongoing evaluation for the next budget cycle.

Jones and Trentin (1971) have suggested that budgets be used as the primary tools for planning and controlling a program. This approach helps athletic trainers differentiate between the concepts of budgeting and forecasting. As mentioned in chapter 2, forecasting is the process of predicting future conditions based on various statistics and indicators that describe the past and present situations. Typically, only a few people near the top of the organizational chart perform forecasting. Because budgeting is a type of planning, however, it requires input from

The Small Business Administration's management series is available from the Superintendent of Documents, U.S. Government Printing Office, Washington, DC 20402, or at www.sba. gov/.

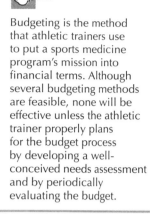

Budgeting is the method that athletic trainers use to put a sports medicine program's mission into financial terms. Although several budgeting methods are feasible, none will be effective unless the athletic trainer properly plans for the budget process by developing a well-conceived needs assessment and by periodically evaluating the budget.

the grass roots of the sports medicine program. An effective budget will consider the input of all employees about using the financial resources to meet documented program needs as opposed to simply allocating funds according to past traditions.

Types of Budgets

Most sports medicine budget planning is based on one of six budgeting models (Ray 1990). The six most common budgeting methods are zero-based, fixed, variable, lump-sum, line-item, and performance budgeting. Each of these methods can be an effective way to help athletic trainers plan the financial activity of their programs, depending on the particular circumstances and nature of the programs they direct. Depending on the financial health of the program and its parent institution, each budgeting method will normally be coupled with either permission to increase spending or a mandate to reduce spending.

The **spending-ceiling model**, also known as the *incremental model* (Wildavsky 1975), is the budgeting circumstance most often desired by sports medicine program directors. Stan used this model to determine his budget in the opening case. This method requires justification only for expenditures that exceed those of the previous budget cycle. Budget increases are most often linked to the inflation rate, which presents problems for sports medicine programs because prices for medical goods and services typically rise faster than inflation does. Athletic trainers who use this method are usually able to balance financial resources and expenditures for two or three years but often fall behind after that because of the difference between the inflation rate and the increasing cost of medical goods and services.

Sports medicine programs in financial crisis are often forced to combine their primary budgeting method with the **spending-reduction model**. Stan will have to adopt this model because of the financial problems in his school district. Under the spending-reduction model, department heads, including directors of sports medicine programs, are required to reduce their budgets to preserve institutional funds. For obvious reasons, this method requires the most imagination and creativity of all the budget models. Because financial resources tend to be reduced periodically in most sports medicine settings, the wise athletic trainer should identify those goods and services that could be cut without seriously affecting the program. If a financial crisis does arise, the athletic trainer will be prepared.

Each of the following budgeting methods can be used in either a spending-ceiling or spending-reduction mode:

■ **Zero-based budgeting. Zero-based budgeting** is an administrative method that requires unit directors to justify every expense without reference to previous spending patterns. This method requires close attention to documentation of actual program needs. Stan is being forced to adopt a combination of the spending-reduction and zero-based methods in the opening case. Although it requires more effort on the part of the athletic trainer, zero-based budgeting can be an excellent tool for developing priorities in a sports medicine program. Zero-based budgeting requires athletic trainers to evaluate each subfunction of the program and rank it according to how important it is to the accomplishment of the overall mission. The director should include a rationale for each item in the budget request, explaining why the expense is necessary and what alternatives there are to funding it.

■ **Fixed budgeting. Fixed budgeting** is an appropriate process for sports medicine programs in financially stable environments. This method requires an athletic trainer to project both expenditures and program income, if any, on a month-by-month basis to determine total program costs and revenues for the fiscal year. This exercise is useful because it can help the athletic trainer determine the likely cash flow of the operation at various points in the year. This type of budgeting is probably most appropriate for large, well-established sports medicine clinics during periods of relative economic certainty. School sports medicine programs rarely use fixed budgeting because most of these programs are not income oriented.

■ **Variable budgeting. Variable budgeting** requires that expenditures for any given time period be adjusted according to revenues for the same period. Unfortunately, the athletic trainer who coordinates the activities of a sports medicine clinic will rarely be able to predict the monthly balance of expenditures to revenues with perfect accuracy. Assume that the clinic director budgeted $25,000 for expenses in June, anticipating that revenues would be approximately $50,000. Under the variable budgeting system, if actual revenues were only $40,000, the clinic director would be required to reduce expenditures by 20% for that month. Like fixed budgeting, this method is rarely used in school-based programs.

■ **Lump-sum budgeting.** In **lump-sum budgeting,** a parent organization provides an athletic trainer with a fixed sum of money and the authority to spend that money any way he sees fit. Most athletic trainers who use lump-sum budgeting like it because it gives them the freedom to spend money where they think it is needed the most. Lump-sum budgeting requires an administrator to hold athletic trainers accountable after the fact.

■ **Line-item budgeting.** **Line-item budgeting** requires that athletic trainers list anticipated expenditures for specific categories of program subfunctions. Typical line items for a sports medicine program include expendable supplies, equipment repair, team physician services, and insurance (see figure 4.3). Line-item budgeting allows a parent organization to retain greater control over the sports medicine program because money budgeted for one line cannot usually be spent on another line without permission. The advantage of a line-item budget is that it is easy to understand and prepare. The disadvantage is that the athletic trainer has limited flexibility in responding to midyear financial crises because funds dedicated to one use cannot be easily transferred to another use.

■ **Performance budgeting.** **Performance budgeting** breaks the functions of a sports medicine program into discrete activities and appropriates the funds necessary to accomplish these

BUDGET COMPARISON REPORT

Acct. No.: 213702   **Dept.: Sports Medicine**   **Responsible person: Stan Curtis**

Object code	Account description	09-10 Expense	11-11 Budget	11-12 Request	Percent change
3110	Travel	229.25	300.00	300.0	0
3205	Supplies	7,632.32	9,000.00	9,475.75	5.3
3305	Printing	89.29	100.00	100.00	0
3315	Speakers	0	1,500.00	1,500.00	0
3320	Stipends	5,997.96	6,300.00	6,300.00	0
3360	Postage	257.65	300.00	300.00	0
3530	Repairs	313.15	500.00	500.00	0
3650	Phone	428.89	475.00	500.00	5.3
3720	Uniforms	430.00	500.00	500.00	0
3850	Periodicals	150.00	150.00	150.00	0
4035	Insurance	200.00	250.00	300.00	20.0
4100	Dues	90.00	100.00	100.00	0
Department total		**$15,818.51**	**$19,475.00**	**$20,025.75**	**2.8**

▶ **Figure 4.3** Sample line-item budget for a school-based sports medicine program.

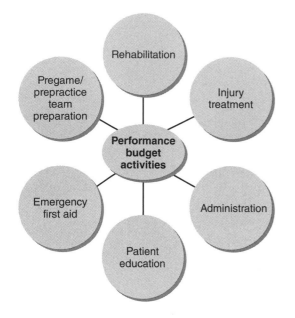

▶ **Figure 4.4**   Performance budget activities.

activities. Examples of activities typically associated with a school sports medicine program include prepractice and pregame team preparation, rehabilitation, injury treatment, administration, patient education, and emergency first aid (see figure 4.4). Expenses for each of these activities can be calculated and used to determine the overall budget. This method is similar to line-item budgeting in that mini-budgets are developed for separate categories of expenditures. Sports medicine programs do not commonly use performance budgeting because of the expense and difficulty of analyzing specific activity costs.

Planning the Budget

The process of budget planning varies depending on institutional budgeting cycles and rules and the type of budgeting system being used. Before Stan faced a budget crisis, he probably used a spending-ceiling, or incremental, budget model to help him plan his fiscal needs.

Needs Assessment

The first step in any budget cycle involves a careful assessment of program needs. Witkin and Altschuld (1995, p. 4) define **needs assessment** as "A systematic set of procedures undertaken for the purpose of setting priorities and making decisions about program or organizational improvement and allocation of resources. The priorities are based on identified needs."

A **need** is the gap between a present state of being and the desired state to which a program should aspire (Kauffman, Rojas, and Mayer 1993). People commonly confuse needs with solutions. For example, suppose that Stan, the athletic trainer in the opening case, was concerned that physicians were referring too many of the student-athletes under his care to outside clinics for their rehabilitation rather than having them complete their recovery in his facility. Underlying his concern was the fact that these services were driving up the cost of the school district's insurance policy. In addition, Stan was also troubled that he and his team physician were out of the loop when return-to-play decisions were made for many of these athletes. The need in this case would be Stan's desire to have all (or, in any case, most) of the injured athletes complete their rehabilitation in-house.

This need should not be confused with the many possible solutions to help meet the need. Stan could develop a closer working relationship with the physicians who are referring the athletes to the outside clinics. He could do a better job of educating the parents about the rehabilitation services and capabilities of his staff. He could improve the rehabilitation facilities in the school where he works. He could hire another staff member whose sole function would be rehabilitation. He might even encourage the school administration to refuse payment for rehabilitation services performed outside the school unless Stan or the team physician approved them in advance. Some of these solutions will have budgetary consequences, and some won't. The important thing to recognize for the purpose of the needs assessment, however, is that none of these options is a need. Each is a potential solution that might help eliminate the need in this case. Stan does not *need* a new rehabilitation facility, but the program does need to keep more of its patients in-house.

Needs assessment as it relates to budget planning should generally include the following three phases:

Phase 1: Exploration

During this phase, an athletic trainer should

- identify the needs of the sports medicine program,
- decide what information to collect for each of the identified needs, and
- decide where and how to collect the information.

Phase 2: Information Gathering

During this phase, an athletic trainer should

- collect as much information as possible for each of the identified needs,
- prioritize needs, and
- determine causes for each of the needs.

Phase 3: Decision Making

During this phase, an athletic trainer should

- develop alternative solutions for each need,
- determine budgetary implications for each solution,
- prioritize solutions, and
- integrate solutions into the program budget.

Funding Source Decisions

The next step in planning a budget for a sports medicine program is for the athletic trainer and the division head (for example, athletic director, chair of the academic department, general manager, or principal) to agree on which fund will provide the various items that the athletic trainer needs. This discussion should cover all of the program's projected expenses. Too often, athletic trainers focus only on the costs associated with supplies and equipment during the budget planning process, to the exclusion of other items important for running the program, including services, telephone, photocopying, and so on. After the athletic trainer and the division head have identified all program costs, they should allocate each to a particular budget. Protective pads, for instance, might fall into the sports medicine budget or the equipment budget. The health services budget might cover costs associated with physical examinations. Expenditures for travel to professional meetings might be part of the parent department's travel budget instead of the sports medicine budget. These decisions will depend on both the working relationship and the financial philosophies of the individuals involved.

Which fund these expenditures fall under will affect who controls the funds. If Stan's travel to professional conferences is covered under the director of cocurricular activity's overall travel budget, Stan will probably be required to justify each meeting he wishes to attend. In addition, he will likely be subject to all the restrictions on travel that apply to other district employees who report to the same director.

Another important decision involves whether the purchase of certain injury-protection equipment should be covered by the sports medicine budget or the budget of the team that will be using the equipment. If only one team will use an item, it makes sense to include that item in the team's budget rather than the budget of the sports medicine program. If such items are placed in the budget of the sports medicine program, other teams might develop false expectations of the sports medicine staff.

For example, if Stan purchases knee braces to be used specifically by football players, then other coaches might expect Stan to purchase knee braces or similar devices for their athletes. The sports medicine program will probably be unable to continue to support this expense. A more rational approach would be for the football coaches to include the expense of the knee braces in their own budgets. Only in this way will Stan be able to avoid setting a precedent that he won't be able to afford for long.

Improved Budget Planning

The first year a budget is planned for the sports medicine unit is often the most difficult because of the lack of a precedent on which to base financial plans. The process of budgeting for the first year of operation most closely approximates the zero-based budgeting model, because a rationale for each purchase must be developed without reference to established spending patterns. The presence of such spending patterns facilitates subsequent budget planning, which then approximates the spending-ceiling, or incremental, model. Athletic trainers can enhance their budget planning for sports medicine goods and services by following these guidelines:

- Keep a running inventory of all consumable and nonconsumable supplies.
- When budget submission time comes, calculate the amount of each type of consumable supply that has been used. Project and estimate how much more of the supply will be needed to complete the fiscal year, taking into account the different needs of the sport seasons yet to come.
- On the basis of estimates of how much of each type of supply will be needed to complete the fiscal year, and taking into account any changes that will take place during the next fiscal year (for example, new varsity sports, longer seasons), estimate the amount of each type of supply that will be needed for the next fiscal year.
- Consult with several vendors to obtain estimates of how much prices are expected to rise for the next fiscal year. With this information, develop anticipated prices for all the consumable supplies that will be needed for the next fiscal year.
- Establish long-term relationships with vendors and negotiate bulk rate purchasing opportunities.
- Be knowledgeable regarding the guidelines for bidding and purchasing.
- Consider partnering with other programs for greater purchasing leverage.

Capital Equipment and Improvements

Budget planning for nonconsumable capital equipment and capital improvements is often more difficult than budget planning for consumable supplies that are typically reordered every year. Therapeutic modalities, ice machines, and rehabilitation equipment are examples of nonconsumable capital equipment. These items are expensive, and many sports medicine directors are not able to include them in their annual supply budgets. Planning for acquisition, repair, and replacement of such items requires careful coordination between directors of sports medicine units and higher-level decision makers. Renovations, additions, or modifications to existing facilities are known as capital improvements. Because the capital budget is often unrecoverable once spent, multiple levels of authority must screen purchases and projects of this type and ensure that such expenditures are consistent with accomplishing the mission of the sports medicine program (Jones and Trentin 1971). Maintenance of durable medical equipment can become a necessary task. Planning to cover the costs of maintaining equipment can range from in-house services to outsourced contractual agreements (Cashmore 2006). The following suggestions will help budget planners meet the needs of the sports medicine program in this area:

- Treat equipment repair as a consumable supply and include it as a line item in the annual operating budget. If the institution will agree to roll over the unused balance of this account from year to year, it can serve as a fund for capital equipment purchases.
- Develop priority lists for capital equipment and improvement requests complete with documentation of need. Suggest possible funding alternatives to decision makers.
- Make institutional fund-raisers aware of the priority list and the documentation of need so that they can keep those needs in mind when soliciting funds from contributors.
- Consider answering grant requests from funding agencies or engaging in research projects funded by industry. For example, Hope College became a testing site for a new analgesic cream, which brought the sports medicine unit over $25,000. The college now uses the money to fund capital equipment purchases for the sports medicine program.

Budget Evaluation

Most directors of sports medicine units either ignore budget evaluation completely or perform it reluctantly. Evaluation of the budget, however, is important in the overall budgeting process, because it allows administrators to reach informed judgments on how well the institution is spending its financial resources. The following three relatively simple steps can help athletic trainers evaluate how well the budget process is working.

- **Maintain dual accounting systems.** Besides monitoring the accounting done in the sports medicine unit, request computer printouts from the institution's business office to make sure that expenditures are being charged to the proper funds.

- **Evaluate service contracts.** Evaluate service contracts, such as for ambulance service, insurance, team physicians, and student athletic trainers, each year to make sure that pay rates are competitive for the work being done. Keep a running log of all activities of each contractor, including the number of hours worked and the type of work performed.

- **Compile statistical information.** Periodic statistical reports of how consumable and nonconsumable supplies and equipment are being used can help an athletic trainer justify financial resource deployment. For example, treatment records are an excellent source of information about how often and on whom therapeutic modalities are being used. Many computer software packages can help develop statistical reports.

PURCHASING SUPPLIES, EQUIPMENT, AND SERVICES

After the sports medicine budget has been approved, the process of budget implementation can begin. **Purchasing** is the process that athletic trainers use to implement the budget plan. Methods of purchasing supplies, equipment, and services are critical to the cost-effective operation of the sports medicine program. Creative purchasing strategies can reduce expenditures for sports medicine supplies by up to 40% (Ray 1991b).

Basic Steps in the Purchasing Process

The six basic steps in purchasing (Wright 1983) include request for quotation, negotiation, requisition, purchase order, receiving, and accounts payable. Each is a critical element in organizing a well-supplied sports medicine program. Nowadays, it is not uncommon to complete an entire bidding and purchasing process through an online procedure.

Request for Quotation

The first step in the purchasing process involves sending a request for quotation to a variety of vendors. A **request for quotation (RFQ)** is a document that accompanies a bid sheet and provides instructions for vendors to bid on the supplies, equipment, and services needed by a sports medicine program (see figure 4.5). The use of RFQs is known as **bidding**, and it is the most effective way to reduce costs for expendable sports medicine supplies (see figure 4.6). Certain questions should be considered before supply bid sheets are distributed to vendors (see table 4.1).

> Athletic trainers implement the budget when they purchase equipment, supplies, and services for the sports medicine program. Although bidding is usually the most cost-effective purchasing method for consumable supplies, other purchasing options can be more effective for capital equipment and services.

■ Six Basic Steps in the Purchasing Process

1. Request for quotation
2. Negotiation
3. Requisition
4. Purchase order
5. Receiving
6. Accounts payable

Grant Public Schools

Department of Sports Medicine

Request for Quotation
(This is not an order)

Submit Bid To: Stan Curtis, Head Athletic Trainer
Grant Public Schools
Municipal Stadium
Grant, CA 98201

If additional information is required, contact Stan Curtis at 415-555-7708.

Date Mailed: April 11, 2012   Closing Date: May 2, 2012

Goods must be able to be delivered before: August 1, 2012   Billing not before: July 1, 2012

In order to receive consideration, one copy of the "Request for Quotation," with your bid properly filled in, must be signed and returned by the specified closing date.

All prices and conditions, including freight charges, must be shown. Additions or conditions not shown on this bid will not be allowed.

Contracts or purchase orders resulting from this quotation may not be assigned without the consent of the Head Athletic Trainer, Grant Public Schools.

The seller agrees to protect the purchaser from all damages arising out of alleged infringements of patents.

Unless otherwise specified, the right is reserved to accept or reject all or any part of your proposal.

Delivered F.O.B. to specific address in Grant, California 98201. Seller assumes all freight and delivery expenses.

If given an order for item(s) specified on the attached "Grant Public Schools Sports Medicine Bid Request," bidder agrees to furnish the items at the price(s) specified and under the conditions indicated.

Bidder to complete:

Bidder's name and address:

_____

_____

_____

Telephone Number:

1-800- _____ and/or

Area Code (_____) _____

Prices will be good for _____ days.

Delivery will be made _____ days after receipt of order.

Signed by _____

Printed name _____

Title _____ Date _____

▶ **Figure 4.5** Sample request for quotation form to accompany bid sheet.

Grant Public Schools Sports Medicine Bid Request

Please complete and return within three weeks of receipt to Stan Curtis, Head Athletic Trainer, Grant Public Schools, Grant, CA 98201.
Phone 415-555-7708 or fax 415-555-7922

All bid prices should include the following factors:
    —Cost of shipping to Grant, CA
    —Billing no sooner than 7/1/12

*If listing a substitute item, please specify brand name, packaging quantities, and product codes. If no brand is specified in the *Item* column, please specify the brand you are bidding in the *Substitute* column.

Item	*Substitute	Quantity	Bid price/unit	Total
1.5-inch J & J Coach tape (no substitute)		110 cases		
3-inch elastic tape (Elastikon or substitute)		10 cases		
2-inch elastic tape (Conform or substitute)		10 cases		
3-inch underwrap		5 cases		
6-inch elastic wraps (irregular if available)		20 dozen		
3-inch elastic wraps (irregular if available)		4 dozen		
1/8-inch adhesive felt (6" × 36")		20 pieces		
1/8-inch adhesive foam (5" × 72")		10 pieces		

▶ **Figure 4.6** Sample bid sheet to accompany request for quotation.

TABLE 4.1 Factors to Consider in the Bidding Process

Question	Consideration
Will brand names be specified or are generic products acceptable?	Products for which a brand name is required should have a "no substitute" notation clearly marked on the bid sheet.
How many and which vendors will be invited to bid?	The suggested minimum is three. Vendors who have a reputation for excellent service should be considered over those who do not.
Will the institution or the vendor be responsible for paying shipping costs?	Most suppliers of consumable products are willing to pay shipping if specified on the bid.
What types of products will be purchased via bidding?	Consumable supplies and some types of durable equipment are good candidates for bidding. Most services should be bid only with great caution because the quality of service may be reflected in lower prices.
When should RFQs be sent to vendors?	This depends on the institution's purchasing process. If athletic trainers are required to purchase supplies through a central purchasing department, a minimum of three months from RFQ to delivery should be allowed.

Negotiations

Negotiations are an important part of the purchasing process, because their effective use can help safeguard the interests of a sports medicine program. Athletic trainers should negotiate in the following three categories of purchases.

1. Capital equipment. This is the expensive, durable equipment that often makes up the bulk of the rehabilitation and therapeutic modality inventory for a sports medicine program. Purchases are infrequent and costly.

2. Medium-priced annual rebuys. These are usually purchases of services that require annual renegotiation. Examples include salaries, physician consulting fees, ambulance services, and athletic medical insurance.

3. Lower-cost consumable supplies. These items constitute the bulk of the sports medicine supply budget. Although some supplies will have to be reordered throughout the year, careful planning will allow the athletic trainer to place only one major supply order for the entire year. This method will strengthen the athletic trainer's negotiating position because of the discounts normally associated with quantity purchasing.

Although negotiation on the price of a supply, item of equipment, or service is common, athletic trainers should also consider other areas in which they can realize cost savings through negotiation. The athletic trainer should also negotiate the way in which the goods will be supplied, their quality, shipping costs, and support after the purchase.

■ **Price.** Price is the most obvious point for negotiation in purchasing sports medicine goods and services. The use of the RFQ is the first step in price negotiation for consumable supplies, but it isn't the only option available. Vendors are often willing to negotiate price reductions after submitting the RFQ. But if athletic trainers use excessive price negotiation after vendors have returned the RFQ, a poor working relationship and higher prices in subsequent years are likely to result. Athletic trainers have an ethical responsibility to avoid the practice of playing one vendor against another to achieve the lowest possible price. Most vendors understand that they will be most competitive if

■ Types of Services Commonly Purchased by Athletic Trainers

- Team physician
- Consulting physician
- Ambulance
- Liability and malpractice insurance
- Athletic accident insurance
- Drug screening
- Laboratory and radiology
- Equipment service contracts
- Nutritional services
- Counseling services
- Radiology
- Pharmacology
- Durable medical equipment

they keep their prices low. In addition, they understand that athletic trainers will use bidding to try to keep their costs as low as possible. But playing one vendor against another after the bids have been returned is frowned upon and is sure to damage relationships with vendors. Price negotiation is usually the most effective when one is purchasing services, for which bidding is less common.

■ **Supply.** Among the most common points for negotiation between athletic trainers and vendors are delivery and payment schedules for purchased goods. Because many educational institutions have fiscal years that begin on July 1, common practice is for athletic trainers to order supplies for the next school year in May, take possession in June, and defer billing until after July 1. This allows athletic trainers time to restock and prepare for their fall seasons during one fiscal year and pay for the supplies during the subsequent year. Negotiation over delivery and billing is even more important for sports medicine clinics, where fluctuations of cash flow have a greater effect.

■ **Quality.** Athletic trainers typically negotiate for the quality of the goods they purchase by specifying brand names or generics on the bid sheet. A point of negotiation particularly applicable to large capital improvement items is the warranty. Although an **implied warranty** should accompany every product, the athletic trainer is free to negotiate an **express warranty** that affirms the performance characteristics of the product. See figure 4.7 for an example of an express warranty.

For the period of:	We will replace at no cost to you:
One year from the date of the original purchase	Any part of the ultrasound unit that fails due to a defect in materials or workmanship. During this one-year period we will also provide, free of charge, any necessary labor to replace or repair the defective component.
Five years from the date of the original purchase	Any part of the generator or crystal that fails due to a defect in materials or workmanship. During this five-year period we will also provide, free of charge, any necessary labor to replace or repair the defective component.
Seven years from the date of the original purchase	Any part of the plastic housing that fails due to a defect in materials or workmanship. During this seven-year period we will also provide, free of charge, any necessary labor to replace or repair the defective component.

What this warranty does not cover:

- Improper installation
- Failure of the product if it is abused, misused, or used for a purpose other than that for which it was intended
- Damage to the unit caused by flood, fire, or natural disasters
- Damage to circuit breakers or electrical systems
- Incidental damage caused by failure of this unit
- Routine maintenance or calibration

▶ **Figure 4.7** Example of an express warranty for an ultrasound unit.

■ **Shipping.** The two primary points for negotiation about shipping purchased goods are payment of shipping costs and the freight-on-board (FOB) point. The wise athletic trainer will include a statement in the RFQ stipulating that the vendor will assume all costs associated with shipping and handling the product. This common practice clarifies the cost of supplies for athletic trainers by allowing vendors to factor the costs of shipping into their bids. The **FOB point** specifies the place at which title for the sports medicine supplies will pass from the vendor to the purchaser. Generally, athletic trainers should specify their institutions or clinics as the FOB point to provide greater protection against loss or damage during shipping.

■ **Support.** Negotiation for technical support is especially important for high-technology capital improvement items. Computers and isokinetic testing and rehabilitation devices are two examples of the type of equipment for which athletic trainers might require technical support. The cost of this support is often negotiable and will become an important factor in the overall cost during the life of the equipment.

Requisition

The next step in the purchasing process is completing and submitting a **requisition** for needed supplies, equipment, or services (Wright 1983). This step can either be formal or informal depending on the authority level of the athletic trainer in the overall institutional bureaucracy. The requisition is simply a written request to expend institutional funds for needed resources (see figure 4.8).

Grant Public Schools				Purchase requisition		
Suggested vendor		Previous supplier? Yes ☐ No ☐		Date		
Ship to: Attn:				Date needed		
Quantity	Description			Unit		Total
Requested by:	Requested for:		Acct. no.	Approved by:		
For purchasing department use only						
Date ordered	P.O. No.	Ordered from:		Ship via:		

▶ **Figure 4.8** Sample purchase requisition form.

Purchase Order

Once an athletic trainer has approved requisitions in hand, purchase orders can be produced and sent to vendors. A **purchase order** is a document that formalizes the terms of the purchase and transmits the intentions of the buyer to purchase goods or services from the vendor (see figure 4.9). The purchase order should be completed and transmitted only after the RFQs have been received from the vendors. An important decision is whether to award purchase orders to vendors based on the low bid for the entire supply order or to make the award based on the low bid for each individual item. Athletic trainers will save the most money if they make the award based on each item. This method, however, has drawbacks. Most vendors have a minimum-order policy. A vendor awarded a purchase order for $4.95 out of a possible $10,000 RFQ will be unlikely to negotiate favorable terms in the future. One possible solution is to award purchase orders only for amounts over a certain critical level, usually around $200. This procedure breaks the total supply order into packages that will save the athletic trainer money and ensure a reasonable profit margin for the most competitive vendors.

Vendor's copy

Grant Public Schools

Purchase order no.

To:

This number must appear on all invoices ↑

↓ Ship to Grant Public Schools, Grant, CA

☐ Memorial Stadium, 225 Stadium Dr.

☐ Central Administration, 321 Pine St.

☐ Physical Plant, 5436 Elm Ave.

Bill to: Grant Public Schools
           Grant, CA 98201

Account number:	Order date:	Ship via:		
Quantity	Description		Unit price	Amount
Please send duplicate invoices.	Approved by:			

▶ **Figure 4.9** Sample purchase order form.

Receiving

Receiving is the process of accepting delivery of goods purchased from vendors. When goods are received, they should immediately be checked to make sure that the packing slip matches the contents of the shipping container and to determine whether all the goods specified in the purchase order have been received. All goods should be inspected for damage. If any damage is discovered, it should be reported to the vendor immediately. Most vendors have a policy of replacing damaged goods only if reported within a given period. It is a good idea to always save the packing slips when an item is received for institutional records in case proof of receipt is ever requested.

Accounts Payable

Payment for sports medicine supplies and equipment is usually due within a specified time period after the receipt of the goods or the invoice, whichever occurs last. Athletic trainers who work in educational, professional, or industrial settings should submit invoices to their respective business offices as soon as they receive them to take advantage of early-payment discounts offered by most vendors. Those athletic trainers who work in independent sports medicine clinics should evaluate the terms of the early-payment discount. If the finance charge is lower than the current cost of money, stretching the payments as far as possible into the payment term would make sense. For example, assume that you are in charge of an independent sports medicine clinic that needs to borrow money from a bank to cover supply purchases during certain times of the year when cash flow is predictably slow. If a particular vendor charged 0.5% per month (6% annual percentage rate) on the unpaid balance of your account and the bank was charging you an annual rate of 8%, you could pay off your account with the vendor over the maximum time allowed and spend the 2% you will save on another program need.

Alternative Purchasing Strategies

Besides the traditional method of bidding for sports medicine supply purchases and paying for them with institutional funds, athletic trainers should consider three other potential sources of cost savings: pooled buying consortia, alumni and booster organizations, and external funding organizations and programs.

Pooled Buying Consortia

A **pooled buying consortium** can be an effective method for purchasing certain types of sports medicine supplies. Schools that are members of an athletic conference should consider pooling their adhesive tape orders, for example, to receive a quantity discount. This method can be effective for many different types of supplies, including bandages, ice bags, paper cups, elastic wraps, and crutches. Coaches and athletic directors have used pooled buying consortia for many years to purchase balls and other athletic equipment for less than it would cost to purchase such supplies individually.

Alumni and Booster Organizations

Alumni and booster organizations can be helpful in offsetting the costs of large capital expenses that would usually lie outside the normal budget of the sports medicine program. Treatment and rehabilitation devices are expensive items that booster clubs are often willing to buy for the sports medicine program. Athletic trainers, however, must work in conjunction with the institutional development officer when making such requests of booster clubs. Many institutions have policies designed to ensure that all philanthropy passes through the development office to maximize the ability of the institution to obtain such gifts. In some cases, programs can establish naming rights to facilities in an effort to fund-raise for a sports medicine program. For example, universities will have procedures in place whereby a donor can contribute an amount of money in a restricted manner toward an athletic training program and in return the program will name its educational classroom or athletic training room after the donor.

■ External Funding Sources

Contact the following sources for information on external funding:

- National Athletic Trainers' Association Research and Education Foundation
- American College of Sports Medicine
- Gatorade Sports Science Institute
- National Institutes of Health
- National Science Foundation
- National Operating Committee on Standards for Athletic Equipment

The Foundation Center is an outstanding source of information for persons interested in applying for financial support from one of the thousands of public or private funding sources. See its website at www.foundationcenter.org for complete online information about how to get started, how to develop a proposal, where to apply, and other important information on grant proposal development.

External Funding Organizations and Programs

Many private and public sources of funds are available to athletic trainers for certain narrowly defined purposes (The Foundation Center 1997). These organizations and agencies provide money to help offset the costs of research and education for a variety of problems related to sports medicine. Grants from organizations generally pay for expenses associated with specific projects and are not intended to fund the routine expenses associated with operating a sports medicine program. For example, a college with an accredited athletic training education program that wanted to begin a lecture series might consider applying to a funding agency to help offset the cost of the series for a specific period. An athletic trainer who needs a particular piece of equipment to conduct a research project might also consider applying for a grant. External funding often supports the initiation of drug and alcohol education programs.

Athletic trainers interested in obtaining a grant from a funding agency will have to prepare a comprehensive grant application according to the exact specifications outlined in the application instructions. Most grant programs are competitive, and only the most worthy projects receive funding. An athletic trainer should select a funding agency whose goals are in congruence with the project for which she is seeking support. Some organizations and agencies have funding programs that are national in scope. Many states, cities, and local school districts also have either public or private foundations that support worthy projects. Some businesses will offer grants of either cash or products for sports medicine-related projects (Margolin 1983). Most universities have an office dedicated to helping their employees identify potential sources of external funding for specific projects.

■ Reasons Grant Proposals Fail

Anyone who has ever written a grant proposal knows that the proposal may be rejected. Grant proposals do not receive funding for many reasons (Locke, Spirduso, and Silverman 1993). The granting agency will probably reject a late or incomplete application. Similarly, if the proposal does not meet the granting agency's specifications or is poorly written, it will likely be rejected. Even well-written proposals that are submitted on time may be denied if the project is of insufficient importance for advancing the field. If the budget is unrealistic or the proposed methods are inappropriate, the granting agency is unlikely to fund the request. Additionally, the grant application may fail if the project is of a low priority for the granting agency. Finally, in challenging economic times, competition from investigators seeking external funding is likely to increase.

■ Relative Merits of Leasing

Advantages

- Possible tax advantages
- Decreased risk of obsolescence
- Lower initial costs
- May include repair service

Disadvantages

- Higher overall costs
- No ownership
- Higher effective interest rate than traditional financing

Capital Equipment—Buy or Lease?

Once a decision has been made to acquire an expensive piece of equipment, the athletic trainer and the organization's business manager must decide whether to purchase the equipment or lease it. Many expensive rehabilitation devices and other therapeutic modalities can be leased rather than purchased. Obviously, each method has advantages and disadvantages. The primary advantage of purchasing over leasing is cost, especially if the equipment is being purchased outright as opposed to being financed. The other advantage of purchasing is that the sports medicine program owns the equipment. Ownership can become a disadvantage, however, if the equipment relies on technology that becomes obsolete before the equipment is fully depreciated (Kess and Westlin 1987). One of the advantages of leasing is that an institution can use its capital in other ways because it has not devoted large amounts to equipment purchases. In addition, some tax advantages may be available to sports medicine clinics when they lease their equipment rather than purchase it.

Purchasing Services

Purchasing services is different in several ways from purchasing supplies or equipment. The first, and most obvious, difference is that the quality of a service can be more difficult to assess than that of a product. It is important to monitor all service-related contracts for quality assurance (Kujawa and Short 2005). Meticulous record keeping on services performed and repairs or upgrades should be maintained with dates and the names of the technicians who performed the work.

For example, assume that a large university sports medicine program contracts with a local radiology clinic for all its X-ray, MRI, CT, and nuclear medicine needs. The athletic trainers at the university will probably find it more difficult to determine the quality of these diagnostic services than they would, for example, the quality of the athletic tape they buy. This circumstance arises, in part, because they have to rely on the professional judgment of another person in the case of the radiology services. They don't have the expertise to make an informed judgment on the quality of every aspect of the service. The problem can become more acute if only one radiology service is available in the community. The athletic trainers cannot compare the service they receive from one radiology practice with what another might be able to offer. Athletic tape, on the other hand, is easier to evaluate. Many brands and styles are available from many vendors. A straightforward exercise can determine which brand is best for the money.

Nevertheless, athletic trainers can employ several methods to take some of the uncertainty out of purchasing services:

■ **Try to get the service free of charge.** Most team physicians volunteer their time. Many ambulance companies are willing to park at the site of an athletic contest free of charge. Some service providers are willing to donate their time in exchange for an advertisement in the game program.

■ **If you can't get the service free of charge, try to employ cost sharing whenever possible.** For example, your team physician might not be willing to see injured athletes in his office for free, but he might be willing to accept only what the athlete's insurance will pay.

■ **When more than one provider is available for a particular service, be sure to evaluate, in advance, what each is willing to provide and at what price.** For example, if two ambulance services operate in your community, speak with each to find out how much they charge for event standby and transport. Find out which hospitals they are willing to transport patients to. Ask them about their mean response time. Will they participate in your emergency plan drills?

▪ **Investigate the service provider's reputation with other athletic trainers.** If you are searching for an orthopedic surgeon to serve your athletes, ask other athletic trainers whom they use and why. Discussions with other athletic trainers can also help you attain equitable services.

▪ **Develop a contract or memorandum of understanding that specifies your expectations of the service provider.** This document can help improve communication between the sports medicine program and the service provider and prevent problems in the future. The contract should specify a period, usually no more than two years, for which the contract will be in effect. It may also include termination clauses and renewal options.

▪ **Develop a database for each service provider.** How many injured or ill athletes did your team physician see last year? How long do your athletes have to wait before the orthopedic consultant sees them? What is the rate of false-positive drug screens reported by the laboratory you employ? Only by answering those kinds of questions and comparing the answers with the cost of retaining the services will you be able to judge the value of this aspect of your program.

▪ **Involve other departments.** It is possible that other departments may be utilizing the services of the same vendor as the sports medicine department. Communication between areas of your institution or organization can bring about greater awareness and possibly contribute to collaborative service benefits.

▪ **Perform annual reviews.** To ensure ongoing satisfaction with services, it is a good idea to perform annual reviews of service agreements. Any concerns should be addressed formally.

INVENTORY MANAGEMENT

The U.S. Small Business Administration publication *Business Basics: Inventory Management* (1980a, pp. 2-3) defines **inventory management** as follows:

▪ Acquiring an adequate supply and variety of inventory to meet production and sales needs

▪ Providing safety stocks to meet unexpected demand or delays in inventory replenishment

▪ Investing in inventory wisely so that excessive capital is not tied up, excessive space is not required, and unnecessary borrowing and interest expense is not required

▪ Maintaining accurate and up-to-date records to help identify and prevent shortages and to serve as a database for decisions

Inventory management, one of the most important aspects of increased efficiency in a sports medicine program, is equally important for large and small operations. Large operations, such as professional athletic teams and universities with National Collegiate Athletic Association Division I football programs, have big investments in sports medicine supplies that they should manage wisely and prudently. Larger programs are more likely to operate multiple facilities, making the control and distribution of sports medicine supplies more difficult and requiring more attention to inventory techniques.

Inventory control is important for small programs as well, because errors in inventory and supply management result in more financial hardship for programs with smaller budgets. Another problem athletic trainers in smaller programs face is that coaches, athletic administrators, and physical education teachers often have access to the athletic training room and the sports medicine supplies in it.

Athletic trainers have a financial responsibility to maintain control over the inventory of sports medicine equipment and supplies. They can usually accomplish this by inventorying regularly, centralizing storage of supplies, automating the inventory process, restricting access to storage areas, and implementing reminder systems.

Stiefel (2002) describes an inspection and prevention maintenance program (IPM) consisting of five key elements:

1. Maintain an up-to-date list of all equipment owned or leased.
2. Inspect only those items that actually require periodic inspection.
3. Inspect all equipment prior to its first use, and record identifying information, purchase order number, cost, warranty information, physical inspection, electrical inspection, and applicable performance tests.
4. Establish an inspection schedule for each piece of equipment based upon its failure rate.
5. Keep track of completed inspections.

The following suggestions should help athletic trainers improve their ability to track the location and rate of use of their supplies.

■ **Inventory regularly.** Compile a complete inventory of expendable supplies at least once a month. Institutions that operate multiple athletic training rooms should inventory the stock in each facility every week. Compile the inventory reports for these satellites in the primary training room and use them to develop the monthly inventory report.

■ **Centralize storage.** Wherever possible, centralize the storage of sports medicine supplies to make them easier to manage. If you need to stockpile supplies in several locations, send the smallest amount that will suffice for a reasonable period, preferably one week. This system requires athletic trainers to be attentive to inventory levels and helps prevent sudden or unexpected shortages.

■ **Automate the inventory process.** Develop and implement a continuous monitoring system that allows for a quick check of inventory levels at any time. One effective method uses a computerized inventory record based on standard spreadsheet software. When removing supplies from the central storage site, the athletic trainer fills out a small form indicating the date, type, and amount of supply being taken and the amount remaining after the withdrawal (see figure 4.10). At the end of each day, a student or secretary enters the information on the forms into the computer record. This system allows the athletic trainer to track the status of the inventory on a daily basis.

SPORTS MEDICINE SUPPLY CHECKOUT FORM

Date _____

Supply type _____

Quantity _____

Supply destination _____

Amount remaining in storage _____

Person taking the supplies _____

Person recording the withdrawal into the computer _____

▶ **Figure 4.10** Sample inventory control form.

- **Restrict access.** Unauthorized access to the athletic training room and the supply room where sports medicine supplies are kept is the primary cause of inventory control breakdown. Institutions should develop policies and procedures that specify who has access to the sports medicine facility and under what circumstances. As few people as possible should have keys to the facility; access should be limited to those who are responsible for and have a legitimate need to use it. Policies should clearly state the responsibilities of anyone issued keys to the facility.

- **Keep a reminder system.** Each type of supply should be marked with a sign that reads "Reorder when *X* amount remains" to remind athletic trainers to reorder supplies when they reach a critically low level.

APPLICATIONS TO ATHLETIC TRAINING: THEORY INTO PRACTICE

Apply the concepts discussed in this chapter to the following two case studies to help you prepare for situations you might face in actual practice. The questions at the end of the studies are open-ended—many possible correct solutions exist.

■ Case Study 1

Tammy Jenkins had just arrived at Los Ranchos College after being appointed the school's first certified athletic trainer. It was mid-June, and Tammy knew she had quite a bit to do to get ready for the arrival of the fall sports athletes in August. She decided to start by approaching the athletic director.

"Coach," Tammy began, "I need to order the sports medicine supplies as soon as possible if we expect to be ready to go in August. I need to know a few things. First, how much money do I have to work with? Second, are there any specific purchasing procedures I need to follow? I'd really like to get busy with this today if I could."

The athletic director informed Tammy that she didn't have a specific budget for sports medicine supplies. In the past, sports medicine supplies were paid for out of the general athletics budget, which he controlled. "You just put your list together, and I'll take a look at it," he told her. "Oh, I almost forgot," the athletic director continued, "I wanted to make sure we at least had the tape here in time, so I went ahead and ordered it. It should be delivered some time in July."

Although Tammy was uncomfortable about not having a specific budget, she knew she wouldn't be able to change everything right away. She spent the rest of the day compiling an inventory of the supplies on hand. That evening she put together a list of the supplies she thought she would need to get through the first year, along with an estimate of each item's cost.

When she presented it to the athletic director the next day, he told her she would need to cut the proposal by 25%. "I think this list is fairly modest," Tammy said. "I'm not sure I can cut that much out of it." After further discus-

sion, the athletic director told Tammy that the cost of the tape, when added to the total cost of her supply list, was just more than he could afford. When Tammy asked how much he had paid for the tape, she was astonished to find out that it was 100% higher than the price she paid at the school where she used to work. "Where did you order the tape from?" asked Tammy. The athletic director replied, "We get all our supplies from Acme Sporting Goods downtown. We always have. Anything you need, just call them and they'll take good care of you. The owner is a big supporter of the college." Tammy suddenly realized that she had her work cut out for her!

QUESTIONS FOR ANALYSIS

1. What budgeting system does the Los Ranchos College sports medicine program use? Is it optimal for the conditions? What system would you implement? Why?

2. Why was Tammy so distressed when she found out how the tape had been purchased? What is the likely effect of this purchasing system on Tammy's program? How should she alter the purchasing system?

3. If Tammy changed from direct purchasing at Acme Sporting Goods to a system of competitive bidding, what would be the likely result?

4. What can Tammy do to lower her costs for sports medicine supplies while maintaining the supportive relationship the college enjoys with the owner of Acme Sporting Goods?

5. If you were in Tammy's position, would you have taken the same approach to purchasing supplies? If not, what would you have done differently? Why?

Case Study 2

Diversified Physical Therapy Services (DPTS) is a large rehabilitation services corporation that operates a string of clinics in a 10-county area in eastern Iowa. Besides operating the clinics, DPTS supplies rehabilitation professionals to 12 hospitals. DPTS recently acquired contracts at 15 high schools to supply sports medicine services. The contracts provide an athletic trainer for each school for 1,000 hours per year. As an additional service, DPTS purchases all sports medicine supplies for the schools up to a maximum of $2,500 per school.

At a recent meeting of the DPTS partners, one of the owners expressed concern over the plan to provide the schools with sports medicine supplies. Although he liked the idea in general, he was concerned about waste and cost-effectiveness. He also pointed out to the other partners that if each school used less than the $2,500 allotment, the company would be coming out ahead.

The DPTS partners decided to create a central storage site for all 15 high schools. The athletic trainers would be allowed to take what they needed for a two-week period. When they exhausted those supplies, they would have to come to the central storage site, housed in a clinic in the geographic center of the schools' service area, and check out enough for another two weeks. The business manager in the clinic where the supplies were stored would be responsible for auditing supply requisitions to ensure that each school remained below the $2,500 limit.

QUESTIONS FOR ANALYSIS

1. What are the strengths of the central supply plan adopted by DPTS? What are the weaknesses?
2. What alternatives are there to the central supply plan? Would they be superior? If so, why?
3. What are the strengths and weaknesses of the plan to provide up to $2,500 in supplies to each school? Is this a service that most schools would want? Why or why not?

SUMMARY

Budgeting is a process designed to coordinate resources and expenditures and also serves as a tool for estimating receipts and disbursements. Different formal types of budgeting exist: zero-based, fixed, variable, lump-sum, line-item, and performance budgeting. Each of these methods can be an effective way to help athletic trainers plan the financial activity of their programs. Performing a needs assessment assists with setting budgetary priorities and the allocation of resources. Purchasing of supplies, equipment, and services can be a regular task for athletic training managers. Purchasing involves bidding, requisitions, and other legal steps that are required to appropriately obtain goods and services. Once items are purchased, an accurate inventory should be maintained that reflects an adequate supply of items to meet an organization's needs. Proper maintenance of inventory and service agreements requires accurate and up-to-date records.

KEY CONCEPTS AND REVIEW

1. Understand the different kinds of budgeting processes and apply them to an athletic training setting.

A budget is a plan for the coordination of resources and expenditures. It helps ensure that needed services are delivered effectively and on time and that financial resources are expended in accordance with the institutional mission. The six most common types of budgeting systems are zero-based, fixed, variable, lump-sum, line-item, and performance. An organization can use each in either a spending-ceiling (or incremental) or a spending-reduction mode. Careful consideration of which funds will support the various activities of the sports medicine program enhances budget development. Budgeting for the first year of the sports medicine program is the most difficult because of a lack of previous spending patterns. Budgeting for capital improvements is more difficult than for consumable supplies because of the expense involved. Budget evaluation is an important but often neglected activity that will help athletic trainers make informed decisions on how to expend program resources.

2. Coordinate the purchasing of athletic training equipment, supplies, and services to maximize the use of program funds.

Purchasing is the process of budget implementation. The six most common steps in the purchase of sports medicine supplies include request for quotation, negotiation, requisition, purchase order, receiving, and accounts payable. Athletic trainers should attempt to negotiate with vendors over price, supply, quality, shipping, and technical support. Alternatives to purchasing by bidding include pooled buying consortia and the use of alumni and booster organizations. Athletic trainers should consider the relative merits of leasing over buying when shopping for expensive capital equipment.

3. Manage the athletic training program's inventory of equipment and supplies.

Inventory management is an important aspect of administration for athletic trainers. Mistakes in inventory management can have drastic consequences for both large and small programs. Athletic trainers should always be aware of the status of their supply inventory so that they can deliver sports medicine services in a timely manner.

Facility Design and Planning

OBJECTIVES

After reading this chapter, you should be able to do the following:

1. Understand and defend the importance of the design phase in planning and constructing new sports medicine facilities.

2. Understand the facility design and construction process in sports medicine settings.

3. Understand the common design elements of a well-planned sports medicine facility.

4. Describe the sports medicine facility in terms of its specialized function areas.

5. Discuss principles associated with marketing a sports medicine facility and practice.

▶ After meeting with the university president, the whole staff was excited about beginning the planning for a new athletic building. The president informed everyone that the board of trustees had approved the project. The athletic director, the chair of the exercise and sport sciences department, and the vice president for finance were appointed to the planning committee for the new building. After the meeting, the athletic director asked Kelly McCarthy, the director of sports medicine, to submit his ideas for the sports medicine facility in the new complex. Although Kelly was enthusiastic about the prospect of a new facility, he was a little nervous about having to design the new sports medicine center because he had never done anything like that before.

Kelly spent a few weeks toying with some ideas for the new sports medicine center before he finally drew a rough sketch and submitted it to the athletic director. The athletic director thanked him and filed the sketch away in a drawer labeled "New Building." Kelly didn't hear from the athletic director about the new sports medicine center again, so he assumed that his ideas had been accepted.

Six months later construction began. Four months after the groundbreaking, Kelly and the rest of the athletic department staff were given a hard-hat tour of the site to view the progress on the project. When they reached the area that was to contain the new sports medicine facility, Kelly was astonished at how small it seemed in comparison to the sketch he had submitted. When he asked about its size, the construction manager told him that the planning committee had had to shave off a few feet to accommodate the conference and media area in the adjacent basketball coaches' dressing room. The construction manager assured Kelly that the sports medicine facility would look much bigger after the finish work was completed.

When the building finally opened, Kelly and his staff moved into a sports medicine facility that, although brighter and newer than the old facility, was neither bigger nor more functional. He had essentially traded one undersized facility for another.

No architecture is so haughty as that which is simple.

—JOHN RUSKIN

Kelly McCarthy's experience with planning a new athletic building is common among athletic trainers. The opportunity to be involved in the planning, design, and construction of a sports medicine facility usually comes only once during the career of most athletic trainers, who typically have little or no experience in facility planning. Most buildings are designed and constructed to provide service for decades; so decisions made during the planning, design, and construction phase of the sports medicine facility are, for all practical purposes, permanent. Hence, it is understandable but unfortunate when expensive and uncorrectable mistakes occur. This chapter will help athletic trainers understand the basic processes of planning, designing, and constructing a sports medicine center.

CONCEPTUAL DEVELOPMENT

The most important phase in constructing a new sports medicine center is developing an appropriate concept for its design. Whether the facility is intended to serve a school or a professional or private sports medicine clinic, the conceptual development process is essentially the same despite the important differences in layout and funding strategy between these facilities.

At least two arguments support paying careful attention to the conceptual development of the design of the sports medicine center. First, this is the only stage of the project that involves review by the people who will actually use the facility. After the project has begun, many reviews will occur, but primarily construction professionals and municipal employees such as plumbing and electrical inspectors will carry them out. The athletic trainer has input during the design phase of a facility construction project.

In the opening scenario, Kelly McCarthy made a poor decision by assuming that the lack of feedback from the planning committee meant that they would implement his recommendations as submitted. Obviously, Kelly should have checked often to be sure that his ideas were being implemented. The construction of a new building is a political act that involves making choices about how to use limited resources. The time for athletic trainers to exercise their influence is during the design phase.

The second argument for paying attention to design development relates to permanency and cost. Buildings are intended to last a long time. Once the foundation is poured and bricks and mortar are in place, changes based on new thinking about the way the sports medicine facility should be designed become expensive to implement. Although the owners of private sports medicine clinics can always sell the building in the future if they become dissatisfied with its design, school and university officials generally do not have this option, because most campus-based sports medicine centers are part of large, multipurpose buildings.

> The design process is a critical time for athletic trainers to influence the final form of the sports medicine facility. Elements of the process include needs assessment, institutional approval, selecting a construction process, selecting an architect, developing schematics, securing funding, bidding construction, bid analysis, and beginning and monitoring construction.

Design Process

Most athletic trainers will never be involved in selecting an architect. As mentioned before, however, many will be responsible at some point in their career for input into the design of new sports medicine centers. Understanding the processes normally used by institutions during the design and construction phases of a new building can help athletic trainers avoid the kinds of mistakes that Kelly McCarthy made in the opening case. Although the steps described in the following paragraphs are not the only way to design, plan, and construct a new facility, they represent the most common elements of the construction process.

Planning Committee

The **planning committee** is a group of individuals appointed to work with the architect to develop the design of a new building. Planning committees should include people representing the various activities that will take place in the building. Fletcher and Ranck (1991) suggest that the chief executive officer of the institution appoint the members of the planning committee and include employees who will be responsible for operating, maintaining, and using the building. They also recommend that in school and university settings, at least one person from administration, the business office, and the physical plant be assigned to the planning committee. Theunissen (1978) suggests that the most appropriate person to act as chair of the planning committee is the person who leads the department or discipline most responsible for use of the new facility. This person may or may not be an athletic trainer. Hence, athletic trainers must effectively communicate their needs so that the overall design will incorporate them.

The planning committee should reflect a balance between primary decision makers, secondary decision makers, and definers (Dougherty and Bonanno 1985). Among the **primary decision makers** are institutional members with formal authority over large units or subunits of an organization—the people in a position to see the big picture. **Secondary decision makers** are typically professional staff members who deliver a program. In a school sports medicine setting, they include athletic trainers, team physicians, and selected faculty members. **Definers** are the people who will use the facility. In a sports medicine setting, definers would be patients, students, and athletes. Athletic trainers from other institutions might also act as definers by giving advice and asking questions that might not have occurred to the primary and secondary decision makers.

> ### ■ Phases of Design and Construction of a Sports Medicine Center
>
> 1. Conduct a needs assessment.
> 2. Seek approval for the project.
> 3. Select a construction process model.
> 4. Select an architect.
> 5. Develop schematics.
> 6. Secure the required funding.
> 7. Bid the construction.
> 8. Analyze bids and take action.
> 9. Begin construction.
> 10. Monitor construction.

Step 1: Conduct a Needs Assessment

The first step in designing a new sports medicine facility is a comprehensive assessment of future program needs. Information from the needs assessment (see chapter 4, p. 136), combined with a statement of present operating status, is called the **program statement**. The program statement is an important document because it helps the architect determine space requirements for the new facility (Dibner 1982). The process of needs assessment might seem tedious, but without it a competent job of planning for future space needs cannot be accomplished. One of the many mistakes Kelly McCarthy made in the opening case was that he sketched out a design for the new sports medicine center without taking into account future growth patterns. The needs assessment is usually conducted at the departmental or program level and involves asking and answering a series of questions (see table 5.1). If the administrator of a sports medicine program has been doing a good job of programmatic self-study, the needs assessment will be much easier to complete (see figure 2.13 on p. 65).

Step 2: Seek Approval for the Project

After the needs assessment has been completed, assuming it justifies the need for a new sports medicine facility, the people with financial control of the institution must be convinced that the project is necessary. This step is important whether the sports medicine program is in a school, professional, or private clinic setting. Every organization has a person or a group of people who must ultimately decide whether to spend the vast sums required for new construction. An athletic trainer must be willing to document the need for such facilities in detail. Even after presenting such documentation, however, the athletic trainer should not be disappointed if it takes months, or more realistically, years for such a project to gain approval.

Step 3: Select a Construction Process Model

Construction of new facilities usually occurs in one of three ways. **Lump-sum bidding**, the most traditional method, is often used for governmental units like public schools and colleges. In lump-sum bidding, the architect submits schematic drawings to several general contractors. The contractors study the plans and quote a cost based on the instructions provided by the architect. Because some contractors might intentionally underbid a project to secure a contract, it is wise to screen the contractors in advance and send bids only to those with proven records. The importance of this step can't be overemphasized. The temptation to accept the lowest bid without regard for the reputation of the contractor is powerful. The differences in the bids can amount to many thousands of dollars. You might eventually have to spend this money, however, if the workmanship is shoddy or if the contractor has cut corners. A prudent

TABLE 5.1   Sports Medicine Facility Needs Assessment Concerns

Question	Where to look for answers
What is the present clinic caseload? How is it likely to change?	Annual reports, interviews with staff and administrators
Is the present facility adequate? Why or why not?	Building codes, national design standards, literature review, peer consultation
Is the present facility suitable for implementing the strategic plan?	Program and institutional facility strategic plans
Which program problems are related to facilities?	Critical incident reports, interviews with staff, accreditation reports
Can the facility benefit from additional usage by other tenants or providers?	Class space, community education programs

approach is to visit at least one building that each of the contractors has constructed to determine the quality of the work. Be sure to spend some time alone with the owners so that you will feel free to ask questions about the experiences they had with the contractor. Although negative responses to some of the following questions would not necessarily reflect on the contractor's skill, it would be wise to find out if

- the contractor worked well with the architect,
- the project was completed on time,
- the project stayed within the budget,
- all the building systems functioned properly when the project was finished,
- the construction was of high quality,
- the contractor was willing to require subcontractors to correct any mistakes,
- the owners would make any changes to the building if given the chance, and
- the owners would hire this contractor again.

Another construction model that may be used is termed **construction management**. The construction-management approach uses the general contractor as part of the design team; that is, the contractor is on board from the beginning of the project, rather than coming in near the end of the design phase. The construction manager can then advise on building materials, schedules, cost analysis, and necessary subcontractors. A drawback to using the construction-management approach is the manager's fee, which can approach 5% of the total project cost. In addition, the manager will not exert direct authority over the work of the subcontractors, because the owner hires the subcontractors (Snider 1982).

The third construction process method is known as **design-build**. This system uses only one firm to both design and build a sports medicine center. As with the other construction models, there are advantages and disadvantages to the design-build concept. The obvious advantage is that the owners have only one firm with which to communicate. They can take any problems that arise to a single source for redress, allowing for more rapid and potentially cost-saving approaches to solving problems that arise during the construction phase of the project.

The streamlined approach used in design-build is also its weakness. This method involves fewer checks and balances among the various firms normally involved in a construction project. The integrity of the entire project rests on the ability of one firm—specifically on the ability of a few people in one firm. This is a good reason to screen design-build proposals even more carefully than a more traditional construction process model.

■ Advantages and Disadvantages of Lump-Sum Bidding

Advantages
- Results in lowest possible price
- Ensures fairness
- Complies with state and federal statutes

Disadvantages
- Contractors might underbid
- Less control for owner
- Contractor might cut corners

■ Advantages and Disadvantages of Construction Management

Advantages
- Construction manager is part of design team
- More advice on materials, costs, and schedules

Disadvantages
- Construction manager's fee
- No direct control over subcontractors

■ Advantages and Disadvantages of Design-Build

Advantages
- Easier communication
- Ability to fast-track problems

Disadvantages
- Fewer checks and balances
- Greatest potential for major problems

> ### ■ Three Methods for Selecting an Architect
>
> **1.** Ask friends and colleagues.
> **2.** Screen several architectural firms.
> **3.** Commission a design competition.
>
> For more information on how to find an architect, contact the American Institute of Architects at http://architectfinder.aia.org/. For a directory of architects and architectural consultants with experience in designing athletic facilities, visit http://athleticbusiness. com/ and click on "Architectural Galleries."

Step 4: Select an Architect

The owner of a clinic or the chief executive officer of an institution retains an architect to create building designs. The architect should be available to provide advice and guidance from the beginning of a project until the keys to the new facility are handed over to the users. Although the selection of an architect is listed as the fourth step in this text, it frequently comes earlier in the process. In fact, an architect can help with many of the previous steps.

Several methods can be used for selecting an architect (Dibner 1982). The first and easiest way is to contract with a firm recommended by friends or colleagues. For obvious reasons, this might not serve a sports medicine program well. A better method is to develop a list of architectural firms with a variety of attributes—big and small, local and distant, and so on. Interview each firm to determine whether it would be suitable for and interested in taking on the project. A site visit to at least one project each firm has completed is recommended. A third method for selecting an architect is to commission a design competition. This method is typically used only on very large projects because it is costly in terms of money and time.

Whichever method is used, a good match between the client and the architect is essential. Forseth (1986) recommends that architects for sports medicine facilities be selected based on their openness to suggestions and their previous experience in designing similar facilities. *Athletic Business* magazine publishes a directory of architects that have experience in designing athletic facilities. Many of these architects have designed sports medicine facilities as a part of these larger projects.

Step 5: Develop Schematics

Once the program statement mentioned previously has been developed, the architect will develop **schematic drawings** that reflect the relationships among the principal functions of the sports medicine center. One of Kelly McCarthy's errors in the opening case was that he never met with the architect to develop the schematic drawings that were eventually submitted. Had he done so, the architect probably would have been able to help him think in detail about traffic patterns and space requirements—two of the major elements that the schematic drawings should address.

Determining Space Needs Several authors have suggested methods to help athletic trainers determine how much space a new sports medicine center will need. Penman (1977) has suggested that the minimum amount of space required for a bare-bones athletic training room stocked with only one treatment table, one taping table, some counter space, and miscellaneous equipment is 300 square feet. Arnheim and Prentice (2002) suggest that the minimum size of a school or college athletic training facility should be 1,000 to 1,200 square feet. Secor (1984) has expanded on Penman's idea by creating a formula that athletic trainers can use to plan space requirements based on the number of athletes and other physically active patients they expect to serve during peak caseloads:

(Number of patients at peak / 20 per table per day) × 100 square feet = Total square footage

Although these suggestions provide a useful starting point for determining space needs, athletic trainers charged with the design of a new sports medicine center must take into account that varied functions will take place in the sports medicine center and that each of those functions will have different space requirements.

Another factor that influences the overall space requirements of a sports medicine center is the proportion of work that will be done in each of the various sections. The type of client served by the sports medicine center will largely determine this factor. For example, a hospital-based sports medicine center will probably dedicate a greater proportion of its space to rehabilitation. In contrast, the typical college and high school sports medicine facility requires a larger taping and bandaging section than private or hospital-based sports medicine clinics do. Finally, the anticipated growth of the program must be factored into the size estimates for the schematic drawings (Cohen and Cohen 1979). Although forecasting growth is difficult, it is extremely important, especially given the exploding demand for access to sports medicine services.

In summary, the following factors influence the space requirements of a sports medicine facility:

- Number of clients to be served
- Type of clients to be served
- Type of services to be offered
- Amount and kinds of equipment needed
- Number and qualifications of staff
- Projected growth of the program

Traffic Patterns   When working with the architect to develop the schematic drawings, the athletic trainer should determine anticipated **traffic patterns** based on the relationship of the subfunctions of the sports medicine center to each other. This step in the design phase is crucial. Attractive, functional sports medicine facilities are characterized by smooth traffic flow among all parts of the facility. If the design does not anticipate the traffic patterns that develop once the facility is built, the result is likely to be a sports medicine center that seems noisy, congested, crowded, or all three. Muther and Wheeler (1994) suggest that the best way to ensure smooth traffic flow is to identify each of the subfunctions of the sports medicine center and to justify the space that they will occupy by placing them on a **relationship chart** (see figure 5.1). The architect in consultation with the athletic trainer usually completes this task. The relationship chart can seem confusing at first glance, but it's actually quite simple. The chart is constructed so that the row for each special area intersects the rows for all the other areas. The athletic trainer's task is to decide how close each area should be to any other area and to justify her reasoning for each decision. For example, it is generally undesirable for the hydrotherapy area to be in proximity to the storage area because moisture could easily damage sports medicine supplies that require a cool, dry environment for maximum shelf life. The intersection of the rows for these two areas would be coded with an "X" and a "7," indicating that these areas should be kept apart for climate control purposes. Conversely, the hydrotherapy area should be close to the office so that someone can directly observe patients at all times. The intersection of these two rows would be coded with an "A" and a "1." Once charted, the physical relationships of subfunctions to each other become less conceptual and more concrete.

After the space relationships have been established, coded, and justified on the relationship chart, the next step is constructing a **bubble diagram**. The bubble diagram illustrates the spatial relationships among the subfunctions of a sports medicine center based on the proximity factors established in the relationship chart. Although the bubble diagram is by no means a floor plan, it is the first step toward being able to understand visually how all the parts of the sports medicine center will be laid out (see figure 5.2).

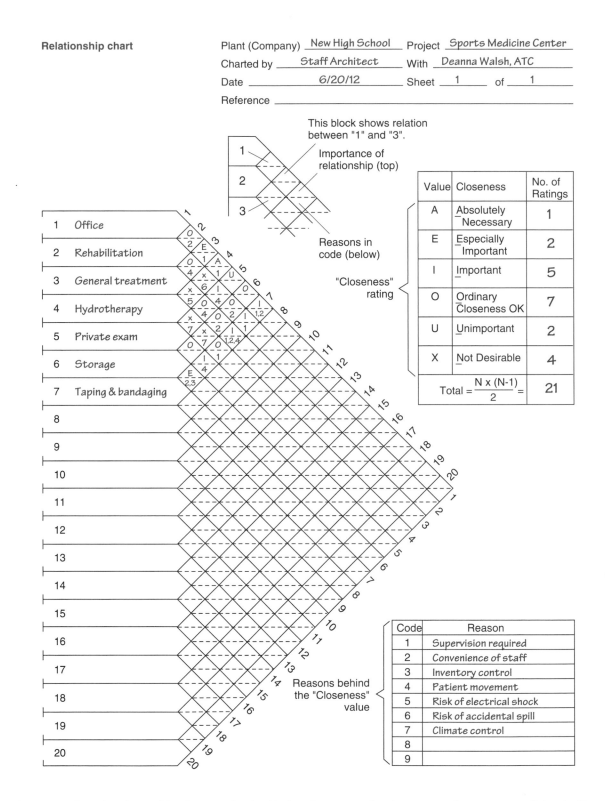

▶ **Figure 5.1** Sample relationship chart used to justify the placement of various spaces in a sports medicine facility.

Adapted, by permission, from R. Muther and J.D. Wheeler, 1977, *Simplified systematic layout planning* (Kansas City, MO: Management & Industrial Research). Extended copyright 1990 by Richard Muther. Adapted courtesy of copyright holder: Richard Muther.

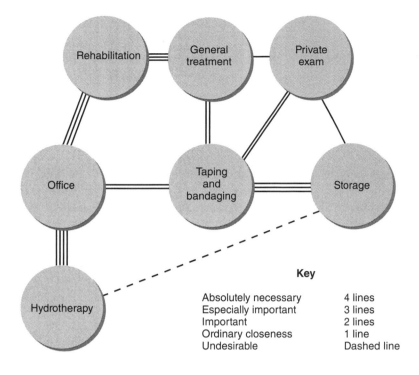

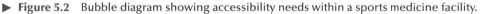

Key

Absolutely necessary	4 lines
Especially important	3 lines
Important	2 lines
Ordinary closeness	1 line
Undesirable	Dashed line

▶ **Figure 5.2** Bubble diagram showing accessibility needs within a sports medicine facility.

Step 6: Secure the Required Funding

Obviously, all construction projects require a source of funding. Many funding options are available for sports medicine center construction depending on the type of institution. Private sports medicine clinics generally have fewer options than do public-sector institutions like high schools, colleges, and universities. Even professional athletic teams have greater flexibility in financing sports medicine facilities than private clinics do, because many of the stadiums that house them are constructed at least in part with public tax dollars. The owners of most private sports medicine clinics will have to secure loans from a bank for new construction.

Athletic trainers who approach a financial institution for a loan should remember that banks are more likely to make loans for the construction of multipurpose buildings. For example, the athletic trainer who wishes to build a sports medicine clinic as part of a larger medical arts building will probably have a better chance of securing a loan than will the person who wants to build a health club that offers sports medicine services. The medical arts building can serve many purposes, whereas the health club would probably require extensive remodeling before resale should the bank need to foreclose. In general, bankers perceive medical practitioners as good risks.

At least two things are usually required of an athletic trainer who applies for a **commercial loan** from a bank for new construction of a private sports medicine facility: an assignment of life insurance (this protects the bank against loss in the event the athletic trainer dies before paying off the debt) and a **business plan**. The business plan is essential because it contains information that the bank will need to project whether or not the clinic is likely to succeed. A business plan for a sports medicine clinic would include the following items:

- A statement of the activities that the clinic will engage in
- A **market analysis** detailing the clinic's competitive advantages, analysis of the competition, pricing structure, and marketing plan
- The credentials of the principal owners and operators of the clinic
- Historical and projected financial statements of both cash flow and income

■ A breakdown of costs associated with the project based on the schematics developed by the architect

■ The amount of personal equity being committed by the athletic trainer

■ The amount of the loan being requested

Sports medicine facilities in the public sector, including private educational institutions that receive state and federal assistance, can be funded in at least three ways other than by a commercial loan.

One of the most common fund-raising methods is the **capital campaign**. A capital campaign is a major institutional response to several needs that the institution intends to remedy over three to five years. People at the very top of the institutional hierarchy usually authorize and direct capital campaigns. The goal of a capital campaign is to secure pledges of financial support from a broad institutional constituency including alumni, faculty and staff, foundations, affiliated institutions such as churches, and friends. Funds for a new sports medicine center will usually be a small fraction of the overall goal for a capital campaign. Nevertheless, an athletic trainer might be heavily involved in helping secure pledges under the direction and supervision of the institutional development officer.

Another way in which public-sector institutions and some hospitals secure funding for the construction of sports medicine facilities is through the sale of **tax-exempt bonds**. The sale of such bonds is usually authorized either by public vote (as in the case of public school construction) or by a bonding authority established by the states. Bonds are usually sold in one of two ways: publicly, usually to friends of the institution, or privately to a bank or other financial institution as part of its investment portfolio. A common practice is for similar institutions to pool their projects and sell bonds together under one issue. This practice is useful because it lowers the overhead costs associated with conducting a bond issue.

The third common method that institutions use to finance new sports medicine facilities is to borrow internally from their **endowments**. An institution's endowment is the sum of its assets in cash and investments. Institutions usually hesitate to borrow from endowments because the interest earned from an endowment can account for a significant percentage of the annual operating budget. If the endowment is large, however, and the sports medicine building project is relatively modest in relation to it, this is probably the easiest method of financing such a project.

> The following websites are useful sources of information on how to develop an effective business plan:
>
> www.businessplans.org/
>
> www.bplans.com/
>
> www.businessplanarchive.org/
>
> www.business-plan.com/
>
> www.brs-inc.com/

Methods for Funding Public-Sector Sports Medicine Facilities

■ Capital campaigns

■ Bond sales

■ Borrowing from endowment

■ Commercial loans

Step 7: Bid the Construction

If an athletic trainer is using the lump-sum bidding model, this is the time to bid the construction. Before the actual bids are sent to the contractors who will compete for the job, the architect will develop the **construction documents** (Dibner 1982). The construction documents are highly detailed technical drawings that the contractors will need to determine a realistic estimate of construction costs. The construction documents are the drawings that the contractor will use to guide construction of the new sports medicine center.

The architect will then prepare and send a packet of **bidding documents** to acceptable contractors. The bidding documents include an invitation to bid, the bid form, and special instructions from the architect. The bidders must submit their bids within a specified time, and all bids are opened at the same time. Normally, administrators hire the contractor who submits the lowest bid. In many states, law requires public institutions to allow all qualified contractors to bid for new construction projects. In addition, a certain percentage of the construction budget might have to be reserved for contractors of historically underrepresented minority groups.

Step 8: Analyze Bids and Take Action

After the sealed bids have been opened, the planning team must carefully analyze each one. First, the athletic trainer–architect team must make sure that the information on the returned bids is consistent with the project described in the bidding documents. If a contractor changes any item of the project, producing a lower bid, and the change goes unnoticed, legal problems could result. Another reason to screen the bids carefully is to ensure that the costs quoted by the various contractors are somewhat consistent. If one contractor's quotation is significantly lower than all the others, the athletic trainer and architect should ask for an explanation. Obviously, the quality of the finished facility will suffer if the contractor cuts corners to secure the contract.

If the returned bids exceed the available funding, four possible courses of action can be pursued (Biehle 1982). The first is to delay the project and raise additional funding. If excessive time is needed to raise the funds, the total project cost will probably rise because of inflation. The second option is to negotiate a lower price with the contractor. This approach usually involves eliminating certain features that were part of the original design or using less expensive building materials. The third option is to ask the architect to develop an alternative design. This approach is costly in both time and money. Finally, the project can be abandoned. If this happens, the athletic trainer should realize that most architects' contracts include termination fees in excess of the compensation the architect will be owed for the time and energy already spent on the project. In addition, the architect might retain the rights to the drawings. If the athletic trainer plans to use them for a future project, he should negotiate the right to do so before signing the architect's contract.

Step 9: Begin Construction

This step is self-explanatory. After the contractor's bid has been accepted, the architect works with the athletic trainer's (or the institution's) attorney to draw up the construction contract. The architect will have access to several standardized contract forms for this purpose.

Step 10: Monitor Construction

Several people play important monitoring roles during construction. The first is the **general contractor**, who is responsible for coordinating the work of the various **subcontractors** and for ensuring the quality of their workmanship. The architect represents the athletic trainer or the institution and ensures that construction is proceeding according to the standards developed by the architect. If the workmanship does not comply with the standards enumerated in the contract and construction documents, the architect has the authority to reject the work (Dibner 1982).

The athletic trainer and the planning committee have important roles to play during the construction phase. They should be present on the job site as often as possible to make sure that the design features agreed upon are being implemented. The frequent presence of the athletic trainer at the construction site can ensure that the contractor and subcontractors are implementing the details as planned. The athletic trainer should know the sports medicine facility better than anyone else.

If the athletic trainer suspects that the contractor or subcontractor is not properly implementing the architect's design, she should quickly inquire into the situation. The athletic trainer must address all concerns to the architect, not to the contractor or subcontractors. As the agent of the athletic trainer or the institution, the architect will investigate and mediate a solution to the problem.

To realize a fully functional space for a sports medicine program, an athletic trainer should plan for the following elements: size, location, ergonomics, electrical systems, plumbing systems, ventilation systems, lighting, specialized function areas, and accessibility.

ELEMENTS OF SPORTS MEDICINE FACILITY DESIGN

Athletic training facilities should meet the standards of any modern health care facility (Accreditation Association for Ambulatory Health Care 2010). An athletic trainer must consider at least nine elements when working with an architect to design a new sports medicine facility: size, location, ergonomics, electrical systems, plumbing systems, ventilation systems, lighting, specialized function areas, and accessibility (see figure 5.3). The section on developing schematics discussed size and space estimates. This section addresses the other eight design elements.

Location

A sports medicine center that is intended to serve the general population should be located near other health care providers. Patients will appreciate, for example, not having to travel far for X-ray or laboratory services. Proximity to referring physicians is another practical feature. The ideal location for a private sports medicine clinic is in a medical office building that houses those other health services—physicians, laboratory, and X ray.

Having athletic facilities nearby is useful for observing a rehabilitating patient's functional capacity in running or other sports skills. If the clinic sees many student-athletes, a location close to the school makes travel convenient for students.

As mentioned earlier, school-based sports medicine centers for student-athletes are usually housed in large multipurpose athletic, physical education, or recreation buildings. The placement of the sports medicine center within the facility is an important decision. Most experts agree that it should be as close as possible to both the men's and the women's locker rooms (Fahey 1986). Although some suggest that each locker room have direct access to the sports medicine center, problems of security and privacy may intervene. Athletes and other physically active patients should not have to cross through another activity area to reach the sports medicine center.

Another consideration is the position of the sports medicine center relative to outside entrances. An injured athlete should not have to walk or be carried through many doors—ideally, a door should lead directly from the outside playing fields into the sports medicine center. Wherever the center is located, it should have extra-wide doors that will accommodate two people assisting a nonambulating athlete. (Wide doors will also be able to accommodate a stretcher, spine board, or gurney.)

In a multistory building, a ground-floor location is most accessible to clients who ambulate with difficulty. If the sports medicine center cannot be located on the ground floor, it should be close to an elevator.

Having an institution's facilities for health services and sports medicine services adjacent has several advantages. First, cooperation can be enhanced if athletic trainers and other

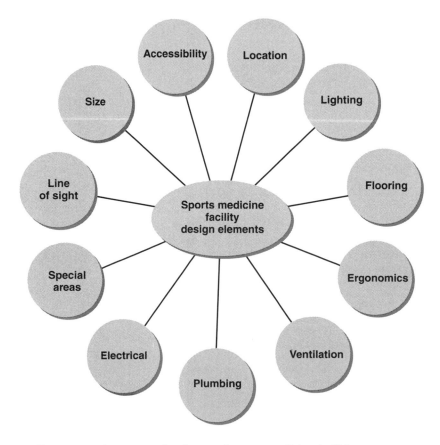

▶ **Figure 5.3** Elements in the design of sports medicine facilities.

health professionals work together daily. Second, placing these two facilities next to each other means that they can share certain operations, often resulting in savings of time or money. For example, if health services and sports medicine services are adjacent, medical records can be stored in a single location (the health service file room). Assuming that procedures protecting student confidentiality are upheld (see chapter 6), medical records are thus more conveniently available and more complete.

Proximity among facilities also enhances the referral process. A student-athlete who reports to the athletic trainer with an illness can be referred immediately to the health service (increasing the likelihood of compliance). Likewise, if a student who is not an athlete comes to the health service with an orthopedic injury, the athletic training staff are readily available for consultation. Perhaps the ultimate argument for this arrangement, however, is financial—costs may decrease because facilities, supplies, and services need not be duplicated. If the health service contains private examination rooms, they don't have to be included in the sports medicine center. The health service and the sports medicine center can share secretarial support as well as certain types of equipment and supplies, such as cast saws and suture kits. Having health services adjacent to the sports medicine center also eliminates the need for athletic trainers to store or dispense medications; health service personnel can more properly handle that function (see chapter 8).

Although this concept generally functions well on small campuses, larger schools might find it difficult to implement because athletic facilities are typically located on the periphery of the campus, whereas student health services are more centrally located. But a combined facility should be considered whenever possible in light of the many advantages.

Ergonomics

Ergonomics is the scientific study of human work. This multidisciplinary field originated when engineers, anatomists, physiologists, psychologists, and health care professionals came together to design optimal working environments for military uses (Reilly 1981). Ergonomics has much wider application today, and many consider it essential in the design of products and work processes and environments, although it has been slow to catch on in health care environments (Scholey and Hair 1989). Pheasant (1991, p. 4) has defined ergonomics as "the science of matching the job to the worker and the product to the user." The purpose of considering ergonomics in the design of a sports medicine center is to enable athletic trainers to work more productively, safely, and comfortably. Athletic trainers do not perform all their work in the sports medicine facility, of course. They perform a variety of tasks requiring a sound ergonomic basis on the field, in the gym, and in the office. Athletic trainers employed in industrial settings are frequently called on to suggest workstation design changes based on ergonomic problems. The discussion here is especially important for industrial settings. Many ergonomic considerations are beyond the scope of this text.

One of the prime tenets of ergonomic design is that people, including athletic trainers, come in different shapes and sizes. Therefore, in a new sports medicine facility, the design should include spaces, furniture, and fixtures that are as adaptable as possible. Pheasant (1991) has identified four errors in design thinking that athletic trainers would do well to avoid as they plan their facilities.

■ Four Ergonomic Errors in Design Thinking

As you plan the design of the sports medicine facility, be sure to keep in mind the following erroneous assumptions about ergonomic elements.

1. This design works for me, so it will work for everyone.
2. This design works well for the average person, so it will work well for everyone.
3. Because people vary so much, we can't worry about designing the facility for everyone—people will just have to adapt.
4. Style and appearance are more important than ergonomic function.

Although other sections of this chapter cover some ergonomic considerations in the design of a sports medicine facility (see the sections on lighting and ventilation, for example), a few ergonomic design issues do not fit neatly into other sections and so are included here.

■ **Tables.** Treatment and taping tables typically come in one height, even though the stature of the athletic trainers using the tables is highly variable. Consider installing taping tables of several different heights. If a taping counter is planned, plan for three sections ranging in height from 32 to 40 inches (81 to 102 centimeters). The ideal treatment table, from an ergonomic standpoint, would be adjustable so that the user could raise or lower it depending on the task to be accomplished (just as a dentist's chair can be raised or lowered depending on the height of the patient and the procedure to be performed).

■ **Shelves and cupboards.** Equipment should be stored on shelves or in cupboards that are easy to reach. It should not be stored on the floor where the athletic trainer will have to stoop to lift it. Some equipment can be hung on pegs fixed to the wall. Step stools should be available near the equipment storage area so that short athletic trainers can access the equipment without having to reach too far overhead.

■ **Stools.** Adjustable-height stools should be available at every treatment station so that athletic trainers can administer treatments in a sitting position if necessary. Adjustable-height stools are especially important when treatment tables are not adjustable, as most are not, and the athletic trainer is tall.

■ **Carts and dollies.** Rolling carts, dollies, and laundry bins should be available so that athletic trainers can move equipment and supplies from one place to another with minimum effort.

■ **Flooring.** The kind of flooring installed in the athletic training facility has ergonomic consequences for both the patients and the staff. The harder the surface, the more difficult it will be for staff to stand for long periods. Floors that have an excessively high or low coefficient of friction will present slipping or tripping hazards.

Electrical Systems

The electrical system is one of the few elements that, if improperly installed, could cause injury or death. Three-pronged hospital-grade plugs and electrical outlets (characterized by a green dot), along with circuit breakers, are useful in preventing damage to electrical equipment; but because electrical shock can cause severe burns or cardiac arrest (see figure 5.4), all electrical outlets in a sports medicine center should also be equipped with a **ground fault interrupter (GFI)**, designed to interrupt the flow of electricity if a surge of 5 milliamps or more is detected (Porter and Porter 1981). Ground fault interrupters can be installed either as part of the electrical outlet or as part of the circuit breaker, and they are required equipment in rooms in public and private buildings where water is present. Some medical and therapeutic durable medical equipment, such as isokinetic machines, may require a different voltage output (220 volts) as compared to the typical 110 volts.

Another issue in electrical design is the location of electrical outlets. Secor (1984) recommends that electrical outlets be spaced every 4 feet (1.2 meters) throughout the facility. This spacing gives the athletic trainer flexibility to move equipment as the program changes. Electrical outlet placement should always consider potential future changes related to space utilization; therefore it is a good idea to design a facility with more outlets than necessary at the time of planning. In general, place electrical outlets at least 3 feet (.9 meters) from the floor to keep power cords off the floor. This placement reduces danger in the event of an accidental spill or flood and allows the athletic trainer to move therapeutic modalities more easily, especially if space between treatment tables is limited. To reduce the probability of overload, a single circuit should service a limited number of modality outlets.

0-8 milliamps = Safe
8-100 milliamps = Painful
100-200 milliamps = Fibrillation
≥200 milliamps = Muscle contraction and tissue burns

▶ **Figure 5.4** Effects of 60-cycle electric current on human tissue.
From Porter and Porter 1981.

The number will depend on the type and number of appliances that will be used simultaneously. Outlets can be placed within a support beam or on the floor if the open space area is too large to permit use of wall-based outlets for equipment that is best located in the center of the open space.

Many sports medicine centers, especially those located in hospitals, have designed treatment stations with pull cords that patients can use to shut off electrical power. This feature is especially useful when patients' electrical stimulation treatments become painful. Rather than wait for the athletic trainer to cross the room to adjust the dosage, the patient can simply pull the cord and stop the flow of electricity to the modality. Athletic trainers can also choose to place remote power switches for hydrotherapy units in their offices to prevent accidental shock. An extension of this concept would be to have a master switch in the athletic trainer's office for every outlet to which a therapeutic modality could be connected for rapid shutoff in case of emergency.

Keep in mind that it is estimated that 30% to 60% of equipment problems are due to operator error (Ritter 1990). All electrical equipment should be carefully checked during setup, and the operator's manual should be reviewed before any service calls are initiated. There are three reasons, however, to immediately remove any equipment from patient use: electrical shock, a burning odor, and smoke coming from a device.

Plumbing Systems

Placement of water outlets and drains is an important consideration in the design of a sports medicine center. A mistake in the design of the plumbing system, which is usually installed inside walls and under floors, is expensive to correct.

Like the electrical system, plumbing systems should be designed to be easily expandable. As a sports medicine program grows and changes, the need for water or drainage in different parts of the facility might change as well. Outlets for both hot and cold water should be provided in every section of the sports medicine facility. Some of these outlets should drain into sinks, and others should be free standing to fill hydrotherapy tubs. Floor drains should be placed at several strategic points around the facility. The floor should be sloped at least 1% toward the drains (Penman 1977).

If the facility is to contain an ice machine, a separate cold water line and floor drain should be provided for it. Whenever possible, the built-in drain of each hydrotherapy tank should connect directly to a dedicated floor drain. The drain faucet of tanks that use a pump drain should be connected to a **standpipe drain** by a hose or similar device to prevent splashing. In every case, a hydrotherapy tank should have an overflow prevention drain.

A plumbing contractor will be able to offer a variety of fixtures. **Plumbing fixtures** used in a sports medicine center can be relatively simple and inexpensive, but athletic trainers might find three exceptions desirable. The first is a **mixing valve**, which allows precise water temperature by combining hot and cold water and eliminates the need for separate controls. Mixing valves often have built-in thermometers and are especially useful for filling hydrotherapy tubs. Another plumbing enhancement athletic trainers might choose is a **foot-pedal activator** for hand-washing stations. These devices are especially useful for athletic trainers who use massage and perform other activities in which the hands are covered with lotions, ointments, or similar products. Finally, the athletic trainer might choose to connect hydrotherapy tanks directly to the water source. The advantage of having a dedicated source of hydrotherapy water is that accidental spills are much easier to prevent. On the other hand, using hoses to fill hydrotherapy tanks provides greater flexibility for each water outlet.

A common mistake is to pay a great deal of attention to designing the plumbing systems and then overlook associated accessories. For instance, built-in liquid soap dispensers next to hand-washing stations are extremely useful. Paper cup dispensers are desirable. The planning team could choose paper towel dispensers and wastepaper containers that are recessed into the wall—they're usually more expensive, but they save space and are more aesthetically pleasing. Finally, a drinking fountain will require a dedicated water line and drain and an electrical outlet so that the water can be chilled.

Planning for installation of plumbing systems should consider areas such as bathrooms, physician examination room, changing and locker rooms, and possible drug-testing rooms or facilities. Each of these types of rooms would require a sink or shower area. Even minor renovations of health care spaces can result in substantial upgrades of mechanical, electrical, and plumbing systems (Kesler and Fagan 2005).

Ventilation Systems

Little has been written about the ventilation of sports medicine facilities. But if a sports medicine center is improperly ventilated, working conditions can become extremely uncomfortable. The two most important ventilation concerns are temperature and humidity control. Penman and Penman (1982) recommend a maximum of 0.75 feet per second draft factor with between 8 and 10 changes of air per hour during peak loads. They recommend a humidity level between 40% and 50%.

A sports medicine center should have its own **thermostat**. A common mistake in designing ventilation systems is to use a common temperature control for the sports medicine center and adjacent areas, such as locker rooms and shower areas. The result is that the sports medicine center is usually too warm to work comfortably in. If the sports medicine center has several rooms, each should probably have a separate thermostat.

The other major ventilation concern is humidity. Excessive humidity is not only a comfort problem but also a hygiene problem. Viruses, fungi, and bacteria survive more easily on moist surfaces than they do on dry ones. Areas where water is used extensively, such as the hydrotherapy section, should be equipped with exhaust fans that are strong enough to keep humidity to reasonable levels. This is especially important if glass walls separate the hydrotherapy section from the rest of the facility because high humidity levels in the hydrotherapy room may lead to fogging of the glass.

Whether or not to provide air-conditioning is an important decision because it is expensive to install and use. In many areas of the United States, however, the temperature and humidity are so extreme at times when the sports medicine center is used most heavily that air-conditioning is essential. Because air-conditioning cools the air by removing moisture, it is an important feature for both comfort and hygiene.

Lighting

Illumination is another important but often overlooked feature in sports medicine center design. How bright should the sports medicine center be? Arnheim and Prentice (1997) recommend that sports medicine centers be illuminated at 30 foot-candles (a unit of illuminance on a surface that is one foot from a point source of one candle) at a height of 4 feet (1.2 meters) above the floor. Other authors have suggested that a sports medicine facility requires illumination of 50 foot-candles 4 feet above the floor (*Planning Facilities* 1979). Common sense dictates that different sections of the sports medicine center have different illumination requirements. Areas devoted to taping, bandaging, and wound care require more lighting than storage or hydrotherapy areas do. The areas designated for physician examination and treatment of injured athletes and other physically active patients probably require the most intense illumination. Floor lamps can supplement lighting in these areas to provide extra illumination for procedures such as wound debridement and suturing.

In addition to artificial lighting, **natural lighting** from either skylights or windows, and light colors on reflective surfaces like ceilings, walls, and floors, can significantly brighten a sports medicine center (figure 5.5). The design of school sports medicine centers has traditionally lacked windows because of concerns about student-athletes' privacy. The sports medicine center, however, is not a locker room. All patients should be dressed properly when entering the facility, and they should be draped appropriately when receiving treatment. With natural lighting supplied by windows, appropriate drapery or blinds must still be considered for the purposes of patient confidentiality of care. In particular, when care is provided during evening hours with lights on inside the facility, outsiders can see into rooms with ease. Even though patients are wearing proper dress, privacy of medical care must be considered.

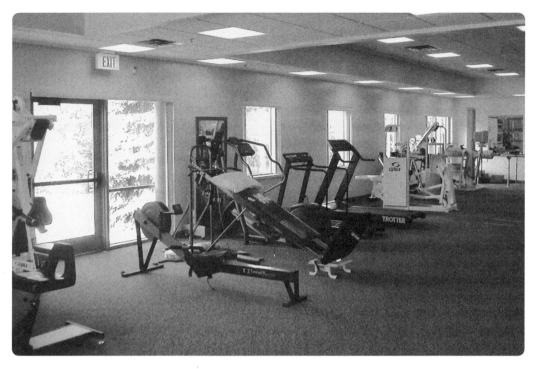

▶ **Figure 5.5** A sports medicine facility that makes good use of natural lighting.

Photo courtesy of Rich Ray.

Specialized Function Areas

Eight specialized function areas are common to most sports medicine facilities: office, taping and bandaging, hydrotherapy, general treatment, rehabilitation, storage, lavatory and changing area, and private examination (see figure 5.6). Many factors determine how much space to devote to each of these functions, including the types and numbers of sports to be served, the number of athletes and other physically active patients to be served, the qualifications and expertise of the sports medicine staff, the operational budget, and the type of client to be served. See figures 5.7 through 5.10 for examples of how to arrange special function areas for different types and sizes of programs.

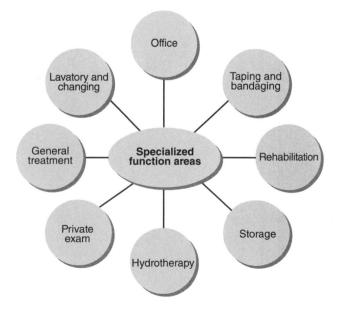

▶ **Figure 5.6** Specialized function areas of the sports medicine center.

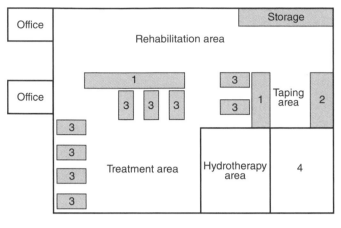

Key
1 Counter
2 Taping bench
3 Treatment tables
4 Therapy pool

▶ **Figure 5.7a** Floor plan for a small college sports medicine facility.

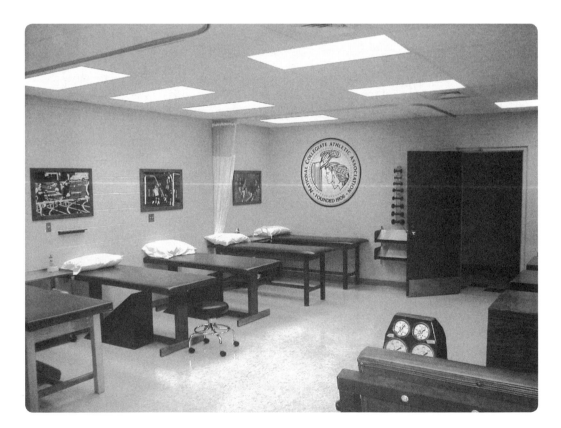

▶ **Figure 5.7b** The treatment area of the small college sports medicine facility shown in the floor plan of figure 5.7a.
Photo courtesy of Rich Ray.

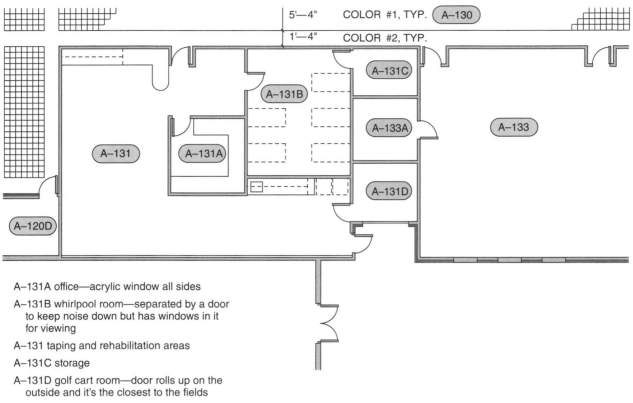

A–131A office—acrylic window all sides

A–131B whirlpool room—separated by a door
to keep noise down but has windows in it
for viewing

A–131 taping and rehabilitation areas

A–131C storage

A–131D golf cart room—door rolls up on the
outside and it's the closest to the fields

A–133A not part of the athletic training room

▶ **Figure 5.8a** Floor plan for a high school sports medicine facility.
Courtesy of Ann Arbor Pioneer High School, Lorin Cartwright.

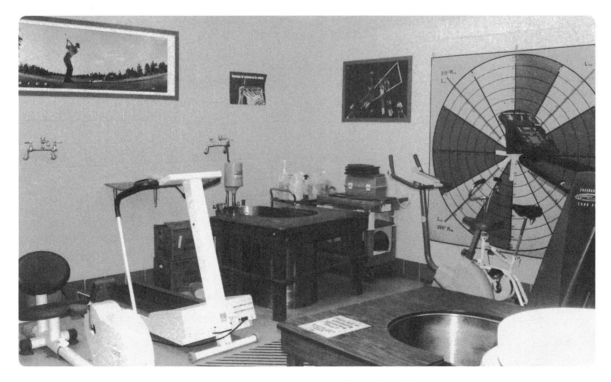

▶ **Figure 5.8b** A view of the sports medicine facility shown in the floor plan of figure 5.8a.
Courtesy of Ann Arbor Pioneer High School, Lorin Cartwright.

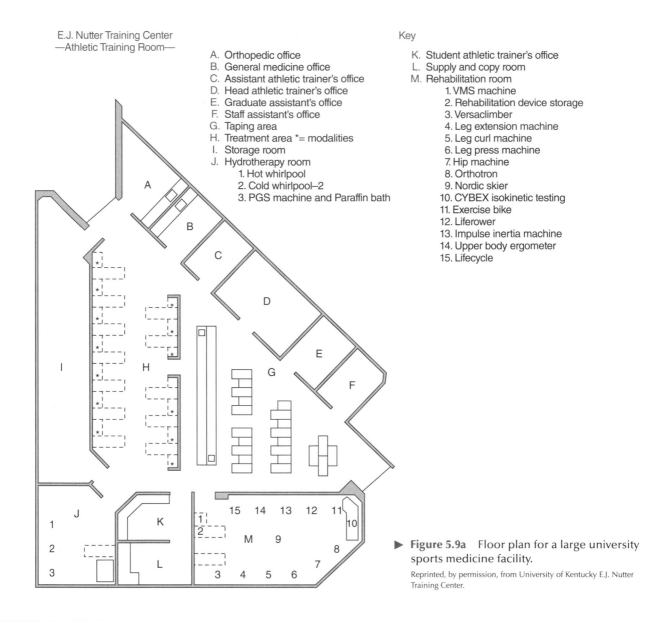

E.J. Nutter Training Center
—Athletic Training Room—

Key

A. Orthopedic office
B. General medicine office
C. Assistant athletic trainer's office
D. Head athletic trainer's office
E. Graduate assistant's office
F. Staff assistant's office
G. Taping area
H. Treatment area *= modalities
I. Storage room
J. Hydrotherapy room
   1. Hot whirlpool
   2. Cold whirlpool–2
   3. PGS machine and Paraffin bath

K. Student athletic trainer's office
L. Supply and copy room
M. Rehabilitation room
   1. VMS machine
   2. Rehabilitation device storage
   3. Versaclimber
   4. Leg extension machine
   5. Leg curl machine
   6. Leg press machine
   7. Hip machine
   8. Orthotron
   9. Nordic skier
   10. CYBEX isokinetic testing
   11. Exercise bike
   12. Liferower
   13. Impulse inertia machine
   14. Upper body ergometer
   15. Lifecycle

▶ **Figure 5.9a** Floor plan for a large university sports medicine facility.

Reprinted, by permission, from University of Kentucky E.J. Nutter Training Center.

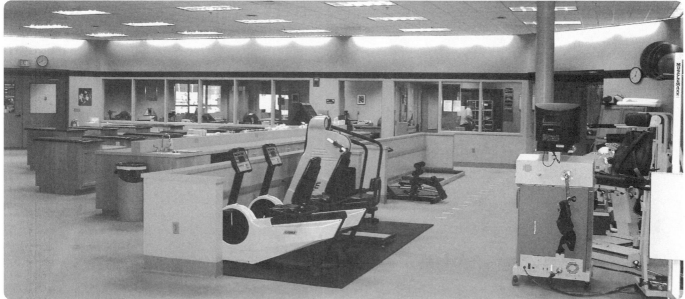

▶ **Figure 5.9b** Rehabilitation and taping areas of the facility shown in figure 5.9a. The offices are in the background.

Reprinted, by permission, from University of Kentucky E.J. Nutter Training Center.

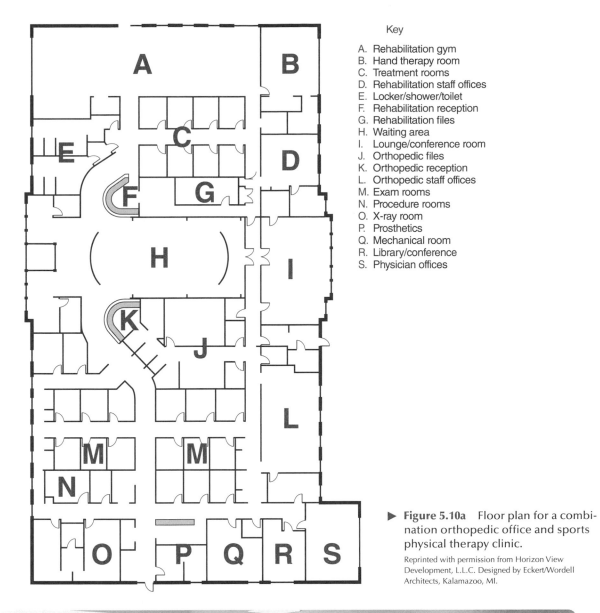

Key

A. Rehabilitation gym
B. Hand therapy room
C. Treatment rooms
D. Rehabilitation staff offices
E. Locker/shower/toilet
F. Rehabilitation reception
G. Rehabilitation files
H. Waiting area
I. Lounge/conference room
J. Orthopedic files
K. Orthopedic reception
L. Orthopedic staff offices
M. Exam rooms
N. Procedure rooms
O. X-ray room
P. Prosthetics
Q. Mechanical room
R. Library/conference
S. Physician offices

▶ **Figure 5.10a** Floor plan for a combination orthopedic office and sports physical therapy clinic.

Reprinted with permission from Horizon View Development, L.L.C. Designed by Eckert/Wordell Architects, Kalamazoo, MI.

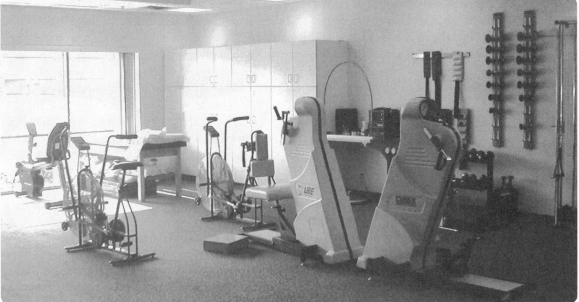

▶ **Figure 5.10b** A section of the rehabilitation gym shown in figure 5.10a.

Photo courtesy of Rich Ray.

Office

In most situations, the athletic trainer's office is located within the sports medicine facility. The athletic trainer's office should serve several purposes. First, it should be the central repository for all program records, including patients' medical files (unless they are kept in an adjacent health service records room as previously discussed), budget information, correspondence, insurance information, product information, and educational materials for students and clients. The athletic trainer's office can also be used for private examinations (although this presents several problems; a separate private examination area is ideal) and counseling if space is limited or unavailable. Finally, the office serves as an administrative work area for the athletic trainer. Adequate office space should be available to accommodate all staff athletic trainers. A common conference area within the office is a useful place for meetings or for students to do their work.

Several design features are important for the athletic trainer's office. First, the athletic trainer should have a clear view of the entire sports medicine facility from the office; windows should allow supervision of activities at all times. If the office must also serve as a private examination and consultation room, it must be equipped with an exam table and blinds for the windows. Obviously, the office should contain a desk, filing cabinets, bookshelves, and a telephone with a line that callers can access without having to go through a building switchboard operator, who might not be on duty after normal business hours. Another useful feature is an extra telephone line for data transfers from a computer. In institutions with networked computer operations, a **data port** should be included as well. The office should also have enough comfortable seating to accommodate several people at one time for those occasions when the athletic trainer must consult with patients, parents, coaches, physicians, and others in groups.

Taping and Bandaging

In school-based sports medicine centers, the taping and bandaging section is often one of the busiest, especially just before practices and games. For this reason, athletic trainers designing school sports medicine centers should carefully consider the location and space devoted to this function. Private and hospital-based sports medicine clinics generally perform much less taping and bandaging, so the area they devote to these needs is usually minimal.

Several design elements are important for a functional taping and bandaging area. First, it must include an adequate number of taping stations. Taping stations can be individual tables or large platforms designed to accommodate several people at one time (Cady 1979). Whichever arrangement is chosen, the taping table should be a minimum of 36 inches (91 centimeters) high, although some athletic trainers will be better served by taping tables that are taller.

Another important design element of the taping and bandaging area is adequate counter space. The counter should have an easily cleaned surface like Formica, should be large enough to allow easy access for all athletic trainers working in the area, and should have electrical outlets every 4 feet (1.2 meters). Although the traditional placement of the counter is along a wall, an attractive alternative is an island counter in the middle of the taping and bandaging area—the island provides taping stations on both sides, allowing easy access for twice as many athletic trainers. The taping and bandaging area should include cupboards and drawers with locks for secure short-term storage of supplies needed routinely. One way to save space in the taping and bandaging section is to combine taping stations with cupboards (Ribaric 1980).

Finally, the type of floor covering to use in the taping and bandaging area can be a difficult problem. Both adhesive sprays and petroleum-based ointments can permanently stain carpeting and vinyl tile. For that reason, it might be wise to contract with a company that provides carpet runners for doorways and entrances. When the runners become soiled, the company will replace them with clean ones.

Hydrotherapy

The hydrotherapy section of the sports medicine center is the one specialized function area that should be physically separated because of water spills and the noisy turbines used to power whirlpool baths. The ideal design would include a glass enclosure around the area, which will contain noise, heat, humidity, and accidental spilling or flooding while allowing the athletic trainer to monitor the activities from another section of the facility.

Besides the sloped floor and expandable plumbing mentioned earlier, athletic trainers should consider other important features when planning the hydrotherapy area. Adequate space should be available for all equipment that uses water, including hydrotherapy tanks, steam pack units, ice machines, freezers, and paraffin baths. In school sports medicine centers, water coolers and portable ice chests are usually stored here as well. Although expensive to construct, operate, and maintain, multistation submersed whirlpools and two-lane training pools can be included in hydrotherapy areas. If so, plans must also include filtration units and water heaters. Ceramic tile similar to what would be found in a shower room or toilet area should cover the floor of the hydrotherapy area. The walls can be constructed from cinder block if they are painted with a high-gloss epoxy paint that can be easily cleaned. From the outset, budgeting for hydrotherapy areas should consider fees for ongoing daily and long-term maintenance of the equipment being planned. In the absence of adequate budgeting for required maintenance, athletic trainers will need to modify their annual sports medicine program budgets to offset the costs incurred by the hydrotherapy equipment.

General Treatment

The general treatment area usually contains a number of treatment tables and any electrotherapeutic equipment and is therefore one of the largest space commitments. You can calculate a square footage estimate for this area by determining the peak caseload at the busiest time of the day and estimating the number of treatment tables necessary to accommodate these patients simultaneously.

Allow approximately 30 inches (76 centimeters) between tables for placing three-shelved carts with therapeutic modalities. Place an electrical outlet next to each treatment table. Provide a fluorescent light immediately above each table, each with its own light switch. Make sure that at least some of the treatment tables have sliding drapes for privacy during treatment. Some treatment tables should be adjustable for elevation of swollen extremities. Treatment tables can double as storage cabinets if you fit them with cupboards, drawers, or shelves.

Materials for walls and floor coverings for this area should be light colored and easy to clean. Vinyl tile works well for this purpose, but it is slippery when wet. Carpet is difficult to clean but provides a warmer, quieter atmosphere (see previous discussion of flooring ergonomics).

Rehabilitation

In most athletic training settings, the rehabilitation area is another section that requires a great deal of space; it might take up most of the space in private and hospital sports medicine clinics. A few commonly used pieces of equipment to rehabilitate injured physically active patients—isokinetic equipment, treatment and exercise tables, treadmills, upper and lower extremity ergometers, stair climbers, and isotonic weight machines—can easily fill a large area. In addition to the space for the equipment, adequate space must exist between exercise stations for safety purposes.

The location of the rehabilitation section is somewhat controversial. Most athletic trainers agree that it should not occupy the same space as the treatment or taping functions. Many athletic trainers have moved the rehabilitation function to a general-purpose weight training facility. Although this has some advantages, exposing unsupervised patients to expensive and potentially harmful devices is probably unwise. The best arrangement gives the rehabilitation area its own room within the confines of the sports medicine center, especially if the institution's weight training facility is nearby in the same building. This scheme allows for careful, supervised rehabilitation of injured physically active patients while maintaining a quiet atmosphere in the general treatment area. When these patients are ready to advance to heavier weights and general-purpose strengthening devices, they can go to the weight room.

Walls should be constructed of a material that allows insertion of hooks and screws, as it is possible to store many rehabilitation tools by hanging them on the wall. A full-length mirror is also useful to give patients visual feedback when they are performing rehabilitation exercises. Ceiling height of the facility should always be considered in the early phases of planning based on the intent of the space utilization. If the area will also encompass functional rehabilitation and sport-specific types of activities, a higher ceiling should be considered.

Flooring

In the athletic trainer's office, a carpeted floor covering usually is the most appropriate type of surface. Likewise, the best alternative for floor coverings in the rehabilitation center is probably carpeting. The largest part of the rehabilitation area might consist of nothing but carpeted floor space to allow for a variety of functional and closed kinetic chain rehabilitation activities. If patients use dumbbells or other free weights, a carpeted floor will absorb the shock and noise more effectively when equipment is dropped. Specially designed rubber-matted flooring pieces can also be used when a large amount of wear and tear is expected in an area that may involve, for example, free weights or jumping-type activities. Nowadays it is not uncommon for sports medicine facilities to also incorporate a functional field or artificial turf area in an effort to simulate weight-bearing activities on a return-to-play surface. If the rehabilitation room is located anywhere other than the ground floor, the architect might need to reinforce the floor to support heavy equipment.

Storage

The storage section of the sports medicine center is commonly overlooked; many administrators may see this large, empty space as a waste of money to build, but it is an important space for the storage of everyday items and one that should be included. Given the cost, several important considerations apply to storage rooms. The storage room should be located within the sports medicine center itself if possible. In addition, the closer the storage room is to the taping and bandaging section, the more convenient it will be for the athletic trainer to restock depleted expendable supplies. The storage room must be cool and dry at all times. Many expendable supplies commonly used in sports medicine, especially adhesive tape, deteriorate in warm, humid environments. Obviously, the storage room should have plenty of shelves and cupboards. To maximize storage space utilization, shelving should be placed as high toward the ceiling as possible; a ladder will enable access to lesser-used items. Access to the storage room should be strictly controlled to prevent unauthorized removal of supplies. Additionally, it is important to consider any pharmaceutical requirements that must be met by the storage room. Storage rooms need to provide a secure environment for both prescription and nonprescription medications that are housed for athletes and patients.

Lavatory and Changing Area

Although many older athletic training facilities lack a lavatory and changing area, this highly desirable design feature is commonly included in newer facilities. This area can be designed to serve both the athletic training staff and the patients who use the sports medicine facility. It should include a handicapped-accessible toilet and sink, along with a shower and lockers. The area should have a shelf for storing towels and a bin for disposal of soiled laundry. In some programs, this area may also be used during drug-testing procedures.

Private Examination

Many situations in sports medicine call for private examination of an injured client to preserve modesty or provide a calm environment. Although the private examination area of the sports medicine center does not need to be large, it should provide a comfortable environment for the client and the athletic trainer or physician. Private examination rooms should include an examination table, a mobile lamp, a sink for washing hands, and a counter and cupboards to hold commonly needed supplies. Any supplies or equipment that the team physician frequently uses should be readily available in the private examination room, as should gowns and drapes for clients. As already mentioned, the private examination room can be combined with the office if necessary.

Accessibility

Title III of the Americans with Disabilities Act of 1990 (ADA) "prohibits discrimination on the basis of disability by public accommodations and requires places of public accommodation and commercial facilities to be designed, constructed, and altered in compliance with the accessibility standards." The law applies to virtually every kind of facility, including public and private educational institutions, health care facilities, and other places of business. The ADA applies not only to new buildings but also to existing facilities, which must be altered to provide access to persons with disabilities except where such alterations would be structurally impractical (Bureau of National Affairs 1990; Parmet 1993). Common design elements that help ensure accessibility include ramps, special parking spaces, railings, modified door handles and automatic opening devices, elevators, lowered drinking fountains, and toilet stalls wide enough to accommodate a wheelchair. Architects, construction managers, facility designers, and building code officials all have training in the elements of ADA compliance. Working with a well-qualified architect who is sensitive to the needs of persons with disabilities is the best way to ensure that the sports medicine facility will be able to serve a broad range of patients.

Marketing a Sports Medicine Facility and Practice

As a provider of health care services, the sports medicine program and its facility should be a recognized operation of high quality, appearance, and reputation. In a not-for-profit environment, such as most secondary schools, colleges, universities, and professional team settings, obtaining such status is often achieved simply through quality of care and interpersonal skills. The reason is that the practitioners already have a customer base that intends to utilize their service, which is mostly free (excluding auxiliary consultations and services), is easily accessible, and is offered for the sole purpose of providing care for the athletes. The circumstances are entirely different in a for-profit type program such as a private practice sports medicine center. When your fiscal survival relies on a business model for remuneration for services, you must successfully recruit a clientele base and provide a level of care and services that have all of the hallmarks of a thriving operation. One of the main tasks in operating a successful for-profit sports medicine program is planning and implementing a marketing strategy. Clover (1997) has outlined the following 11 critical elements that encompass a marketing strategy:

1. **Name.** As previously discussed, the name of a business is very important. Some names will be easier than others to market. For example, naming a facility using the owner's last name, such as "Smith's Sports Medicine Center" may make it easy to remember. However, if the owner's last name is difficult to pronounce or remember, it may not be as easy to market. Catchy logos, slogans, and colors are all part of the naming process that should be considered from a marketing perspective. Names should always be protected through copyright and trademark procedures.

2. **The strategic planning team.** It is always helpful to gather the assistance of stakeholders who can offer objective viewpoints. Those developing a marketing plan should consider including individuals who are viewed as stakeholders at various levels of the organization, though not all necessarily need to be employed by the business. Aside from clinicians employed by the business, area athletic directors, referring physicians, and others who are familiar with either the community or health care in general can offer significant support to your effort to achieve success.

3. The decision-making team. The decision-making team comprises a few key individuals who have the ability to extrapolate all of the input of a marketing plan and turn it into a long-term vision that can be implemented in a practical and cost-effective manner. If a decision-making team is too large, they may find it difficult to agree on a final plan.

4. Environmental assessment. An environmental assessment looks at both internal and external factors related to the marketing plan. Internal environmental factors include the organization's strengths and weaknesses, the types of services provided, staff skill sets, the geographical location of the business, financial status, and staff morale. External environmental factors are those controlled by persons and forces outside of an organization. These may include, but are certainly not limited to, consumer needs, competitors' strengths and weaknesses, third-party payer influences, referral patterns, and population and commercial business growth within the surrounding community.

■ Ideas and Techniques to Promote and Advertise the Clinic

- Brochures
- Newsletter (some type of return information is very important to evaluate the readership of the newsletter)
- Educational pamphlets (e.g., what to do for a sprained ankle, how to access your medical group given the type of insurance one has)
- Direct mail (e.g., special educational programs coming up)
- Media exposure (e.g., well-written news releases about what the clinic is doing)
- Presentations to clients (e.g., physicians, coaches)
- Exhibits (e.g., health fairs, road races)
- Special service events (e.g., chamber of commerce, Junior League)
- Speaker's bureau (e.g., available to speak on sports medicine-related topics)
- Public education forums (e.g., bring in athletic trainers in the area and go over face mask removal using the Trainer's Angel, do a series on injury prevention for different sports, present a taping clinic)
- Phone book (advertisement should stand out on a crowded page and be found in all related parts of the phone book)
- Advertising for program/magazine/newspapers (e.g., information, return request)
- Television (e.g., cable)
- Radio (e.g., spot advertisement: "Snow report brought to you by . . .")
- Signs—where and what type (e.g., ball parks)
- Education (e.g., high school, adult learning, college, first aid training)
- Sponsorship of teams, individuals, athletic events (watch for proper exposure)
- Participate in athletic events (e.g., corporate challenge, road races)
- Establish a tradition (e.g., all-star football game, scholarship)
- Vehicle advertising (e.g., signs on a company van)
- Receptions for physicians
- Barbecues for coaches
- Equipment demonstrations (e.g., different types of knee braces, different types of shoulder pads)
- Member in athletic organizations (e.g., sports medicine consultant)
- Member of local athletic groups (e.g., Chamber of Commerce, athletic council)

Strengths and Weaknesses of Advertisement and Promotional Approaches

TELEVISION (PUBLIC OR CABLE)

Strengths

- High impact
- Audience selectivity
- Schedule when needed
- Fast awareness
- Sponsorship available
- Merchandising possible
- Must be local

Weaknesses

- High production cost
- Uneven delivery by market
- Upfront commitment required
- If not a local station, may have no impact on area

RADIO

Strength

- Low cost per contact
- Audience selectivity
- Schedule when needed
- Length can vary
- Personalities available

Weaknesses

- Nonintrusive medium
- Audience per spot small
- No visual impact
- High total cost for good reach

MAGAZINES

Strengths

- Audience selectivity
- Editorial association
- Long life
- Large audience per insert
- Excellent color
- Minimal waste
- Merchandising possible

Weaknesses

- Long lead time needed
- Readership accumulates slowly
- Uneven delivery by market
- Cost premiums for regional or demographic editions

NEWSPAPER

Strengths

- Large audience
- Immediate reach
- Short lead time
- Market flexibility
- Good upscale coverage
- Information advertising

Weaknesses

- Difficult to target
- High waste
- High cost for national use
- Minimal positioning
- Clutter

POSTERS, BILLBOARDS

Strengths

- High reach
- High frequency of exposure
- Minimal waste
- Can localize
- Flexible scheduling

Weaknesses

- No depth of message
- High cost for national use
- Best positions already taken
- No audience selectivity
- Minimum one-month purchase

Reprinted from J. Konin, *Clinical Athletic Training*, 1997, Slack Inc. Table 10-4, page 117. "Strengths and Weaknesses of Advertisement and Promotional Approaches."

5. Market segmentation. The total number of people in a surrounding area is not a good overall indicator of potential business. Instead, a marketing plan should be able to identify various segments of the population that need services and match the services offered to those in need. Specializing in youth sport injuries in a predominantly retirement-based community may not bode well for a business. Market segmentation is essentially about supply and demand.

6. Objectives, strategies, and goals. Establishing goals and objectives enables formulation of a process for the organization or business to follow in an effort to measure success. For a sports medicine marketing program, objectives that can be measured in terms of a time line, as well as quantitative and qualitative perspectives, are best suited to decision making.

7. The marketing mix. The marketing mix is the fun part of the plan. However, if it is not taken seriously and carefully thought out, it can turn into an overhead expense with no return on investment. Marketing mix involves using products or gadgets to promote your sports medicine practice. There is much more to it than placing a logo on a T-shirt to promote a business. Price assessment, product durability and usage, locations, and forms of promotional advertising are all included in the marketing mix. The sidebars on pages 180 and 181 list promotional ideas along with their strengths and weaknesses.

8. Positioning. Positioning is a simple yet daunting process designed to create a certain type of image or reputation. Positioning involves including all thoughts at all times for the purpose of defining an end product that will be implemented within the overall marketing plan.

9. Patient relations. Patient relations is an ongoing process that involves more than good interpersonal exchanges with patients. Additional actions that have an effect on positive patient relations include timely responses to physician inquiries, a flexible schedule for patients, objective responses to complaints or concerns, and maintenance of short waiting room times.

10. Finalization of plan and review. Prior to the implementation of a marketing plan, the entire plan and its objectives should be reviewed with all stakeholders. This is important to ensure that everyone involved has a clear understanding of the investment and expected return.

11. Evaluation. Periodic evaluation of the marketing plan should be performed and tracked to determine how all parts of the plan are working. Changes can be made if necessary based on findings from the evaluation that would have an effect on the plan as a whole.

APPLICATIONS TO ATHLETIC TRAINING: THEORY INTO PRACTICE

Use the following three case studies to help you apply the concepts in this chapter to real-life situations. The questions at the end of the studies have many possible correct solutions. The case studies can be used in class discussion or for homework or test questions.

Case Study 1

Deanna Walsh is the athletic trainer for a large Wisconsin high school that offers 20 sports for 750 student-athletes. The voters of the school district recently approved a bond issue to build a new $30 million high school. The planning committee asked Deanna to meet with the architect to discuss her ideas for the new athletic training room. Before the meeting, Deanna carefully considered the features she wanted to see incorporated into the new facility. She drew a sketch of the layout she desired and made a list of all the design features she wanted, including

- total size of 2,500 square feet;
- separate but connected rooms for taping, treatment, rehabilitation, office, storage, and private examination;
- a hanging ceiling with acoustical tiles to reduce noise;
- one treatment and taping table for every 10 athletes she would have to service during peak service hours;
- floor coverings of vinyl tile (for the taping, treatment, and storage areas), ceramic tile (for the hydrotherapy area), and carpeting (for the office and private examination room); and
- air-conditioning, with separate thermostats for each of the six rooms.

After considering Deanna's suggestions and attempting to incorporate them into the overall design of the athletic and physical education portion of the building, the architect informed her that the new sports medicine center was too expensive as proposed and that they would have to reduce its cost by one-third.

QUESTIONS FOR ANALYSIS

1. Did Deanna employ the proper planning process when developing her ideas for the new athletic training room? What should she have done differently? How could she build a stronger case for her ideas?

2. What additional features should Deanna include in her list? How can she justify these features?

3. Which features should Deanna modify or eliminate to meet the architect's requirement?

4. Place yourself in Deanna's position and produce your own schematic drawing of the athletic training room you would propose for the new high school. Justify each of the features that you would include.

Case Study 2

Russ Emmons, ATC/PT, operates a successful seven-year-old physical therapy and sports medicine practice. His caseload nearly doubled when three new orthopedic surgeons moved into town a couple of years ago. When the local high school proposed a contractual relationship in which Russ would provide athletic training services for a fee plus referrals, he decided the time had come to expand out of his rented, cramped facility into his own building. Russ consulted a friend who had recently built an auto parts store for advice about hiring an architect. "I know just the architect you want," his friend told him. "He did a great job for me and I'm sure you'll like him." Russ decided to take his friend's advice, and he made an appointment to see the architect. When they met a couple of weeks later, Russ was pleased with his friend's advice. The architect listened carefully to Russ' ideas and offered many helpful suggestions that Russ had not considered. Toward the end of the meeting Russ asked the architect how he should go about locating a contractor to build the new clinic. "You wouldn't necessarily have to find anyone," the architect replied. "My firm could coordinate the construction internally. You'd only have to deal with one person, and we could probably speed the whole construction process up quite a bit." Russ decided he liked the idea, and several weeks later, after reviewing the project with his attorney and a loan officer from the bank, he signed a design-build contract with the architect's firm.

QUESTIONS FOR ANALYSIS

1. What advantages will Russ have in owning his building? What disadvantages?

2. Did Russ make any mistakes in hiring an architect? What could he have done to avoid those mistakes?

3. Russ chose to use the design-build model for developing his new building. Was this a wise decision? What kinds of problems is he likely to encounter? What advantages will he realize?

4. What factors should Russ consider in the location of his new practice?

Case Study 3

Following just the first month at your new job at Ramo Sports Medicine Clinic, the owner, Mr. Ramo, has asked you to lead a team of employees to develop a new and innovative comprehensive marketing plan. The major goal is to take advantage of the skills and expertise of the staff clinicians and increase the number of clients who would seek Ramo Sports Medicine Clinic for rehabilitation. All of the clinicians have an interest in manual therapy skills and injury prevention methods.

Mr. Ramo has annually attempted to reignite his staff's enthusiasm toward marketing efforts. However, he believes that the majority of them have a greater interest in simply treating patients, and that they feel the business side of marketing the clinic is not their responsibility. Knowing this, your task is to propose a plan that is inclusive of the staff yet isn't entirely reliant on their efforts.

While Mr. Ramo is not paying you any additional money for your role of coordinating the marketing plan, he has agreed to release you from 5 hours per week of treating patients. He has not informed you of any budget limitations; all he said was that he wanted you to keep the overhead costs within reason and create a financial plan that would demonstrate how your return on investment will cover all of the marketing costs.

QUESTIONS FOR ANALYSIS

1. What challenges will you have marketing the name of the clinic? With respect to positioning, what type of information would you need to gather before making any suggestions regarding how the clinic should be portrayed by the community?

2. How would you plan to incorporate the ideas and input of the current staff?

3. Which key stakeholders within the community should you consider using in an advising capacity?

4. If Mr. Ramo informs you during your planning process that he has decided to allot you a total of $10,000 for marketing expenses, which can be spent over the course of a six-month period, in what ways do you think it would be best to promote the clinic?

5. Based on your choices for promoting the clinic, what methods would you put into place to measure the success or failure of the marketing efforts?

SUMMARY

Athletic trainers work in a variety of settings that often are already in place when they begin employment. However, it is not uncommon for an athletic trainer to be involved in the planning of a new facility or the renovation of an existing sports medicine center or space. The most effective sports medicine facility is one that has undergone comprehensive planning prior to any building and development. The process of planning includes, but is not limited to, design elements such as spacing, lighting, and accessibility. It is important to consider optimal function in terms of the traffic that will characterize the facility and the usage of equipment. Planning, designing, and constructing a sports medicine center will involve the collaboration of internal and external stakeholders and contractors, as well as financial planning. Once a sports medicine center is built and ready for use, key factors in promoting and marketing the facility will be considered.

KEY CONCEPTS AND REVIEW

1. Understand and defend the importance of the design phase in planning and constructing new sports medicine facilities.

The design and construction of new sports medicine facilities is a task that athletic trainers carry out infrequently but is expensive and important. It is at the design stage of such projects that athletic trainers can exert the greatest influence over the final product. Mistakes during the design phase will increase the facility's cost or decrease its function.

2. Understand the facility design and construction process in sports medicine settings.

Most athletic trainers will work with planning committees consisting of program specialists and high-level administrators to design a sports medicine center. The design process involves 10 steps: assessing needs, approving the project, selecting a construction model, selecting an architect, developing schematic drawings, securing funding, bidding the construction, analyzing bids and reacting to them, commencing construction, and monitoring construction.

3. Understand the common design elements of a well-planned sports medicine facility.

Nine factors must be considered in the design of a sports medicine center: size, location, ergonomics, electrical systems, plumbing systems, ventilation systems, lighting, specialized function areas, and accessibility.

4. Describe the sports medicine facility in terms of its specialized function areas.

The specialized function areas of most sports medicine facilities include an office; areas for taping and bandaging, rehabilitation, general treatment, hydrotherapy, storage, and lavatory and changing; and a room for private examination of patients.

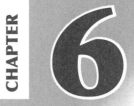

CHAPTER 6

Information Management

OBJECTIVES

After reading this chapter, you should be able to do the following:

1. Understand the importance of documentation as part of a complete information management system in sports medicine.

2. Understand and describe the different methods of athletic injury and treatment documentation.

3. Understand and describe the different types of information to be managed in a typical sports medicine program.

▶ Karen Thompson is the certified athletic trainer at Central City High School, besides having a three-fifths appointment as a physical education and biology teacher. Two months ago she requested a computer for the school's athletic training room as part of a large grant proposal by the school district titled "Computers Across the Curriculum." She hoped that a computer would help her with record keeping. Because she is the only athletic trainer at the school and has to spend most of her time taking care of injured student-athletes, she usually has to bring paperwork home in the evening to keep up.

One day in September, after teaching her classes, Karen saw several large boxes on a treatment table in the athletic training room. Her computer had arrived! Because student-athletes were already starting to line up for taping and treatment, Karen moved the boxes to the corner of the room that doubled as her office. "Now that I finally have the equipment," she told herself, "I can start to think about how I can use it to improve our record-keeping system."

A week later the boxes were still there. When Karen called the school district's business manager to inquire about setup and training, he informed her that the grant covered only the equipment. He suggested that she consult with her colleagues if she had questions or problems. Karen was familiar with most common computer uses but didn't have any experience with the kind of database that she wanted to use to manage her injury and treatment records. She then realized that she had many hours of trial and error ahead of her.

*The newest computer can only compound, at speed,
the oldest problem in the relations between human beings,
and in the end the communicator will be confronted
with the old problem of what to say and how to say it.*

—EDWARD R. MURROW

Like many athletic trainers, Karen Thompson perceives her primary mission as providing high-quality health care to injured student-athletes. She is frustrated not because she must meticulously document the care she administers, but because she believes that an excessive shift has occurred away from patient care to documentation for its own sake. Her view of the computer as a solution to her information management problems, whether valid or not, is common.

This chapter provides athletic trainers with the basics about information management in the athletic health care setting. We are working in an information society. The 2000 census revealed that over 40 million workers performed jobs that involve accumulating and transferring information. Athletic trainers will increasingly be expected to be effective managers of information.

As health care professionals, we do not have the luxury of deciding whether or not we will manage information. The question is not "Will I choose to manage information and communicate effectively?" but rather "What skills and tools do I need to manage information and communicate effectively?" For many reasons, athletic trainers are expected to document every patient care activity and the response to it. Athletic trainers must gather and disseminate the information necessary to accomplish a number of goals, including improvement of patient care, professional development, and improvement in education and counseling. Finally, athletic trainers are increasingly expected to be competent leaders of the sports medicine programs in their institutions. Athletic trainers who lack the information management skills to assume these leadership positions will quickly become frustrated. Their jobs, like Karen Thompson's, are likely to be characterized more by problems than by creative solutions.

To learn more about population demographics in the United States, visit the U.S. Census Bureau website at www.census.gov.

WHY DOCUMENT?

Although documentation is only one of the information management tasks that athletic trainers must accomplish, it is common to all employment settings. Why is this skill so important? Why should busy athletic trainers concern themselves as much as they do with this task? There are many reasons.

- **Legal protection.** Medical documentation helps protect the legal rights of both the physically active patient and the athletic trainer by providing a written record of the care that the athletic trainer provided. Medical records are often the only defense that athletic trainers have when aggrieved patients take legal action. The adage "If it isn't written down, it didn't happen" is an increasingly appropriate guiding principle for all athletic trainers (Hawkins 1989; Panettieri 2000).

- **Memory aid.** Medical documentation acts as a memory aid for athletic trainers and other professionals involved in the care of injured athletes and other physically active patients. Human memory is a poor substitute for accurate recording of medical facts, especially because a patient's medical record might not need to be referred to for months or even years.

- **Legal requirements.** In many cases, the law requires medical documentation. For example, athletic trainers in professional sports are required to document player injuries for the Occupational Safety and Health Administration (OSHA). Athletic trainers in various practice settings might be required to provide medical documentation for legally mandated workers' compensation insurance.

- **Professional standards.** Medical documentation is required to meet professional **standards of practice**. The Board of Certification (BOC) *Standards of Professional Practice* requires documentation of physician referral, initial evaluation and assessment, treatments, and dates of follow-up care for all athletes cared for in a *service program* typical of most educational settings. The requirements for athletic trainers working in *direct service programs,* typically in sports medicine clinics, are more rigorous. Besides meeting the service program standards, an athletic trainer in this setting must provide a program plan with estimated length, methods, results, revisions, and a discontinuation or discharge assessment and summary. Other professional organizations have different documentation standards. For example, the Joint Commission on Accreditation of Healthcare Organizations (JCAHO) publishes minimum standards for health care documentation that apply to athletic trainers who work in hospitals and similar health care institutions (Marrelli 1992).

- **Improved communication.** Medical documentation improves the quality of communication among the various professionals involved with the physically active patient's case (Kettenbach 1995). Often, the only communication an athletic trainer has with the team or family physician is in writing. If the quality of the documentation is poor, either in content or in writing style, misunderstandings can result between athletic trainer and physician.

- **Insurance requirements.** Reimbursement decisions by third-party payers, such as insurance companies and health maintenance organizations, are based on medical documentation. This rationale is especially relevant for private or hospital-based sports medicine clinics, but it can also be important in professional, high school, and college sports medicine programs.

- **Discharge decisions.** Medical documentation should be part of the basis for deciding when to discharge a patient from an athletic trainer's care (Kettenbach 1995). The medical record should act as a map to guide a reader unfamiliar with the case through the entire injury, treatment, and rehabilitation process. The reader, whether a physician, athletic trainer, or physical therapist, should be able to determine by reading the record whether the patient is ready to be discharged.

- **Improved care.** When properly organized, medical documentation helps direct the athletic trainer to deliver better care. Well-written and well-organized medical documentation should serve as a tool for problem solving in difficult cases (Makoul et al. 2001).

Effective documentation of athletic training interventions serves at least 10 purposes: legal protection, memory aid, legal requirements, professional standards, improved communication, insurance requirements, discharge decisions, improved care, injury surveillance, and outcomes assessment.

For the complete text of the BOC *Standards of Professional Practice,* visit www.bocatc.org. For the JCAHO standards related to documentation, visit www.jcaho.org.

■ **Injury surveillance.** Thorough documentation allows an athletic trainer to review medical records and tally findings as they relate to the types of injuries reported, sports associated with more injuries, body parts injured most, and many other aspects pertaining to trends of injury incidence and intervention.

■ **Outcomes assessment.** As discussed in chapter 2, the formal assessment of outcomes plays a critical role in determining one's effectiveness. Effective documentation can be designed to serve as a vehicle for assessing the interventions by athletic trainers, including the effectiveness of sports safety equipment (Hrysomallis and Morrison 1997).

Medical documentation forms the raw material for program quality assessment. An athletic trainer should set both short- and long-term goals for the care of every injured patient. If the medical record shows care inconsistent with these goals, athletic trainers should be concerned that injured athletes and other physically active patients are being discharged without receiving all the care they need to function competitively.

TWO KINDS OF INFORMATION

Athletic trainers must differentiate between medical records and program administration records. The two types of records are separate entities, and with a few exceptions little overlap should occur between them.

Medical Records

A patient's medical record is a written outline of his health history during the time he was under an athletic trainer's care. **Medical records** are patient specific, and only data that relate directly to the patient's health should be included. Information not related to health, such as news clippings or academic information, has no place in the medical record and should be stored elsewhere. Marrelli (1992, pp. 11-12) recommends the following guidelines:

- Write legibly or print neatly. The record must be readable.
- Use permanent ink (appropriate ink color depends on hospital policy).
- For every entry, identify the time and date, sign it, and provide your title.
- Describe the care provided and the patient's response.
- Describe findings objectively (that is, in terms of behaviors).
- Write entries in consecutive and chronological order with no skipped lines or gaps.
- Write entries as soon as possible after care is provided.
- Be factual and specific.
- Use patient (or family or caregiver) quotes.
- Document patient complaints or needs and their resolution.
- Write out what you are saying, avoiding potentially confusing abbreviations.
- Chart only the care that you provided.
- Promptly document a change in the patient's condition and the actions taken based on that change.
- Write the patient's, family's, or caregiver's response to teaching.

Finally, Schneller and Godwin (1983) recommend that you not erase errors. Instead, draw a line through the error, enter the proper information next to the error, and date and initial the correction.

Where and how should medical records be stored? The answer, of course, depends on the environment in which the sports medicine program operates. Two principles are fundamental. First, the athletic trainer must be able to access medical records easily at the time they are most needed—when the injured athlete or physically active patient is present in the sports medicine facility. The second principle is that records storage should be centralized to the greatest extent possible so that all those with a need to access the records are able to do so. These two principles can be difficult to reconcile in certain environments. For example, a university sports medicine program might operate several facilities on a campus covering a large geographic area. Similarly, a hospital-owned satellite sports medicine clinic might be part of a larger rehabilitation services department but be physically located many miles from the hospital. How can a university athletic trainer working in an arena have immediate access to a basketball player's medical record when the files are maintained in the central athletic training room in the stadium? How can an athletic trainer in a sports medicine clinic access her patient's records when they are maintained in the central records depository of the hospital 5 miles across town? Regardless of how these challenges are overcome, privacy of information should always be considered and medical records should be stored securely.

Solutions to these dilemmas exist. One option for centralized records maintenance in decentralized sports medicine settings is the use of carbonless forms. With this system, one copy of every part of the patient's record is maintained in the facility where that patient's needs are primarily served. Another copy is included in an identical file in the central records storage facility. The advantage to this system is that it is relatively easy to maintain. The disadvantage is that each entry into the patient's record must be filed at least twice, thus increasing clerical time and costs.

Another option for centralization of medical records in decentralized settings is the use of electronic record keeping (Ray 1997). Files are maintained in a computer database that anyone with authorization can access from computers linked to the central computer network. Entries into the record are made in one of three ways. Some entries are dictated directly into the system through telephone links or by voice recognition software from one of the computers linked to the records network. Other entries can be made into existing electronic forms built into the computer database. Finally, records that do not lend themselves to either of these methods, such as communications from physicians, can be scanned into the medical record. The advantage of this system is that authorized users can easily access records from a variety of locations. But the system has several disadvantages. It is expensive to operate and maintain. Computer technology is evolving at such a rapid pace that systems built on technology quickly become obsolete. A second disadvantage is that computerized medical records require scrupulous attention to security measures. The confidentiality of this information is only as safe as the systems designed to prevent unauthorized access. Finally, computerized record keeping has the potential to decrease the quality of athletic trainer–patient interaction. The athletic trainer with a file folder in his hands can easily review a patient's history while asking questions regarding the patient's present complaint. This discussion is more difficult when the medical information is stored on a computer in another part of the room or in the athletic trainer's office. Examples of the types of information contained in the medical record follow.

Physical Examination Forms

The physical examination results should come first in the medical record (see chapter 10). The physical exam normally occurs first chronologically, and the results can be a quick reference for athletic trainers or physicians. Some states mandate the use of specific physical examination forms for high school student-athletes. In other states and settings, athletic trainers can choose from a wide variety of forms. The form chosen should call for the following information (see figure 6.1):

- Personal data (e.g., name, address, date of birth, e-mail, cell phone)
- Health history (past and current, family)
- Vital signs
- Physician's review of systems
- Special procedures (blood and urine analyses, X rays, echocardiograms, and so forth)
- Functional tests (joint strength, aerobic capacity, and so forth)

HOPE COLLEGE HEALTH CLINIC
ATHLETIC PHYSICAL EXAMINATION SUMMARY

1. Name _____ (M or F) _____ Age _____ Date _____
2. S.S. # _____ Year in school   Fr   So   Jr   Sr
   Sport _____ E-mail _____ Cell phone _____

MEDICAL HISTORY SURVEY

3. Do you have now or have had in the past, problems with:	YES	NO
a. Headaches - needing treatment		
b. Heart problems of any kind		
c. Breathing (e.g., asthma)		
d. Abdominal pain		
e. Dizzy spells		
f. Family members with heart disease		
g. Eyes (except glasses)		
h. Hearing or ears		
i. Racing heart or skipped heart beats		
j. Joint pain, swelling		
k. Knees - injury, giving out, swelling		
l. Spine - back or neck		
m. Broken bones		
n. Kidneys or bladder		
o. Chest pain		
p. Diabetes		
q. High blood pressure		
r. Cancer		
s. Operations or surgery		
t. Severe viral infection like mono or myocarditis		
u. Skin disorders		
v. Other major injuries		
w. Drug allergies		
x. Eating disorder		

4. If you answered yes to any of #3 - give details below - identify by letter.

5. Have you ever been knocked unconscious?   Yes____ No____
   If yes, explain:

6. Have you ever had a cervical spine injury?   Yes____ No____
   If yes, explain:

7. Do you have any permanent handicap or disability?   Yes____ No____
   If yes, explain:

8. Are you under a physician's care at the present time?   Yes____ No____
   If yes, explain:

9. Are you taking any medication or drug at this time?   Yes____ No____
   If yes, explain:

10. Year of last tetanus. _____

11. Women - Do you have a monthly menstrual period?   Yes____ No____
    Date of last period. _____
    If no, explain:

12. Do you have an intense fear of gaining weight?   Yes____ No____

(FOR EXAMINING PHYSICIAN ONLY)

13. Eyes:
    Rt. Eye _____ Lt. Eye _____

14. General information:
    HT _____ WT _____ B/P _____ Pulse _____

Examination	Normal	Abnormal
15. Head		
16. Eyes		
17. Nose & throat		
18. Ears		
19. Neck		
20. Lungs		
21. Heart		
22. Abdomen		
23. Hernia		
24. G - U		
25. Extremity		
26. Shoulders		
27. Knees		
28. Other:		
29. Nervous		
30. Knee laxity		

31. Rt. _____ MCL_____ LCL _____ ACL_____ PCL_____
    Lt. _____ MCL_____ LCL _____ ACL_____ PCL_____

PHYSICIAN'S STATEMENT

32. Approved for sports   Yes _____   No _____

33. Approved pending further study
    Explain:

34. Approved with limitations
    Explain:

35. Disapproved
    Comments:

36. Date _____
    Signature _____

▶ **Figure 6.1** Sample of a physical examination form.

Reprinted by permission of the Hope College Health Clinic, Holland, MI.

Injury Evaluation and Treatment Forms

Injury evaluation and treatment records should provide a concise account of the athlete's or physically active patient's progress from time of injury until time of discharge. These forms often constitute the bulk of the medical record. Although many athletic trainers maintain separate records of injury evaluations and treatments, each treatment should be easily linked to a documented injury. Athletic trainers can choose from five methods for documenting injury evaluation and treatment data.

Problem-Oriented Medical Record (POMR)

The **problem-oriented medical record (POMR)** is a system of medical record keeping that organizes information around the physically active patient's specific complaints (Berni and Readey 1978). A cover sheet in the POMR summarizes the patient's past medical, social, and family history, as well as any personal habits that might affect the patient's health. A list of the patient's problems, along with a brief description of the plans implemented to ameliorate those problems, is also on the POMR cover sheet (see figure 6.2).

Problem-Oriented Medical Record Cover Sheet
Database

Past Medical Hx.	Family Hx.
Social Hx.	**Habits** Tobacco: Alcohol: Drugs: Seat belts: Exercise: Nutrition:

Problems — Dates

1. ______
2. ______
3. ______
4. ______

Plans — Dates

1. ______
2. ______
3. ______
4. ______

Follow-Up: See SOAP notes in record.

▶ **Figure 6.2** Cover page for problem-oriented medical record.

Another important component of the POMR is the **SOAP note** (see figure 6.3). The POMR cover sheet should reference each SOAP note. *SOAP* is an acronym for the following documentation parameters:

S: *Subjective evaluation of the patient's problem.* The subjective portion relates to how the patient conveys symptoms. It would include recording the patient's statement "My right knee popped and gave out." The subjective portion may also reflect statements of others who may have seen an injury occur.

O: *Objective evaluation of the patient's problem.* The objective portion of the evaluation includes physical data observed and measured by the athletic trainer during evaluation. It would relate information such as the presence of intra-articular effusion, 2+ Lachmann sign, and AROM –15 degrees in extension.

A: *Assessment of the patient's problem.* Assessment is the athletic trainer's judgment and professional opinion of the nature of the problem based on the subjective and objective evidence. Using the same knee injury case, a reasonable assessment of the problem would be internal derangement of the right knee with probable anterior cruciate ligament disruption. Statements of both short- and long-term goals for the athlete or physically active patient should be included for quality assurance.

P: *Plan of action that the athletic trainer will implement to resolve the problem.* This section should emphasize any specific treatment interventions to be performed, as well as identify any precautions or contraindications for future clinicians to adhere to. The plan may also include statements regarding interval progressions.

Individual Injury Evaluation and Treatment Record

Name: *Jones, Mike*   Sport: *Basketball*   Body part: *R-Ankle*

Date injury occurred: *2/5/12*   Date injury reported: *2/6/12*

Primary complaint: *R-ankle pain*   Secondary complaint: *None*

Subjective data: *Pt. inverted R-ankle while playing basketball. Reports "a loud snap." No previous hx. of ankle injury. Otherwise normal medical hx. Pain w/walking is 5/10. Pain at rest is 3/10. Pain to palpation over the ant. talofibular ligament. No other bony or soft tissue tenderness noted.*

Objective data: *Moderate swelling over lateral malleolus. No discoloration or deformity. Ankle is warm to touch. Lacks 5 deg dorsiflexion and 10 deg plantar flexion in both AROM and PROM compared to L-ankle. Strength is 4+/5 for DF, PF, Inv. & Ev. compared to 5/5 for L-ankle. Anterior drawer test is remarkably positive w/ mushy end point. Talar tilt test equivocal due to swelling. Neg. Klieger's test. Pt. walks w/a noticeable limp and cannot bear wt. on the R-foot w/out assistance. Applied RICE for 20 minutes. Issued compression sleeve and ankle brace. Fitted crutches and provided instruction in crutch walking. Educated pt. on RICE techniques for home program. Provided pt. w/ ankle home care brochure. Pt. indicated he understood instructions.*

Assessment: *Probable 3° ATF sprain.*

Plan: *Will refer to Dr. Smith. Appt. arranged for 3:00 pm today. Applied RICE for 20 minutes. Issued compression sleeve and ankle brace. Fitted crutches and provided instruction in crutch walking. Educated pt. on RICE techniques for home program. Provided pt. w/ankle home care brochure. Pt. indicated he understood instructions.*

Evaluator's signature: *David Black*

Date	Treatments and progress
2/6/12	*RICE × 20 min. Instructions for home care program. Crutches w/instructions. Compression sleeve and ankle brace. Pt. tolerated tx. well. Pain at rest 2/10. Swelling reduced.* **DB**

▶ **Figure 6.3** Sample evaluation and treatment form using SOAP note format.

Focus Charting   **Focus charting** is a less cumbersome alternative to the POMR medical record-keeping method (Iyer 1991a, 1991b). Typical focus charting forms list pertinent data about the injury in the first column, describe the action the athletic trainer will take in response in the second column, and present the response to the athletic trainer's action plan in the third column (see figure 6.4). As in all other forms of medical charting, each entry should be signed and dated, and time notations should be entered if appropriate.

Charting by Exception   **Charting by exception**, as its name implies, is a method in which only patient responses that vary from predefined norms are noted on the record (Murphy and Burke 1990). This method makes record keeping more efficient and less time-consuming. Although charting by exception is obviously inappropriate for recording initial injury evaluation, it has many potential uses for recording treatments and rehabilitation. This method, however, requires maintaining tightly controlled and frequently monitored treatment protocols.

For more information on this topic see chapter 2, "Principles of Examination," in the Athletic Training Education Series text *Examination of Musculoskeletal Injuries* and chapter 4, "Evaluation and Examination," in the Athletic Training Education Series text *Therapeutic Exercise for Musculoskeletal Injuries.*

Sports Medicine Focus Chart

Name: **Jones, Mike**   Sport: **Basketball**

Date	Data	Action	Response
2/6/12	Probable 3° R. ATF sprain	RICE × 20 min. Compression sleeve, ankle brace, crutches issued.	Pain decreased to 2/10. Patient understood home care instructions.
2/7/12	3° R. ATF sprain	Cold whirlpool with AROM × 20 min. Form walking × 10 min. JOBST compression pump × 30 min.	Decreased limp with walking. Increased DF ROM to 5°.
2/8/12	3° R. ATF sprain	Cold whirlpool with AROM × 20 min. BAPS in PE in seated position. JOBST compression pump × 30 min.	Discarded crutches. Swelling reduced to minimal level. PF/DF ROM equal to L. ankle.

▶ **Figure 6.4** Sample focus chart for use in recording injuries (data), treatments (action), and progress (response).

Computerized Documentation   The use of computers for keeping sports medicine records was described as early as 1982 (Abdenour 1982), and the products available to athletic trainers have been increasing in number and utility ever since. As the power and capacity of computers have increased and their price has decreased, athletic trainers have gradually shifted from using large, centralized mainframe computers toward using stand-alone and networked personal computers.

Athletic trainers see computerized record keeping as a way to decrease time spent documenting athletic injuries and treatments, thereby increasing time available for hands-on care of injured athletes and other physically active patients. But the switch to a computerized system of medical record keeping will probably result in an initial increase in time spent on record keeping. Athletic trainers will need time to learn to use the computer. In addition, record keeping and procedural changes will probably have to occur to adapt to the new technology (Allan and Englebright 2000).

As mentioned earlier, another potential problem is maintaining the confidentiality of computerized records. Safeguarding digitally stored data is more difficult than safeguarding data on paper in locked file cabinets. The use of passwords can sometimes slow unauthorized retrieval of medical records, but thwarting a motivated computer hacker is extremely difficult. Finally, depending on the limitations of the computer software, computerized record keeping can limit the athletic trainer's ability to describe the case as fully as might be desirable.

Nevertheless, athletic trainers should welcome the computer as a tool for effective and efficient medical record keeping in sports medicine. Computers allow athletic trainers to retrieve only those parts of the medical record desired for a specific purpose—we no longer need to search physically through a 100-page medical record for a single entry. Nonprofessional clerical staff can perform some of the data entry, freeing the athletic trainer to spend more time with injured athletes and other physically active patients. Athletic trainers can pull information from many individual medical records for writing reports. By using this feature, they can quickly prepare year-end injury and treatment summaries that used to take weeks to complete.

When one is planning to incorporate an electronic documentation system for medical records, there are two additional considerations to take into account. First, what is the life expectancy of the software program? Will it require upgrades anytime soon? How frequent are the upgrades, and will they be provided at no cost or will they carry additional fees? Second, institutional policies or procedures may exist regarding the addition of software to a network or computer. The athletic trainer should always consult with the instructional technology department to seek their expertise in purchasing and installing a new software program.

Narrative Charting   **Narrative charting** involves a more lengthy prose entry into the medical record. This is the most traditional method of medical record keeping. Athletic trainers make entries in paragraph form preceded by the date and time of the entry, relying little on abbreviations or medical shorthand (see figure 6.5). **Dictation** is useful in narrative record keeping. Although clerical transcription can be expensive, dictation can significantly reduce the amount of time required to document injuries, treatments, and progress notes. Voice recognition software is now available that allows health care professionals to dictate directly to an electronic file in their computer through a microphone, thus avoiding the expense of using a transcriptionist.

Dictation, like writing, is a skill that takes practice to perfect. The following suggestions will help improve the effectiveness of dictation:

- Organize the data to be dictated by taking notes in medical shorthand while interviewing the patient. Use these notes to dictate a more comprehensive entry into the medical record.
- Speak clearly and slowly into the dictation machine. If possible, avoid dictating in a noisy room.

- Spell all proper names and medical terms that are used infrequently. This practice is especially important if the transcriber is inexperienced in medical transcription. Consider providing a medical dictionary to the transcriber.

- Review and initial all dictated narrations before filing them in the medical record.

- If you are planning to use voice recognition software, be sure to buy a package designed for medical environments. Allow plenty of time (up to several hours) for the software to imprint your voice patterns and thereby reduce the number of errors.

Reports of Special Procedures

Reports of all special procedures should be included in the medical record. Although special-procedure reports should be entered into the medical record chronologically, each should be annotated to refer the reader back to an initial injury or illness assessment report. Special procedures include but are not limited to the following:

- Isokinetic strength tests
- Blood tests
- Urinalysis
- X rays or other imaging procedures
- Surgical reports
- Cardiac assessments (echocardiogram, graded exercise tests, thallium uptake scans, and so forth)

Smith, Jon

April 7, 2012

Jon is a sprinter on the school's track team. He came in today to be evaluated for pain that he has been experiencing in his anterior shins for the past three weeks. He has been icing his shins prior to and after every track practice in order to relieve the pain, but the problem has progressed to the point where it is very uncomfortable to run. He also experiences some pain when he walks. He has some pain while lying in bed at night. The pain is a dull ache unless the anterior shin is touched, when it becomes a sharp pain.

Visual examination is unspectacular. No swelling, discoloration, or deformity is noted. Palpation reveals point-specific tenderness over the anterior surface of the distal one-third of both tibias. A mild elevation in local temperature is palpable. No crepitus is noted. The gastroc and soleus are both tight bilaterally, allowing only 6° of passive dorsiflexion.

It is my impression that Jon may be suffering from bilateral tibial stress fractures. Jon is a member of an HMO and his physician while he is in college is Dr. Van Notten. I called Dr. Van Notten this morning to discuss Jon's case and was instructed to obtain a bone scan of Jon's tibias bilaterally. Jon is scheduled for the bone scan at Holland Community Hospital tomorrow morning at 9:30. He will be kept out of practice until Dr. Van Notten reviews the bone scan. He was placed on crutches and instructed to apply ice to his shins for 20 minutes every 2 hours while awake. He was told to return to the athletic training room tomorrow after his bone scan.

Signed: *Lydia Sanchez, A.T., C.*

▶ **Figure 6.5** Example of the narrative charting method of injury documentation.

Communication From Other Professionals

An athletic trainer commonly receives written documentation of a patient's medical status from physicians, physical therapists, and other health care professionals involved with the case. One type of documentation is the referral form (Gabriel 1981) sent with an injured athlete when she is sent to the physician's office or the emergency room (see figure 6.6). The injured athlete referral form provides legally defensible proof that the athletic trainer consulted with a physician as required by the *Standards of Professional Practice* and, in many states, by law. In addition, it improves communication between the athletic trainer and the physician by taking the burden of having to relay information off the injured athlete.

The referral form should include the athlete's name, sport, injury date, and appointment date and time. It should allow space for the athletic trainer to document the initial evaluation findings. The form should provide space for the physician to write a diagnosis and orders for treatment or rehabilitation. The athletic trainer and physician should date and sign their notes. Finally, the form should include a section that complies with the Health Insurance Portability and Accountability Act (HIPAA) (see the later section, "Release of Medical Information"). The athlete signs the form, authorizing the physician to share the athlete's medical information with the athletic trainer or other members of the sports medicine team. Athletic trainers have three means of ensuring that referral forms are returned. The most obvious is to ask the injured athlete to bring the form to the next appointment. Athletic trainers can ask the physician to mail the form back, but this method delays direct feedback from the physician. Finally, the athletic trainer could ask the physician to fax a response, which provides the information quickly and gets around the possibility of the athlete's losing or forgetting the form.

A second method for communicating with other health care professionals is through the common professional courtesy of sending letters or copies of office notes to referring health care colleagues. Athletic trainers should enter these notes, often a useful source of information and documentation of the injured athlete's status, into the medical record. Athletic trainers should request a letter from all physicians and other health care professionals to whom they frequently refer injured athletes.

Emergency Information

Athletic trainers in high schools and colleges must frequently contact an injured student-athlete's parents or guardians, which is an urgent responsibility if the athlete has a serious accident or illness. To do so, the athletic trainer usually uses the emergency information form in the medical record (see figure 6.7). This form should include athlete information, such as name, address, phone number or numbers, date of birth, and Social Security or student identification numbers. The form should also include parents' names, addresses, and telephone numbers (home and business). Some athletic trainers have suggested that the form contain the athlete's insurance information as well (Miles 1987). This form should be readily accessible in the medical record, perhaps affixed to the inside cover of the athlete's folder. Emergency information forms could also be organized according to sport and placed in three-ring binders that teams can take with them wherever they go. Some athletic injury and treatment database programs have the capability to store this information on a handheld computer as well.

Permission for Medical Treatment Forms

A widely recognized legal principle is that persons (or their parents in the case of minors) must consent to medical treatment. Any consent forms should be maintained in the medical record (see figure 6.8). Although the use of such forms has been standard operating procedure in most hospital sports medicine programs, their use in school-based settings has been limited. Consent forms are especially important in the high school setting because most of these injured student-athletes are still minors.

HOPE COLLEGE SPORTS MEDICINE MEDICAL REFERRAL

Name _____   Sport _____

Date _____ Time _____   Physician _____

Athletic Trainer's Impression _____

_____

_____

_____

Physician's Diagnosis & Recommendation _____

_____

_____

_____

Recommended Activity Level (Check All That Apply):

Bed Rest _____   Attend Classes Only _____   Practice as Able _____

No Practice or Competition _____   No Restrictions _____

Limited Physical Activity as Noted Above _____

Follow-Up Appointment _____   _____
                                        Date   Time

_____
Physician's Signature

PLEASE INSTRUCT THE STUDENT TO RETURN THIS FORM TO THE ATHLETIC TRAINING ROOM

I hereby authorize _____ to release all records related to the injury/illness specified above to Richard Ray, Meg Abfall, Dr. Patrick Hulst, Dr. John Schloff, the Hope College Health Clinic, or any other representative of the Hope College medical staff. I further authorize the above-named health care provider to discuss my case with any representative of the Hope College medical staff. I waive any and all claims against the above-named health care provider, Hope College, and any of its employees or contractors in connection with the communication and disclosure of such information.

_____
Student's Signature

_____   _____
Date   Witness

▶ **Figure 6.6** Sample medical referral form.

Reprinted by permission of the Hope College Health Clinic, Holland, MI.

Emergency Information

Name: _____   Sport: _____

Date of birth: _____   Address: _____

Social Security or ID number: _____

Phone: (Home) _____   (Work) _____   (Cell) _____

Parents' names: _____

   Address: _____

   Phone: (Home) _____   (Work) _____   (Cell) _____

Person to contact in an emergency: _____

   Relationship: _____   Phone: _____

Name of insurance company: _____

Policy numbers: _____

Is this insurance company a health maintenance organization (HMO)?   Yes _____   No _____

If so, list the HMO telephone number: _____

▶ **Figure 6.7**   Sample emergency information form.

Adapted, by permission, from B.J. Miles, 1987, "Injuries on the road: Good information reduces problems," *Journal of Athletic Training* 22(2).

Along with permission forms, signed releases from patients or their parents that waive all future legal claims against the athletic trainer or the employing institution are commonly used. These **exculpatory clauses**, with few exceptions, are legally unsupportable (Herbert 1987). The primary legal argument against them is that such clauses are contrary to public policy and are therefore legally invalid. Because the public has a stake in quality health care, the courts have been hesitant to allow negligent practitioners to hide behind prospective waivers. In addition, in many states, parents cannot sign away the rights of their children. Any athletic trainer planning to use a prospective waiver with exculpatory language should first have an attorney and liability insurance carrier thoroughly evaluate it.

Release of Medical Information

Another commonly understood legal principle is that health care providers may not release a person's medical records without consent. This principle has been written into the federal legal code in the form of two laws: the Family Educational Rights and Privacy Act of 1974 (sometimes referred to as the *Buckley Amendment*) and the Health Insurance Portability and Accountability Act of 1996 (HIPAA).

Family Educational Rights and Privacy Act   The **FERPA (Family Educational Rights and Privacy Act)** requires educational institutions to receive formal written consent from students (or, in the case of minors, their parents or guardians) before they can disclose educational records to a third party. The law also requires educational institutions to make available to students all records relating to their enrollment unless they specifically waive the right on a

---

Permission to Provide Medical Treatment Agreement

I HEREBY give my permission for my son/daughter, _____ ,
to undergo medical treatment for any injury or illness he/she may sustain or acquire while engaged in interscholastic athletics at Eagletown High School. I understand that the medical personnel of Eagletown High School, including athletic trainers, nurses, and team physicians, will perform only those procedures that are within their training, credentialing, and scope of professional practice to prevent, care for, and rehabilitate athletic injuries. In the event that more serious medical procedures are required, such as surgery or other invasive procedures, I understand that attempts will be made to contact me for my consent. I understand that if my child suffers a potentially life-threatening injury or illness, and in the event I am unable to be contacted within a reasonable period of time, that I authorize any duly licensed medical practitioner to perform such procedures as may be medically necessary to alleviate the problem.

I have had the opportunity to ask questions regarding this release and all of my questions have been answered to my satisfaction. Having understood the above agreement, I freely sign this Permission to Provide Medical Treatment Agreement.

_____   _____
Date   Signature of Parent or Legal Guardian

▶ **Figure 6.8** Sample agreement form for the parents or guardians of minors to grant permission to provide medical treatment.

case-by-case basis. Several exceptions to the rule exist. For example, employees of educational institutions may legally disclose information regarding students, without their consent, to safeguard their health in an emergency. Health records created or maintained by a physician, psychiatrist, psychologist, or other recognized professionals or paraprofessionals are not considered educational records under FERPA and are therefore not covered by the law. Student-athletes do not have a legal right under FERPA to access the content of their health records. Nonetheless, good practice in health care includes receiving informed consent from patients before sharing information regarding their health with a third party.

> For the most recent FERPA information, visit www2.ed.gov/policy/gen/guid/fpco/ferpa/index.html.

Health Insurance Portability and Accountability Act HIPAA was enacted to help employees transfer their health insurance when they switched employers, to ensure that their health information would remain private, and to give people more access to their own health care information. The privacy portion of the law was, in part, a reaction to the fact that much health care information is now transmitted electronically and is therefore more vulnerable to unauthorized release. HIPAA applies only to "covered entities." The law may cover athletic trainers in some settings but not those in other settings. In general, athletic trainers are working in environments subject to HIPAA rules when each of the following three conditions applies:

- The person, business, or agency furnishes, bills, or receives payment for health care in the normal course of business.
- The person, business, or agency conducts covered transactions. Covered transactions are those activities normally associated with billing.
- The covered transactions are transmitted in electronic form.

Athletic trainers working in covered entities should be most attentive to seven areas with regard to HIPAA rules:

1. Obtain consent for treatment. Athletic trainers must provide patients with a written "Notice of Privacy Practices" that delineates the manner in which the health care agency intends to use and disclose a patient's health information. Patients must acknowledge in writing that they received this information, except in emergencies that render the patient unable to provide written acknowledgment.

2. Obtain authorization to release health information. Athletic trainers working in covered entities must receive written authorization to share a patient's health information with persons who are not part of the chain of health care providers, including coaches, athletic administrators, scouts, and the media. The athletic trainer must obtain authorizations for each instance of information release; a blanket release signed at the beginning of the year or even at the initiation of the treatment will not suffice (for athletic trainers not covered by the law, a blanket authorization is permissible). A valid authorization must include

- a description of the information to be disclosed,
- the persons authorized to disclose information,
- the persons to whom the information may be disclosed,
- the purpose of the disclosure,
- the expiration date of the authorization,
- the patient signature and date, and
- if signed by a representative, a description of his or her authority to act for the patient.

Furthermore, authorizations are not valid under the HIPAA rules unless they include each of the following:

- A statement that the individual may revoke the authorization in writing, instructions on how to revoke the authorization, and a reference to the Notice of Privacy Practices mentioned earlier.
- A statement that treatment, payment, enrollment, or eligibility for benefits may not be conditioned on obtaining the authorization; or, if such services are conditioned on the authorization, a statement that details the consequences of refusing to sign the authorization.
- A statement that informs patients that the persons to whom the information is being provided could disclose their health information.

3. Release only the minimum necessary information. HIPAA requires that athletic trainers and other covered entities limit the amount and frequency of information release to the minimum required to accomplish the purposes for which the information is being released. Although this part of the rule does not apply to health care providers involved in the chain of an individual's care, it definitely applies to nonmedical entities such as coaches, administrators, and insurance companies.

4. Safeguard patient information. Although HIPAA allows for certain incidental disclosures of patient information (for example, someone in the clinic overhearing a conversation between two athletic trainers regarding a patient case), the rules require that reasonable efforts be made to safeguard such information. Good practices require maintaining charts and other patient documents in a secure manner.

5. Observe state laws governing the treatment of a minor's health information. Because HIPAA defers authority for access to the health records of minors to the individual states, athletic trainers must be familiar with their state's laws governing minors and their health records.

6. Do not combine authorizations except for research purposes. The HIPAA rules generally require that the patient sign a separate authorization for each purpose for which patient information will be used or released. This rule does not apply when the information will be used for research purposes.

7. Business associates must safeguard patient information. Athletic trainers who refer patients to other entities must ensure that the entity to whom the referral is being made has policies in place to safeguard the patient's health information. The athletic trainer must have contracts with these entities that specify the nature of the safeguards. For example, if an athletic trainer refers patients to a private practice nutritionist, he must have a contract with the nutritionist specifying that the nutritionist may not release the athlete health information without written authorization from the athlete.

Many parties will want access to the athlete's medical records, including coaches, the press, insurance companies, and professional sport organizations. Before providing information, the athletic trainer should make certain that the athlete has formally agreed to the release by signing a properly formatted authorization. If the athlete is a minor, a parent or legal guardian must also sign the waiver. The athletic trainer must be certain to release only the information authorized by the athlete. Each time an athlete's medical information is released, the medical release form should show the content, purpose, and receiver of the information (see figure 6.9).

To find out if you or your employer is a covered entity under the HIPAA statute, visit www.cms.hhs.gov/HIPAAGenInfo/.

Insurance Information

Financial documents such as patient invoices and insurance claim forms are not medical records. They have different purposes and uses, and the laws governing confidentiality protect them in different ways. Insurance information in the medical record should be limited to the following (Glondys 1988):

- Expected payer or payers
- Insured's name
- Patient's relationship to the insured
- Employment data and insurance numbers

Correspondence with insurance companies and other third-party payers should be maintained separately from the medical record. Letters and copies of insurance forms often contain information directly related to the description of the injury circumstances. Copies of medical records used to document claims should not be maintained in the insurance folder; to protect confidentiality, a note referring to the supporting portion of the medical record should be used. This method protects the confidentiality of the medical record by ensuring that unauthorized individuals do not gain access through the insurance claims process.

Program Administration Records

Much of the information that athletic trainers must manage is administrative. Whereas medical records are specific to only one athlete or physically active patient, **program administration records** are more general and are usually organized around subfunctions of the sports medicine program. The absolute standards for confidentiality that apply to medical records are usually, but not always, significantly relaxed for many types of program administration records. Whenever program administration records deal with specific individuals, however, confidentiality should be maintained. Examples of various types of program administration records follow.

Reports to Coaches

A common practice of most athletic trainers who work in professional, high school, and college settings is to provide coaches with daily written reports of the health status of their athletes (see figure 6.10). Daily reports can help improve communication between the athletic trainer and the coach. Coaches appreciate timely information about the health status of their athletes because they can then plan more effectively. Another important benefit of the daily report to coaches is that athletic trainers can easily document recommendations for participation status.

Release of Medical Information Authorization

I, _____, DO/DO NOT give consent for the team physician, athletic trainer, or other medical personnel employed by _____
College to release such information regarding my medical history, record of injury or surgery, record of serious illness, and rehabilitation results as may be requested by either the representatives of any professional or amateur athletic organization seeking such information.

I understand that the representatives of a professional or amateur athletic organization have made representations to the team physician, athletic trainer, or other medical personnel employed by
_____ College that the purpose of this request for my medical information is to assist the organization being represented in making a determination as to offering me employment.

I understand that a record will be kept of all individuals requesting information and the date of the request. This information is normally confidential and except as provided in this Release will not be otherwise released by the custodian of the information. This Release remains valid until revoked by me in writing.

I have had an opportunity to ask questions regarding this Release and the process by which my medical information may be released. All of my questions have been answered to my satisfaction. Having read and understood the above, I freely sign this Release of Medical Information Authorization.

_____   _____
Date   Signature of Student-Athlete

_____   _____
Date   Signature of Parent or Legal Guardian (for minors)

_____   _____
Date   Signature of Witness

- -

Medical Information Release Log

Date of Release	Released to	Form of Release	Content of Release	Released by
1.				
2.				
3.				
4.				

▶ **Figure 6.9** Sample authorization form and log for release of medical information.

For example, assume that the athletic trainer recommends in the daily report that an athlete be limited to noncontact football drills because of a resolving neck injury. If the coach allows the athlete to participate in a full-contact scrimmage and the athlete is reinjured, the athletic trainer can at least document that he recommended a reduced activity level for the injured athlete.

Should athletic trainers be concerned about violating their legal and ethical duty to hold athlete's medical information and health status in confidence—even from their coaches? This

DAILY COACH'S REPORT

Sport: Football   Date: October 14, 2012

Name	Injury	Date injured	Date reported	Comments
Smith, Tim	L-wrist/old fx. pain	10-12-12	10-12-12	Seen by Dr. West
Funk, Roger	L-shldr. sublx.	10-12-12	10-12-12	Seen by Dr. West, rest
DeHaan, Dirk	R-AC contusion	10-12-12	10-13-12	Treatment, seen by Dr. West
Russell, Bob	R-ankle sprain	10-12-12	10-13-12	Treatment, rest
Fernandez, Scott	Neck strain	10-12-12	10-13-12	Seen by Dr. West, treatment, play as able
Jones, Rick	L-arm contusion	10-10-12	10-11-12	Seen by Dr. West, rest

No participation	Play as able	Removed from list
Funk, Roger	Smith, Tim	Nick, Art
DeHaan, Dirk	Fernandez, Scott	Rios, Manny
Russell, Bob		
Jones, Rick		

▶ **Figure 6.10** Example of a computer-generated daily coach's report.

is a thorny issue for a variety of reasons. First, as mentioned in the section on HIPAA, the legal responsibilities associated with confidentiality of a patient's record will vary depending on whether the athletic trainer is a covered entity under HIPAA. Second, although athletic trainers have an ethical responsibility to obtain authorization from the athlete before disclosing information to a coach, common practice in school, collegiate, and professional sports for many years has been for athletic trainers to report on the health status of athletes to their coaches (for all the reasons enumerated in the previous paragraph) even in the absence of explicit authorization. Many injury situations occur in such a way that the coach is a witness to the injury or is the agent of referral to the athletic trainer. In situations like these, the coach is already an informed party. Even when the coach doesn't know about an injury, most athletes just assume that the athletic trainer will speak to the coach about the situation. Conversely, most athletic trainers have had cases in which athletes have specifically requested that the athletic trainer not inform their coaches about an injury or illness—for a variety of reasons. The question is complicated even further when athletic trainers, as agents of management of professional athletic organizations, are required by the terms of their contracts to disclose the health status of all athletes to a coach or general manager.

Thompson and Sherman (1993) recommend that formal agreements should exist that specify the extent to which the athletic trainer will share information with team personnel. In the absence of such agreements, the athletic trainer should hold all information in confidence. In addition, the following guidelines are recommended for dealing with this issue:

■ Inform all athletes in writing that you will share with the coach health information that affects their ability to participate fully in team activities or when their safety might be at risk, except when an athlete makes a specific request to withhold the information. Obtain athletes' written consent for this at the beginning of each season.

- Remind athletes during their initial assessment that as part of their treatment plan you will be discussing their status with their coaches. If HIPAA classifies you as a covered entity, obtain written authorization for this.

- Counsel athletes who are reluctant to allow you to discuss their case with a coach about the advantages and disadvantages of withholding the information.

- If athletes request that you hold information in confidence before you have had an opportunity to evaluate the information ("I want to tell you something, but you have to promise me you won't tell the coach"), inform them that you can't make such a promise and that you'll have to hear what they tell you first. If they won't tell you without such an assurance, offer to refer them to another health care provider not associated with the team or institution.

- Disclose to coaches only the information they need either to plan team activities or to structure a safe participation environment for the athletes in question. Suppose, for example, that an athlete has a sexually transmitted disease and must see the physician at 4:30, thus having to miss practice. We recommend that you tell the coach only that the athlete is ill and will miss one day of practice.

- Document in the medical record the extent of disclosure made to a coach. In cases in which the athlete will not authorize disclosure, document this as well.

Budget Information

Athletic trainers with financial authority must maintain accurate records of all financial transactions. In school, college, and professional settings, financial reports usually include monthly budget statements (produced in-house or sent from the institutional business office), purchase orders, and invoices. Documents that support budgetary decisions and **requests for proposals (RFPs)** should also be maintained in the program administration record system.

Nonmedical Correspondence

Nonmedical correspondence comprises letters and memoranda not associated with a specific patient's health status. Unlike medical correspondence, which must be meticulously recorded and preserved, much of the routine nonmedical correspondence can be discarded after action is taken. Nonmedical correspondence that must be retained should be filed under the appropriate subject heading and not in a separate folder labeled "Correspondence."

Equipment and Supply Information

Equipment and supply inventories and catalogs from medical supply vendors are another kind of program administration record. Institutions often require administrative units to keep an inventory of nonexpendable capital equipment on file. This inventory usually includes the type of equipment, the amount or number of units, and the serial numbers. Some institutions assign their own identification numbers for nonexpendable equipment, which should also be included as part of this record. Athletic trainers in all settings are frequently called on to purchase or recommend the purchase of sports medicine products. A well-organized file of appropriate catalogs can be useful. Warranties and equipment maintenance records should also be filed in the program administration records.

Personnel Information

Information on sports medicine staff members' employment constitutes an important part of the program administration record-keeping system. Like an individual's medical record, the personnel record is confidential, and only those with a documented need for the information should be able to access it. Personnel information should be kept in a secure place, preferably a locked filing cabinet. Records on athletic training students' performance should be treated similarly. Examples of the kinds of records normally associated with the personnel function include

- performance evaluation records;
- salary and promotion records;
- employment application information, including application forms, resumes, and letters of recommendation; and
- employment contracts.

Reporting Information

Athletic trainers are often responsible for documenting the activities of a sports medicine program either for institutional or for outside accreditation purposes. The information required to compile such reports constitutes another aspect of the program administration record-keeping system. Documentation of patient caseloads and summaries of any special program accomplishments are often compiled in an annual report. Accreditation agencies require access to different kinds of information, depending on their purpose. Hospital accreditation agencies generally request summary statistics on patient outcomes and evidence of compliance with professional standards of practice. Agencies that accredit educational programs require data related to student outcomes such as graduation, certification, and employment rates.

Another kind of reporting information is required by law to show compliance with the **OSHA Bloodborne Pathogen Standard**. Part 1910 of Title 29 of the Code of Federal Regulations requires that employers develop programs that protect employees, including athletic trainers, from occupational exposure to bloodborne pathogens (Occupational Safety and Health Administration 1991). These rules have significant record-keeping requirements. Records kept to comply with the OSHA rules must be retained for three years. Documents that must be entered into the employee's medical record, however, must be maintained for the duration of the employee's employment *plus* 30 years.

> Training materials and forms related to compliance with the OSHA Bloodborne Pathogens Standard are available at www.osha.gov (search for "bloodborne pathogens standard").

Patient and Student Education Information

All athletic trainers should maintain an up-to-date database of article reprints, handouts, and other educational materials that they can provide to both patients and student athletic trainers. The maintenance of such a database as another type of program administration information is important because the body of knowledge in athletic training and sports medicine is changing rapidly.

FILING SPORTS MEDICINE RECORDS

Although it might seem rather basic, an appropriate and effective system for filing sports medicine records is important. Like Karen Thompson in the opening case, most athletic trainers are too busy to spend time searching for important documents in poorly organized files. Although different sports medicine settings will require different filing systems, the following recommendations should prove useful in most cases (Needy 1974):

- Develop a **master outline** of files contained in the system organized under major subject headings.
- Maintain confidential files, such as medical records and personnel folders, in their own locked cabinets.
- Organize files according to major, primary, secondary, and, if needed, tertiary classifications. A budget file classified in this manner would look like this:

Major classification	*Budget*
Primary	2005
Secondary	Expendable supplies
Tertiary	Invoices

- Use file labels of different shapes or colors to differentiate between the various filing classifications.
- Do not overfill file folders. When a folder has reached its capacity, usually 3/4 inches, begin a second folder.
- Organize material within a folder chronologically or alphabetically.
- Develop separate filing systems for temporary and permanent files.
- File records promptly.
- Go through all files yearly. Discard unneeded records and update the master outline.

APPLICATIONS TO ATHLETIC TRAINING: THEORY INTO PRACTICE

Apply the concepts discussed in this chapter to the following two case studies to help you prepare for situations you might face in actual practice. The questions at the end of the studies have many possible solutions. The case studies can be used for homework, as test questions, or in class discussion.

Case Study 1

When Charles Olson, the athletic trainer at Eagletown High School, met with his student staff at the beginning of each school year, he always covered documentation procedures for injuries and treatments. He required all students to use the following procedures:

- Injury evaluation forms were to be completed only by the head athletic trainer. Students were expected to file the forms in individual medical files every Monday, Wednesday, and Friday.
- All treatments were to be recorded by students on the daily treatment log as soon as the treatment was administered. On Monday, Wednesday, and Friday afternoons, the students were to copy all treatments from the daily treatment log onto the bottom half of the injury evaluation report. After a page of the log had been transferred, it was thrown away.

One day Charles was surprised to find a subpoena in his mail for all medical records related to a former student-athlete who had graduated five years earlier. At first, Charles could not find the student's file. Finally, after several hours of digging through boxes in a storage closet

in the gymnasium, he found the file. When he looked up the injury evaluation form for the case in question, he was shocked to see that the treatment records were sloppy, often not dated, and usually illegible because they had been written with a fountain pen that had left blotches of smeared ink on the page. Although Charles complied with the subpoena and submitted all the requested records, he had an uneasy feeling about the quality of those records.

QUESTIONS FOR ANALYSIS

1. What are the advantages of the injury and treatment recording system used at Eagletown High School? What are the disadvantages?

2. What kinds of problems is the Eagletown High School system likely to foster? How could those problems be overcome? What kinds of resources would be required to implement these solutions? How much would it cost?

3. What are the legal implications for this record-keeping system? Which legal issues should Charles address when considering changes in the system?

Case Study 2

Randy Waters is an athletic trainer for an AA minor league professional baseball team. Besides his duties as athletic trainer, Randy is also equipment manager and traveling secretary for the team. Because of his many duties, Randy doesn't have a lot of time for record keeping. He usually discusses the health of individual players with the team's manager over coffee and rolls each morning. Randy informs the manager of any new injuries, and the manager can ask any questions he has.

One day in August, as the playoffs were rapidly approaching, Randy was unable to have coffee with the manager and the other coaches because he had to make arrangements for an upcoming trip. During the game that night, the star pitcher's knee suddenly buckled after a pitch, and he fell to the ground. He had to leave the game, and the team physician evaluated him in the locker room. After the game, the physician told the manager that the knee would be fine in a couple of days but that in the future the manager should rest players for a day or two following an accident like the one the pitcher had suffered. "What accident?" asked the manager with a puzzled look. The physician related that during his exam the player told him he had twisted his knee in the parking lot the previous evening. He had gone to the athletic trainer and gotten some ice for it, and in the morning the knee felt better. The manager immediately went to Randy and demanded to know why he hadn't been informed.

QUESTIONS FOR ANALYSIS

1. Why is the manager so upset with Randy? Is his anger justified?
2. What steps could Randy have taken to avoid this situation? How should Randy modify his information management system to avoid problems like this in the future?
3. What legal risks does Randy's system pose, both for the club and for himself?
4. If Randy decided to use a computer to help him with his information management needs, what kinds of hardware and software might serve him best?

SUMMARY

Athletic trainers now practice in a society overwhelmed with information. The need to document in a timely and accurate manner is essential for all athletic trainers regardless of the setting they practice in. Documentation of information typically falls under one of two categories: medical records and program administration records. Reasons for the importance of documentation include legal protection and requirements, professional standards, communication, insurance company requirements, outcomes measurement, and overall potential for improved delivery of care. The Family Educational Rights and Privacy Act (FERPA) of 1974 and the Health Insurance Portability and Accountability Act of 1996 (HIPAA) are examples of legislation that specifies certain privacy standards related to documentation of information. Various methods can be used to document, including problem-oriented medical records (POMR), SOAP notes (Subjective, Objective, Assessment, Plan), and narrative formats, to name a few.

KEY CONCEPTS AND REVIEW

1. Understand the importance of documentation as part of a complete information management system in sports medicine.

To succeed as professionals in an information society, athletic trainers must manage and communicate information effectively. Documentation is a central task in the athletic trainer's information management role. Medical documentation helps ensure legal rights, acts as a memory aid, satisfies laws and professional standards, and provides data with which to make informed decisions.

2. Understand and describe the different methods of athletic injury and treatment documentation.

The five methods for documenting injury evaluation and treatment data are problem-oriented medical records, focus charting, charting by exception, computerized documentation, and narrative charting.

3. Understand and describe the different types of information to be managed in a typical sports medicine program.

Information in sports medicine is usually made up of medical records and program administration records. Medical records are confidential and should contain injury and treatment reports, physical examination data, reports of special procedures, communications from other health care professionals, emergency information, permission to treat and medical waiver forms, release of medical information forms, and certain kinds of insurance records. Program administration records include reports to coaches, budget information, nonmedical correspondence, equipment and supply information, personnel information, patient and student education information, and information required for writing self-studies and other kinds of evaluative reports.

Reimbursement for Health Care Services

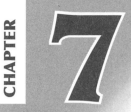

OBJECTIVES

After reading this chapter, you should be able to do the following:

1. Understand the difference between medical, health, and accident insurance.

2. Understand the advantages and disadvantages of self-insurance, primary coverage, and secondary coverage.

3. Define the types of injuries covered by most athletic accident policies.

4. Understand the basic legal responsibilities associated with third-party reimbursement.

5. Understand the role of procedural coding in the third-party reimbursement system.

6. Organize a claims-processing system for a sports medicine program in an educational setting.

7. Understand the steps required to file a claim for reimbursement from a third-party payer.

8. Evaluate and purchase an athletic accident insurance policy for an educational institution.

▶ Sven Olaf, a recent transfer student and star of the New Amsterdam High School soccer team, was racing down the sideline during a game against the crosstown rivals when he collapsed in pain. The school's certified athletic trainer, Jennifer Smith, ran onto the field and discovered that Sven was suffering from severe spasm of the paraspinous musculature. The cause of the spasm was unknown, and the lower extremity neurological examination was normal. Because Sven was in great pain, Jennifer decided to have him transported to the local hospital by ambulance. While waiting for the ambulance to arrive, Sven's parents and the team's coach gathered around to provide support and reassurance. As Sven was being placed onto the spine board, the coach took Sven's father, who was unemployed, aside and told him, "Don't worry about the bills. The school has insurance for this kind of thing and I'm sure we'll be able to take care of it because it was an athletic injury." Two days later, Sven was discharged from the hospital after incurring a bill of over $5,000.

Because Sven had no personal medical insurance, Jennifer submitted the entire bill to the school's athletic accident insurance company. Three weeks later, Jennifer received a letter from the company denying the claim because the injury was substantially linked to a preexisting condition. Although Sven had never told Jennifer, he had suffered a similar injury two years earlier while a student at another school. The emergency room physician obtained this information during the examination and provided it to the insurance company in the medical records needed to process the claim. Because the athletic accident policy excluded preexisting conditions, the company denied the claim.

When Jennifer contacted Sven's parents and informed them that the insurance company had denied the claim, Mr. Olaf angrily told her that the coach had said the school would pay the bills. "The coach promised me!" he shouted over the phone. Jennifer told Mr. Olaf that she would consult with the school administration and call him back. When Jennifer informed the athletic director of the problem, he immediately called a meeting with the coach, the school principal, and Jennifer to determine where they would find $5,000 to pay the bill that the coach, as an agent of the school, had promised they would pay.

What can't be cured must be insured.

—OLIVER HERFORD

Athletic trainers with any experience should be able to sympathize with Jennifer Smith's situation. Athletic administrators have long felt a moral responsibility to prevent the cost associated with athletic injury from barring access to school sports programs. The soccer coach's promise to Sven's father was simply an expression of that sense of responsibility. His promise probably would have been easy to keep in the 1970s, when the parents of most student-athletes had their own comprehensive medical insurance. Unfortunately, this is no longer true. Stein (1996) reported that in 1979, 85% of the population was covered by some form of private health insurance. By 1999, however, this figure had dropped to approximately 71% and by 2009 to approximately 63% (see figure 7.1). Access to private medical insurance is declining, and the terms of medical insurance policies are becoming increasingly restrictive. For example, between 1982 and 1984 alone, the number of companies that required deductibles for hospitalization doubled from 30% to 60%, while the number of employers that required employees to make a contribution to the cost of their insurance premiums also increased (Fein 1986). Nearly all health insurance plans now require such contributions.

The cost of health care became an important political issue during the early and mid-1990s. Several proposals intended to produce significant changes to the health care reimbursement system went before Congress. These proposals ranged from minor reforms of the private health insurance system to schemes that would create a national health care system similar to the Canadian model. Although no significant federally mandated changes in the health insurance system occurred, this national discussion on health care was useful because it pushed the marketplace to develop new, more efficient health care delivery systems that—at least for a few years—helped hold down the rate of cost increase of medical goods and services.

In the meantime, schools and colleges have faced greater financial risks from medical costs than at any time in the past. This chapter therefore provides athletic trainers with the information they need to manage insurance systems and more effectively safeguard the resources of the institutions they represent while living up to the moral responsibility to remove financial barriers from our nation's playing fields. In addition, the chapter examines the third-party reimbursement process to help athletic trainers working in hospitals and clinics understand how they receive payment for what they do.

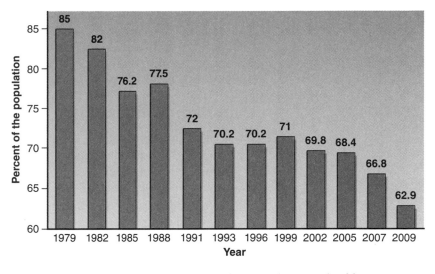

▶ **Figure 7.1** Percentage of the U.S. population with private health insurance.
Data from Health Insurance Association of America 2010.

INSURANCE SYSTEMS

Medical insurance is a contract between the holder of a **policy** and an insurance company to reimburse a percentage of the cost of the policyholder's medical bills, usually after the policyholder has paid a deductible (Rowell 1989). **Health insurance**, on the other hand, is generally more comprehensive, because it often includes provisions for maintaining good health rather than simply paying for illnesses and injuries.

Both of these insurance classifications should be distinguished from the type of policy most educational institutions buy for their student-athletes: **athletic accident insurance**, which is usually intended to supplement a student's family insurance plan and reimburses the cost of athletic accidents only (Chambers, Ross, and Kozubowski 1986). The insurance industry defines *accident* differently from the concept of *injury* as understood by most athletic trainers, coaches, parents, athletes, and other physically active patients. To an insurance company, accidents usually include acute, traumatic injuries, independent of any other cause or preexisting condition, that occur during practices and games. Specific **exclusions** in most accident insurance plans include injuries caused by overuse (tendinitis, bursitis, stress fractures, and so on), illnesses, and degenerative conditions. Some athletic accident insurance companies offer **riders** to cover the costs of chronic conditions, but riders generally increase the **premium** significantly.

A fourth type of coverage is **catastrophic insurance**, which usually takes effect after the first $75,000 in medical bills has been reached and provides lifetime medical, rehabilitation, and disability coverage for athletes who have suffered long-term or permanent handicaps as a result of athletic injuries (National Collegiate Athletic Association 2010). Member institutions of the National Collegiate Athletic Association (NCAA) have received catastrophic insurance at no cost since 1991. Catastrophic insurance is also available to non-NCAA institutions and high schools through their national governing organizations.

Disability insurance is also available through many companies. This type of insurance is designed to protect athletes against future loss of earnings because of a disabling injury or sickness that occurred while they were engaged in sport activities. The NCAA sponsors a disability insurance program for exceptional student-athletes in football, men's and women's basketball, baseball, and men's ice hockey (NCAA 2010). The NCAA also sponsors a special

Among the many kinds of insurance are medical, health, athletic accident, catastrophic, and disability. Athletic accident insurance comes in one of three forms: primary coverage, secondary coverage, and self-insurance.

For a complete description of NCAA-sponsored insurance programs, visit the NCAA website at www.ncaa.org.

assistance fund program that may be used to pay for some medical and dental expenses for Division I student-athletes.

Finally, some insurance companies provide coverage for specific kinds of health-related problems. Dental insurance and vision insurance are two examples. These policies can be bought separately or added to broader health care plans as riders.

Experimental Therapy

Regardless of whether an athlete or other physically active patient is covered by medical, health, accident, or catastrophic insurance, the terms of most policies usually exclude **experimental treatments** and procedures (Newcomer 1990). A variety of medical and surgical techniques now common in sports medicine began as experimental therapies. Physicians, athletic trainers, and other health care professionals frequently experiment with new methods to help patients return to physical activity earlier and more safely. Unfortunately, the insurance industry often determines that a therapeutic method has made the transition from experimental to conventional several years after the medical profession does. Insurance companies define *experimental* in different ways, the best way being simply to list in the policy what they consider experimental procedures. Another method that companies sometimes employ is to list the criteria by which they will determine if a procedure is experimental. This method is less exact and more difficult to defend in the courts. The final, and most common, method insurance companies use is to decide on a case-by-case basis which methods are experimental. The case-by-case decision method can be frustrating for patients and health care providers because they don't know what the insurance company will pay for and what it will not.

Surgical procedures that are considered **elective** or **diagnostic** may also be excluded from health insurance coverage policies. Elective surgical procedures are those that are not considered necessary from a medical perspective; instead, having them performed is the individual's choice. As an example, an athlete who has 20/25 vision and is able to read, write, and participate in sports without harmful risk might opt for a vision correction procedure that would improve his vision to 20/20. Though the procedure would clearly improve the individual's visual sense, it might not be considered medically necessary. A diagnostic procedure, performed on occasions when a specific diagnosis cannot be made from clinical findings and would be more accurately identified via a surgical procedure, would enable selection of the appropriate treatment intervention. In past years, the use of arthroscopy as a less invasive surgical technique for exploring joint pathology was found to be beneficial as a diagnostic procedure. Recently, the prevalence of arthroscopic diagnostic procedures has diminished as a result of the surgical risks and liability associated with not knowing a specific diagnosis before performing surgery on an individual.

Usual, Customary, and Reasonable Fees

Another insurance concept that athletic trainers should understand is **usual, customary, and reasonable (UCR)** reimbursement for medical services. The UCR concept is a flexible-fee system originally developed by the federal government to reimburse health care providers through the Medicare system. Most insurance companies now use this system. A combination of the following factors determines the amount of money that insurance companies will pay to health care providers for a particular service under the UCR system:

- The usual fee charged by each health care provider for the particular service
- The customary fee for the geographic area (either the average fee or the **90th-percentile fee**, whichever is lowest)
- The reasonable fee (the lower of either the usual or customary fee)

To reduce the likelihood of having a claim denied, an athletic trainer should make sure that physicians and other health care providers the patient will be referred to will perform only nonexperimental procedures and that they will accept the UCR fee as payment in full for services rendered. If the planned procedure could potentially be considered experimental, the athletic trainer should consult a representative of the insurance company before referral.

Even the most circumspect athletic trainer will have claims denied from time to time for reasons that might not seem fair. Lawsuits to recover the costs of denied claims should be the last option. The following suggestions might help resolve claims denied because of experimental treatment or UCR clauses:

- Find out the exact reasons the claim was denied. The law requires insurance companies to provide this information.

- Obtain a statement from the physician or other health care provider explaining why the treatment was implemented and justifying the fee.

- If the self-insurance fund of a parent's employer covers a patient, correspond with the employer directly. The employer, not the insurance administrator, has final legal authority to reverse the denial.

- Provide evidence from clinical studies to support your claim that the treatment should not be considered experimental.

- Try to convince the physician or other health care provider to waive the portion of the fee above the UCR amount.

- Contact the state insurance commissioner and request assistance in challenging the denial.

Types of Athletic Insurance

Educational institutions can choose from three options when designing a medical insurance system for their student-athletes: self-insurance, primary coverage, and secondary coverage (Hart and Cole 1992). As with any management option, each system has advantages and disadvantages, including cost.

Self-Insurance

Institutions that choose to self-insure are speculating that the amount they pay out for medical expenses will be less than the amount they will pay for insurance premiums. The institution typically purchases no medical or accident insurance except for catastrophic coverage and pays medical bills incurred by student-athletes. Many national governing organizations such as the NCAA have rules that prevent educational institutions from paying for medical expenses not directly related to participation in intercollegiate or interscholastic athletics. Institutions that self-insure must be particularly careful to create and monitor procedures used to ensure compliance with these rules. Compliance and clearly disseminated policies are of particular importance as they relate to off-season conditioning programs and other directed activities performed absent the supervision of official personnel.

Self-insuring offers several advantages. Saving money is possible, because the institution retains the potential profit that an insurance company normally earns. Processing claims is

---

■ Advantages and Disadvantages of Self-Insurance

Advantages	Disadvantages
■ Potential savings	■ High risk for large claims
■ Simplified claims process	■ Risk of bankrupting fund
■ Greater flexibility	■ Institutional dollars tied up

also simplified because there are no insurance claim forms to complete. Institutions have the flexibility to pay for procedures that a normal insurance policy might exclude.

Although cost can be an advantage with self-insurance, it can be a significant disadvantage as well. A large claim can deplete an institution's insurance fund, making it difficult or impossible to pay other, less costly claims. For that reason, it is typically large, financially healthy university athletic programs that employ self-insurance. One method of providing for the possibility of a large claim is to set aside leftover insurance funds in an endowment account that will eventually provide a cushion against large claims. The disadvantage of this method is that it ties up a substantial amount of money that the institution could use for more productive purposes. Institutions that self-insure can decrease their annual expenses by using a student-athlete's personal insurance as the primary source of coverage wherever possible. In this case, the institution becomes a secondary payer. The following sections discuss primary and secondary coverage.

Primary Coverage

Primary coverage is medical or accident insurance that begins to pay for covered medical expenses as soon as the institution pays the deductible. The athlete's (or the athlete's parents') personal medical insurance is not a source for payment of medical bills arising out of athletic participation. Institutions adopt primary insurance plans for a variety of reasons. Some feel a moral obligation to pay for all athletic medical expenses without involving families or their insurance companies. Others have a student population that is substantially uninsured anyway, so it is logical to choose primary coverage. Finally, primary coverage simplifies and accelerates claims processing because the family does not need to be involved.

The disadvantage of primary coverage is the expense. Because the insurance company takes on all the risk for an institution's student-athletes, as opposed to sharing the risk with personal medical insurance, it must charge a substantially higher premium for the coverage. Hart and Cole (1992) point out that the number of schools that purchased primary coverage for their athletic medicine programs dropped from 30% in 1982 to about 5% in 1992. The percentage of educational institutions that purchased primary coverage in 2002 was less than 1% (John Griesbach, conversation with author, July 2003).

Secondary Coverage

Secondary coverage, also known as *excess insurance,* is a policy that pays for covered medical expenses only after all other insurance policies, including the athlete's personal medical insurance, have reached their limit. Most institutions select this type of insurance plan (Lehr 1992). The most obvious benefit of this approach is that institutions can lower their costs by spreading the risk associated with athletic injuries to other potential payers. Because personal insurance companies share the risk, the cost of secondary coverage can be as much as 60% lower than the cost of primary coverage. Another, less tangible benefit is that this approach, if used properly, can help develop a sense of shared responsibility for safety in an athletic program. Most parents want to provide a safe environment for their children. Presumably, their interest rises when they have a financial interest as well. An additional advantage of the secondary approach is that it encourages athletic administrators to find ways to reduce and control medical costs. See the following section for an expanded discussion.

■ Reasons for Purchasing Primary Insurance Coverage

- Sense of responsibility for paying all medical expenses
- Large percentage of uninsured student-athletes
- Simplified and accelerated claims processing

The disadvantages of secondary coverage relate to claims processing. Because personal insurance serves as a primary layer of coverage, an institution must spend substantial time and energy communicating with parents and their insurance carriers to move claims along. This process can delay settling insurance claims, which can frustrate medical vendors that the institution wants to keep happy. Another potential problem is that the secondary system requires more communication and understanding about the shared responsibility for paying medical costs. In the opening case, misunderstandings about how the school's policy worked were a major part of the problem. The school found itself in a position in which administrators felt pressured to pay for Sven's medical treatment even though the injury occurred before Sven arrived at the school.

Ethical dilemmas may also arise when organizations institute secondary insurance policies. Parents of student-athletes who use their own insurance as a primary insurance will realize that their claims may rise and thus their future deductibles may also increase. In contrast, if they do not include their son or daughter as a dependent on their insurance plan, then the student-athlete would have no primary coverage, leaving the school to absorb all medical costs associated with claims. In this case, the parents will have recognized that they would not be responsible under their own insurance plan for athletically related medical bills.

Reducing Insurance Costs

Premiums for medical or accident insurance are closely linked to an institution's past claims history, enhancing the incentives for institutions to establish risk management programs and decrease medical costs. Insurance companies track the cost of claims made by an institution and compare those costs to the premium that the institution pays. Because all insurance companies must make a profit to stay in business, they will adjust the premium to help ensure that it will cover the likely cost of the claims, the administration of those claims, and the desired profit margin. Some insurance companies adjust premiums every year in an effort to balance this equation. Others make adjustments less frequently so that over the long term, say five years, they meet their financial goals.

In any case, athletic trainers and other members of the sports medicine team can help their institutions keep insurance premiums to a minimum by instituting the following measures. Keep in mind that institutional philosophy will govern which, if any, of these suggestions the institution will adopt.

- Spread the risk among all concerned parties. The best way to do this is to buy secondary coverage so that the personal insurance of athletes or their parents becomes the primary source of payment for athletic injuries.
- Adopt and communicate policies that limit the institution's financial obligations to those injuries that the school's insurance policy covers. For example, some athletic accident policies exclude certain kinds of conditions (for example, stress fractures). The institution can limit its financial risk if it also refuses to pay for those kinds of injuries. To do otherwise results in institutional expenditures far in excess of the annual insurance

■ Advantages and Disadvantages of Secondary Insurance Coverage

Advantages	Disadvantages
■ Less costly	■ Longer claims process
■ Shared responsibility	■ Requires more communication
■ Promotes cost controls	■ Labor-intensive claims process

premium. Despite clear communication regarding such policies, one should always expect to exercise diplomatic skills with parents and caregivers when such noncovered injuries and illnesses arise. It is not uncommon for people not to pay attention to the details of documents, policies, and procedures prior to the occurrence of an injury or illness. Unfortunately, if they have not acknowledged agreement to guidelines and instead learn of the guidelines only after the occurrence of adverse events, there may be disagreement regarding the policy and who should be responsible for payment.

■ Insist that athletes buy their own personal insurance. Remember, even if the institution has secondary coverage, it will end up paying from the first dollar of the claim for injured athletes without their own personal insurance. Some institutions will not allow students to participate in athletic programs without their own personal insurance. Other institutions provide their students with the opportunity to buy university-sponsored health insurance; unfortunately, most of these policies have relatively low coverage caps and will not pay for injuries associated with intercollegiate athletics. When working at the collegiate level for a program that offers scholarships to student-athletes, an athletic trainer should be prepared to hear the expressed concerns of coaches who feel that requiring an incoming student-athlete to have a primary insurance coverage plan is an obstacle to their recruiting efforts.

■ Pass the cost—or some fraction of the cost—of the athletic accident insurance along to the athletes by requiring them to pay a modest sum for the insurance.

■ Limit the institution's financial obligation for costs associated with athletic injuries to those medical services that an institutional representative, usually the athletic trainer or team physician, has preapproved. In effect, you will be creating your own health maintenance organization, because all injured athletes will have to pass through a gatekeeper to have the school or its insurance company cover the cost of their injuries. Injured athletes could still receive medical care from the provider of their choice, but they would have to pay for it if they did not use the services of the athletic trainer, team physician, or some other approved provider (Ray 1996). Establishing precedent and extremely clear guidelines for any exceptions to this model is critical to the success of an internal gatekeeper-type model.

■ Encourage medical providers to treat athletes from your institution on an "insurance only" basis. If the physician is willing to accept whatever the athlete's personal insurance will pay as payment in full, little or no cost will be passed on to the institution or its insurance company.

■ Require injured athletes covered by managed care plans to use medical providers approved by the plan. Many managed care plans, especially health maintenance organizations, will not pay for medical services provided by out-of-plan physicians. These costs are usually passed on to the institution.

■ Conduct annual risk assessment audits to help reduce the incidence of athletic injuries (see chapter 8).

THIRD-PARTY REIMBURSEMENT

Third-party reimbursement is the process by which health care practitioners receive reimbursement from a policyholder's insurance company for services they perform. A **third party** is defined as a person, in this case a medical vendor, who has no binding interest in a particular contract (the insurance policy). Third-party reimbursement is the primary mechanism of paying for medical services in the United States. Hospitals and private practice health professionals rely heavily on third-party reimbursement to generate the income that keeps their practices in business.

Third-party reimbursement is a growing but still relatively new practice for athletic trainers. Insurance companies, concerned about financial issues, have been slow to cover athletic trainers' services, even though the percentage of the population demanding those services is increasing. One of the main reasons related to lack of athletic training services reimbursement is the attainment of goals set forth with student-athletes by athletic trainers seeking remuneration for services. For example, in the general public sector, a patient may be discharged when she meets her activities of daily living (ADL) goals and is able to return to work. However, with athletes, simply returning to sport may be deemed a minimal-level goal. Treatment interventions may continue well beyond the return-to-play phase, and the services of the athletic trainer may extend daily throughout an athletic season. This can become costly to an insurance company, despite the fact that the athletic trainer may perceive the ongoing care as necessary for a higher level of performance as compared to the performance level of a nonathletic patient. Access to payment for athletic training services through insurance companies is becoming more available now that more states credential athletic trainers. In addition, outcome studies conducted by the National Athletic Trainers' Association (NATA) have demonstrated that athletic training services are cost efficient and effective in the treatment of injuries in physically active populations (Albohm and Wilkerson 1999). As more state athletic trainers' organizations lobby their insurance commissioners and legislators for access to third-party billing (with the help of the NATA), the number of athletic trainers who receive payment for their services in this manner is likely to increase.

Although athletic trainers have historically lacked direct access to third-party reimbursement, they are often responsible for generating significant amounts of reimbursable dollars for the clinics and hospitals that employ them; therefore, they must understand this aspect of insurance. Many athletic trainers employed in sports medicine clinics perform tasks nearly identical to those performed by the physical therapists with whom they often work side by side. Athletic trainers working in high school outreach programs are often responsible for bringing in referrals to the clinics that employ them. Many of these patients will pay for the services they receive by submitting a claim to their medical insurance carriers. While the athletic trainer who better understands third-party reimbursement in the private sector will be valuable to the clinical and business operations, he will also become a more valuable commodity and potentially establish the rationale for earning a higher than average wage for a clinical athletic trainer.

Some athletic trainers in university sports medicine programs seek third-party reimbursement from their student-athletes' personal insurance companies. This practice is controversial, however, and some leaders in the profession have criticized it because it creates the feeling that athletic trainers might prioritize their treatment of student-athletes based on insurance coverage (Godek 1992).

Types of Third-Party Payers

There are several models of third-party payment. Many health plans offer several models to their enrollees. Some companies even develop hybrid plans that mix the characteristics of the following models:

- Private medical insurance companies provide group and individual coverage for employees and their dependents. The medical insurance that these companies provide is typically the traditional **fee-for-service plan**. This insurance model is also known as an *indemnity plan* (DeCarlo 1997). Patients are free to go to the medical provider of their choice. The plan reimburses a portion of the cost of covered services, and the patient is responsible for the copayment or deductible. The managed care models described next are rapidly replacing fee-for-service plans.

- **Health maintenance organizations (HMOs)** provide participating health care practitioners with a fixed fee for services rendered to members. A **capitation** (per person)

Athletic trainers who work in hospitals and clinics might earn a portion of their income through third-party reimbursement. Reimbursement through this system requires knowledge of diagnostic and procedural coding and strict adherence to certain legal requirements on the part of the athletic trainer.

For an excellent summary of the different health care insurance options available to consumers, see the Health Insurance Association of America's website at www.ahip.org/. Click on "Consumer Information" and then on "Consumer Guides."

system usually, but not always, determines fees. HMOs that do not use a capitation system usually reimburse providers based on a fixed-fee schedule. Patients insured by an HMO must use a primary care provider that participates in the HMO. A modest copayment is usually charged. Some HMOs provide services at medical facilities, whereas others provide care through a network of individual medical practitioners (**individual practice associations**, or **IPAs**).

■ **Preferred provider organizations (PPOs)** operate similarly to HMOs but usually allow greater choice of health care providers and pay medical vendors on a fee-for-service rather than a capitated basis. PPOs allow policyholders to choose any health care provider they wish but offer financial incentives for policyholders to use providers identified by the PPO. When patients choose to see a medical provider who does not belong to the PPO, they can expect to pay for a greater percentage of the cost of the services. One variant of the PPO is the **exclusive provider organization (EPO)**; participants enrolled in these can receive benefits only from contracting medical providers (May, Schraeder, and Britt 1996; O'Leary 1994).

■ A **point-of-service plan (POS)** is similar to a PPO. The primary difference between the two is that POS plans assign primary care physicians, who act as gatekeepers by coordinating patient care. Most PPO plans do not.

■ Government-sponsored programs provide coverage for the elderly (Medicare), the needy (Medicaid), and members of the armed forces and their dependents (TRICARE, formally known as CHAMPUS).

Legal Requirements

Among the many legal considerations in third-party reimbursement, one of the most important is the requirement that health care practitioners obtain signed authorization from a patient for release of medical records. Unless the patient authorizes such a release, the patient–practitioner relationship requires the medical vendor to keep information confidential. Third-party payers, however, will not process claims unless they have access to the information to substantiate them.

Another legal issue related to confidentiality of the medical record involves answering an insurance company's questions about a patient's case over the telephone. Athletic trainers should always verify the identity of the caller and be sure that the patient has signed an authorization for release of medical records before answering questions over the phone. Rowell (1989) suggests the following steps:

■ With the patient's claim form in hand, ask the caller to read a portion of the information to verify that the caller has the original.

■ If the caller is requesting a detailed explanation, ask the caller to submit the questions in writing on company letterhead.

■ Ask the caller for the insurance company's telephone number. Call the person back through the company switchboard to verify identity.

■ Never answer questions from attorneys until the authorization for release of information is in hand, even if the attorney claims to have it. The best practice is to correspond by mail with attorneys regarding insurance reimbursement cases.

■ Any medical information requested by a recruiter, scout, coach, agent, or other member affiliated with a college or professional team should be disseminated only after receipt of written permission on a case-by-case basis from the student-athlete, or the parent of the student-athlete in the case of a minor.

Fraud is another legal pitfall athletic trainers must avoid in the third-party reimbursement process. Fraud is a significant problem in the insurance industry. The federal government's General Accounting Office estimates that health care insurance fraud accounts for 10% of all health care expenditures—nearly $100 billion per year (Health Insurance Association of America 1999). An athletic trainer must never change the date of an injury, treatment, or assessment, or fail to record payments from an insurance company on a patient's bill. Other fraudulent acts committed by unscrupulous health care providers include claiming reimbursement for treatments that were not provided and increasing the charges for treatments for patients with insurance. The penalties for medical fraud are substantial and can include fines of $2,000 per occurrence plus twice the amount of the false claim.

Diagnostic and Procedural Coding

Reimbursement for sports medicine and all other medical services is based on the coding system used when submitting claims to third-party payers. Two kinds of codes must be submitted—diagnostic and procedural.

Diagnostic coding is required for all forms of third-party billing. The *International Classification of Diseases (ICD-10-CM)* is a book specifying the code that should be applied to every injury or condition that athletic trainers or other health professionals treat. The system defines each condition as a five-digit code that must be entered on all claim forms. Table 7.1 is an example of the diagnostic code for acute sprains and strains of the ankle and foot.

The **Current Procedural Terminology (CPT)** is a list of codes published by the American Medical Association that represents the vast majority of medical procedures. The person completing a claim form for sports medicine services selects the most appropriate code for each of the services rendered. Some examples of common CPT codes employed in sports medicine settings appear in table 7.2.

The importance of carefully checking the accuracy of the diagnostic and procedural codes listed on the claim form cannot be overstated. Using improper codes will significantly increase the time required by the insurance company to process the claim and might result in denial of the claim.

> Information pertaining to the Current Procedural Terminology is available at www.ama-assn.org. Click on "Coding Billing Insurance" in the "Current Procedural Terminology" section.

TABLE 7.1 ICD-10-CM Codes for the Foot and Ankle

Code	Subcode 1	Subcode 2	Condition
845			Sprains and strains of the foot and ankle
	845.0		Ankle
		845.00	Unspecified site
		845.01	Deltoid (ligament), ankle
		845.02	Calcaneofibular (ligament)
		845.03	Tibiofibular (ligament), distal
		845.09	Other
	845.1		Foot
		845.10	Unspecified site
		845.11	Tarsometatarsal (joint) (ligament)
		845.12	Metatarsalphalangeal (joint)
		845.13	Interphalangeal (joint)
		845.19	Other

> A thorough description of physical medicine and rehabilitation codes used by athletic trainers can be found at www.nata.org/sites/default/files/RehabCodes_0.pdf. Resources for revenue generation for athletic trainers can be found at www.nata.org; click on "Revenue Resources."

TABLE 7.2 CPT Codes for Common Athletic Training Services

Category	Code	Procedure
Evaluation	97005/97006	Athletic trainer evaluation and reevaluation (per visit)
	97750	Physical performance or measurement test with written report (each 15 minutes)
Treatment	97116	Gait training (each 15 minutes)
	97110	Therapeutic exercise (each 15 minutes)
	97112	Neuromuscular reeducation (each 15 minutes)
	97530	Therapeutic activities direct (each 15 minutes)
	97113	Aquatic therapeutic exercise (each 15 minutes)
	97124	Massage (each 15 minutes)
	97530	Body mechanics training (each 15 minutes)
	97140	Manual therapy (each 15 minutes)
	97760	Orthotics fitting and training (each 15 minutes)
	97150	Therapeutic procedures—group (each visit)
	97597	Wound care (each 15 minutes)
	97139	Taping (each visit) 29240 Shoulder strapping/taping 29260 Elbow/wrist strapping/taping 29280 Hand/finger strapping/taping 29520 Hip strapping/taping 29530 Knee strapping/taping 29540 Ankle strapping/taping 29550 Toes strapping/taping 29580 Unna boot
	95831	Manual muscle testing—extremity or trunk
Modalities	97035	Ultrasound (each 15 minutes)
	97032	Electrical stimulation manual (each 15 minutes)
	97033	Iontophoresis (each 15 minutes)
	97032	Constant electrical stimulation—constant supervision (each 15 minutes)
	97034	Contrast baths (each 15 minutes)
	97014	Electric stimulation—intermittent supervision (each visit)
	97022	Whirlpool (each visit)
	97010	Hot packs (each visit)
	97010	Cold packs (each visit)
	97012	Mechanical traction (each visit)
	97016	Compression pump (each visit)

CLAIMS PROCESSING

Filing claims quickly and properly is one of an athletic trainer's most important insurance functions. The claims process for athletic trainers in educational settings is distinctly different from that of athletic trainers in private or hospital-based sports medicine clinics. Athletic trainers in educational settings file all (or nearly all) claims with a single insurance company to pay other medical vendors for services rendered to the institution's student-athletes, whereas athletic trainers in sports medicine clinics file claims with a wide range of insurance companies for reimbursement for services they provide. Some universities operate their athletic training programs like sports medicine clinics by routinely seeking third-party reimbursement. The two settings will be discussed separately, however, because the claims process is usually different in each.

Claims processing is the act of formally communicating with an insurance company or other third-party payer to seek payment for services rendered to an injured patient. The process is different for athletic trainers working in educational settings than it is for those working in sports medicine clinics.

Claims Processing in Educational Settings

An athletic trainer can take preliminary steps to make claims processing easier. One of the most important is to gather insurance information for every student-athlete in the program (Frankel 1991). The athletic trainer can often accomplish this task well in advance of the season. For participants who are not identified until the beginning of the season, the preseason physical exam offers an excellent opportunity to collect the information. Personal insurance information forms should be updated annually. Another preparatory step that will save time and avoid confusion after an injury occurs is to communicate by letter with the parents of all student-athletes, informing them of the limits of the school's accident insurance policy and the steps they will need to take to process an insurance claim (see figure 7.2). If the school has a secondary policy, be sure to explain to parents that they must submit all medical bills to their insurance company before submitting the balance to the school.

Dear Student-Athlete and Parents:

At the beginning of every sports season, the athletic department sends the parents of each student-athlete information regarding our insurance coverage. We hope all participants will be injury free; however, if an athlete is accidentally injured, the following information should be useful.

If a student-athlete is accidentally injured and generates medical expenses associated with the accident, all claims must be filed first with the student's or parents' personal insurance company. If a balance remains after the personal insurance company has paid its maximum, that balance will be submitted to the school's athletic accident insurance company. If covered, the school's insurance company will pay the balance of the eligible medical expenses not covered by the personal insurance company up to the maximum of the policy. This excess insurance program is being used at many of the nation's high schools and colleges.

The school's insurance policy covers only new accidents that are sustained during competition or supervised practice. Any bills related to injuries that fall into the category above should be mailed to the athletic department only after first being submitted to the personal insurance company. Preexisting injuries, off-season injuries, injuries incurred during the season that are not directly related to in-season competition or supervised practice (physical education injuries, intramural injuries, etc.), or routine medical care (eye care, dental care, care for illnesses) are NOT COVERED. Also not covered are injuries or "conditions" caused by overuse, such as tendinitis and stress fracture. We strongly recommend that a personal health and accident insurance policy be maintained for all student-athletes.

If you have any questions regarding the accident insurance program, please feel free to contact us at your convenience. We look forward to serving you again this year and hope that your experience will be enjoyable and accident free.

Sincerely,

Athletic Director   Head Athletic Trainer

▶ **Figure 7.2** Sample letter to parents and student-athletes explaining the athletic accident insurance plan.

When the athletic trainer receives a bill for processing, he should create an insurance file for the student-athlete. Because the status of the claim will change, a useful approach is to color code each file according to its status with adhesive labels. As the status of the claim changes, a different-colored label can be applied over the old one. Consider the following system:

- Red label—bills and other information being collected, claim not yet submitted
- Yellow label—full claim submitted but not yet paid
- Green label—claim paid in full and case closed

Besides creating an individual insurance folder, the athletic trainer should enter each claim on an **insurance claim registry form** (see figure 7.3). This document provides the athletic trainer with a quick reference for determining which claims are paid and which are outstanding.

The athletic trainer should not submit any claim to the school's secondary insurance company before receiving an **explanation of benefits form (EOB)** from the athlete's personal insurance company. The EOB describes how the insurance company paid benefits for the claim. The EOB is proof of which bills the insurance company paid and to whom, either medical vendors or parents, the company wrote the checks (see figure 7.4).

INSURANCE CLAIMS TRACKING FORM					
Patient's name	Social security number	Insurance company	Date claim filed	Amount due	Amount of payment received

▶ **Figure 7.3** Sample insurance claim tracking form.

GOOD Insurance Company

Date:

EXPLANATION OF BENEFITS

EMPLOYEE: SSN:
GROUP: CLAIM #:
GROUP ID: DATE INCURRED:
PROCESSED BY: PATIENT:

TREATMENT DATES	CHARGE AMOUNT	PATIENT COPAY	NOT COVERED	REASON CODE	PPO DISCOUNT	ELIGIBLE CHARGES	DEDUCTIBLE AMOUNT	PCT	PAYMENT AMOUNT

TOTAL INDIVIDUAL DEDUCTIBLE MET $ TOTAL CHARGES $
TOTAL FAMILY DEDUCTIBLE MET $ LESS DEDUCTIBLE $
OUT-OF-POCKET YTD $ PATIENT RESPONSIBILITY $
     TOTAL PAYMENT $
     OTHER INSURANCE/ADJUSTMENTS $

PAYMENT DISTRIBUTION

CODE   PAYEE   AMOUNT   CHECK NUMBER

SERVICE CODE	REASON CODE

MESSAGES

IF THE PARTICIPANT BELIEVES THE CLAIM HAS BEEN IMPROPERLY DENIED, HE OR SHE HAS THE RIGHT TO HAVE IT RE-VIEWED. THE APPEAL MUST BE FILED IN WRITING WITHIN SIXTY (60) DAYS OF RECEIPT OF THIS WORKSHEET. ADDITIONAL INFORMATION ABOUT WHERE THE CLAIM SHOULD BE SENT IS CONTAINED IN THE EMPLOYEE BENEFIT HANDBOOK.

▶ **Figure 7.4** Sample explanation of benefits form.

HMOs, part of a larger concept in the medical insurance industry known as **managed care**, remain the predominant form of health insurance available (see figure 7.5). The Health Insurance Association of America (HIAA) estimated that the overall number of Americans in some type of managed care arrangement rose from 15 million individuals in 1984 to more than 75 million in 1995 (Agency for Health Care Research and Quality 1995). In fact, some form of managed care plan covers over half of all Americans who have health insurance (Health Insurance Association of America 2003a). If a student's personal insurance carrier is an HMO, the student will be required to seek treatment from a physician designated as her **primary care provider** except in life-threatening emergencies. This requirement frequently poses problems for athletic trainers because student-athletes must seek medical treatment from physicians not associated with the school's sports medicine program. Most HMOs refuse to pay for treatment performed by a nonparticipating physician or other health care provider without prior approval. When the athlete is a high school student living in the same town as her HMO physician, the problem is merely an inconvenience. When the athlete is a college student living hundreds of miles from home, however, the problem can become more serious. Most secondary carriers will not pay the full cost of an athletic accident if the student's HMO denies the claim because the student sought treatment from a physician outside the plan. Although some large university athletic programs might be able to absorb the costs incurred by avoiding the inconvenience of using a student-athlete's HMO-approved physician, most school- and college-based programs lack the financial resources to become, in effect, primary coverage providers for these students.

An athletic trainer can take several steps with students who are insured through an HMO:

- Contact the HMO in writing and request information about the procedure to be followed in the event of an athletic accident (see figure 7.6). Do this for all the managed care plans that operate in your area so that you can learn the limitations and rules for each of the policies.

- Place an "HMO ALERT" label on the athlete's medical record as a reminder to contact the HMO in the event of an injury that requires outside medical care.

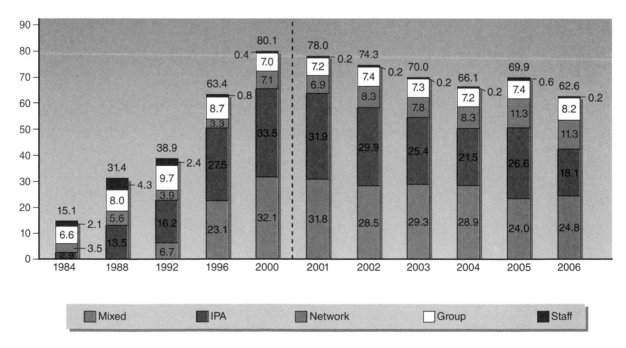

▶ **Figure 7.5** Enrollment in HMOs by model type. Enrollees are in millions.

"HMO Enrollment, by Model Type, 1984-2006", Kaiser Slides, The Henry J. Kaiser Family Foundation, January 2008. This information was reprinted with permission from the Henry J. Kaiser Family Foundation. The Kaiser Family Foundation is a non-profit private operating foundation, based in Mento Park, California, dedicated to producing and communicating the best possible analysis and information on health issues.

- If the student is in college and lives a great distance from the HMO service area, determine if the HMO will assign a physician in the local college community as the student's primary care provider during the time the student is in school.

- If the school's secondary insurance policy will not honor claims rejected by an HMO for noncompliance with the HMO plan, be sure to remind parents of that fact. This reminder should be part of a larger effort to educate parents and student-athletes about the institution's athletic accident insurance. Among the many ways to educate parents and student-athletes are brochures, letters, team meetings, and parent meetings. This educational effort will help prevent confusion and anger later if a claim is denied.

HMO/PPO Authorization Form   Name of Student-Athlete _____

Name of Covered Person _____
                                    (Parent or Guardian)

Name of Employer _____

HMO/PPO Certificate # _____

Dear _____ :

_____ is a student-athlete at _____College and has indicated that he/she is covered under your plan for health and accident coverage while he/she is a student here.

_____ is participating in our intercollegiate sports program and there is a possibility that he/she may suffer an accidental injury while competing. The athletic accident coverage purchased by _____College is an excess policy that requires all medical bills be first submitted to the student's primary health plan for payment before it assumes any liability. It also requires that all student-athletes must follow any procedures required by their HMO/PPO, should they be covered by such a plan.

As the head athletic trainer, it is my responsibility to process any insurance claims that are made by our student-athletes. I am requesting your assistance in properly administering your plan for _____ _____ .

If you have any printed material that would assist in this matter, please send it to me as soon as possible. If there is a phone number that should be called prior to _____ receiving any medical treatment, I request that you send it to me as well. It is most important that I be informed of all medical vendors in the immediate area of _____College that qualify under your plan to treat _____ .

At various times our athletic teams will be several hundred miles from our campus and I need to know the proper procedures for handling any emergency that might take place. I also need to know whether your coverage has a particular definition of "emergency" and whether there are different procedures for treating a life-threatening emergency and a less serious problem such as a fractured leg or dislocated shoulder, that requires the immediate attention of a physician.

Thanks in advance for your help. I look forward to your early reply.

Sincerely,

Head Athletic Trainer

▶ **Figure 7.6**   Sample HMO/PPO authorization form.

Adapted, by permission, from First Agency, Inc. HMO/PPO authorization (Kalamazoo, MI).

Insurance claim forms must be complete and accurate to be processed quickly. Athletic accident insurance claim forms have at least the following elements:

- Student's name and address (home and local when appropriate)
- Student's date of birth, sex, and year in school
- Sport in which the student was injured
- Date, time, and place of the accident
- Description of how the accident occurred
- Nature of the injuries suffered, including specific body parts
- Names and titles of witnesses to the accident
- Parent's medical insurance information

Finally, First Agency (www.1stagency.com/), one of the oldest and largest athletic accident insurers, recommends that athletic trainers avoid the following claims-processing pitfalls:

- Do not wait until an injury occurs to obtain the parent's insurance information from the student-athlete.
- Do not convey the impression that the institution will pay all expenses involving athletic injuries. This was one of the mistakes committed in the opening case study. One of the ways athletic departments can avoid this problem is to appoint a sole spokesperson who is responsible for managing the insurance program. All questions related to the insurance program should be directed to this person.
- Do not take primary responsibility for filing claims with the student's personal insurance company. Either the parents or the medical vendor should file such claims.
- Do not prepay medical vendors from the athletic budget. Prepaying can result in duplicate payments and arouse animosity between physicians and parents.
- Do not delay filing claims with either the primary or secondary insurers. Many policies have time limits beyond which they will not pay.
- Do not assume that medical bills have been filed with the parent's insurance company. Athletic trainers should contact parents soon after an injury occurs to remind them of the process for settling claims. In many cases, parents receive a bill and assume that the institution is taking care of it, causing delays in claim processing that lead to past-due accounts.
- Do not submit incomplete claims. Make sure that bills are itemized and accompanied by the parents' insurance information.

Claims Processing in Sports Medicine Clinics

The claims process in sports medicine clinics is fundamentally different from the process in educational institutions for two reasons. First, the athletic trainer or clinic administrator must integrate claims processing within the context of a larger patient billing system. Because of this arrangement, the livelihood of the sports medicine clinic depends on the ability to secure a steady flow of referrals from primary care physicians and specialists and to obtain reimbursement from third-party payers for patient bills. The second fundamental difference is that sports medicine clinics receive direct payments from third-party payers, whereas in the educational setting the money generally does not pass through the hands of an athletic trainer but goes directly to the medical vendor. This distinction is important, because it means that athletic trainers working in sports medicine clinics face a greater accounting burden than those working in educational institutions do.

One of the most important steps that athletic trainers in sports medicine clinics can take to ensure a smooth claims process is to seek prior authorization from a patient's insurance company before providing treatment. Some third-party payers, such as HMOs and PPOs, require this action; they usually will not provide reimbursement without preapproval by the primary care physician. Some Blue Cross plans will reimburse for rehabilitation and other sports medicine services, whereas other plans might not. The prudent clinic administrator should use the toll-free number provided by Blue Cross to determine in advance the limitations of the patient's policy.

Rowell (1989) suggests the following nine steps for filing insurance claims with third-party payers:

1. Complete the patient's charge slip, listing the patient's name, date of service, type of service, and balance due.
2. Convert all the procedures performed to CPT codes and list prices.
3. List all procedures, charges, and payments in a daily office ledger and the patient's individual ledger.
4. Complete the claim form. Most third-party payers will accept the **CMS 1500** claim form from private practice clinics (see figure 7.7). The **UB-04**, also known as the **CMS 1450**, is the appropriate form for hospitals (see figure 7.8).
5. Obtain the authorized signature on the claim form. In most sports medicine clinics, the chief physical therapist must sign claims. In clinics owned by physicians, usually one of the physicians must sign.
6. Place a copy of the insurance claim form in the patient's record.
7. Enter the claim on the insurance claim registry form.
8. Mail (or transmit electronically) the claim form to the insurance company.
9. Note on the patient's ledger that the claim has been submitted to the insurance company, and mail an informational copy of the ledger to the patient.

The CMS 1500 is available in electronic format from www.cms.gov/. Search "CMS 1500." The UB-04, also known as the CMS 1450, is available in electronic format from www.cms.gov/. Search "CMS 1450."

Medical practice software packages that help automate many of the steps for filing insurance claims are available. In addition, some insurance companies allow medical vendors to submit their claims either in the traditional manner, as just described, or in a scannable format. Preparing the scannable claim form (according to insurance company specifications) allows for quicker claims processing because a scanner automatically enters it into the insurance company's computer system. Claims that require any written explanation, however, will usually be held for review by a processing clerk.

Another option available through some insurance companies allows medical vendors to submit claims electronically using **electronic data interchange (EDI)**. A claim form is completed on the computer screen and then downloaded to the insurance company's computer with a modem and communications software. This method is the quickest way to obtain reimbursement for standard claims because the claim arrives at the insurance company, for all practical purposes, as soon as the clinic sends it.

It is not uncommon to have submitted claims returned with payment denied. This can occur for a variety of reasons; some of these are incomplete or unsigned forms, services rendered by an ineligible provider, lack of medical necessity, services considered to be "maintenance" without expectations for improvement, invoices not submitted within a specific time period, no physician prescription, or a difference in diagnosis from that of the referring physician's office (Konin and Frederick 2005). Providers may take up to 30 to 90 days to pay an invoice even without an initial denial. If a claim is denied, it can be resubmitted as an appeal after corrections are noted by the payer.

The Committee on Revenue of the National Athletic Trainers' Association offers members an excellent guide to help athletic trainers who wish to charge for their services.

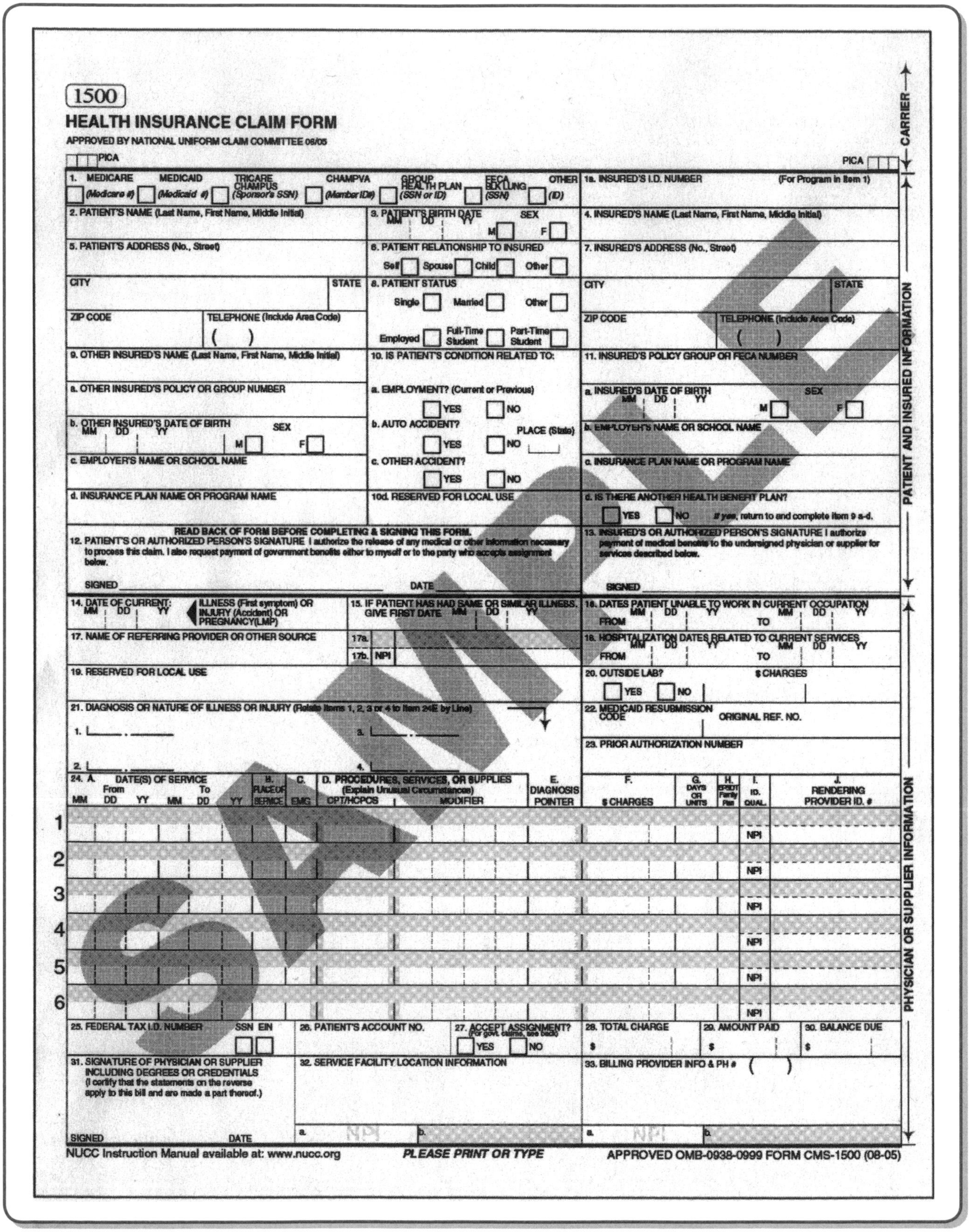

1500

HEALTH INSURANCE CLAIM FORM

APPROVED BY NATIONAL UNIFORM CLAIM COMMITTEE 08/05

PICA | PICA

1. MEDICARE (Medicare #) | MEDICAID (Medicaid #) | TRICARE CHAMPUS (Sponsor's SSN) | CHAMPVA (Member ID#) | GROUP HEALTH PLAN (SSN or ID) | FECA BLK LUNG (SSN) | OTHER (ID)

1a. INSURED'S I.D. NUMBER (For Program in Item 1)

2. PATIENT'S NAME (Last Name, First Name, Middle Initial)

3. PATIENT'S BIRTH DATE MM DD YY SEX M F

4. INSURED'S NAME (Last Name, First Name, Middle Initial)

5. PATIENT'S ADDRESS (No., Street)

6. PATIENT RELATIONSHIP TO INSURED Self Spouse Child Other

7. INSURED'S ADDRESS (No., Street)

CITY | STATE

8. PATIENT STATUS Single Married Other

CITY | STATE

ZIP CODE | TELEPHONE (Include Area Code) ( )

Employed | Full-Time Student | Part-Time Student

ZIP CODE | TELEPHONE (Include Area Code) ( )

9. OTHER INSURED'S NAME (Last Name, First Name, Middle Initial)

10. IS PATIENT'S CONDITION RELATED TO:

11. INSURED'S POLICY GROUP OR FECA NUMBER

a. OTHER INSURED'S POLICY OR GROUP NUMBER

a. EMPLOYMENT? (Current or Previous) YES NO

a. INSURED'S DATE OF BIRTH MM DD YY SEX M F

b. OTHER INSURED'S DATE OF BIRTH MM DD YY SEX M F

b. AUTO ACCIDENT? YES NO PLACE (State)

b. EMPLOYER'S NAME OR SCHOOL NAME

c. EMPLOYER'S NAME OR SCHOOL NAME

c. OTHER ACCIDENT? YES NO

c. INSURANCE PLAN NAME OR PROGRAM NAME

d. INSURANCE PLAN NAME OR PROGRAM NAME

10d. RESERVED FOR LOCAL USE

d. IS THERE ANOTHER HEALTH BENEFIT PLAN? YES NO *If yes*, return to and complete item 9 a-d.

READ BACK OF FORM BEFORE COMPLETING & SIGNING THIS FORM.

12. PATIENT'S OR AUTHORIZED PERSON'S SIGNATURE I authorize the release of any medical or other information necessary to process this claim. I also request payment of government benefits either to myself or to the party who accepts assignment below.

SIGNED ______ DATE ______

13. INSURED'S OR AUTHORIZED PERSON'S SIGNATURE I authorize payment of medical benefits to the undersigned physician or supplier for services described below.

SIGNED ______

14. DATE OF CURRENT: MM DD YY ◄ ILLNESS (First symptom) OR INJURY (Accident) OR PREGNANCY(LMP)

15. IF PATIENT HAS HAD SAME OR SIMILAR ILLNESS. GIVE FIRST DATE MM DD YY

16. DATES PATIENT UNABLE TO WORK IN CURRENT OCCUPATION FROM MM DD YY TO MM DD YY

17. NAME OF REFERRING PROVIDER OR OTHER SOURCE | 17a. | 17b. NPI

18. HOSPITALIZATION DATES RELATED TO CURRENT SERVICES FROM MM DD YY TO MM DD YY

19. RESERVED FOR LOCAL USE

20. OUTSIDE LAB? YES NO | $ CHARGES

21. DIAGNOSIS OR NATURE OF ILLNESS OR INJURY (Relate Items 1, 2, 3 or 4 to Item 24E by Line)

1. ___ . ___   3. ___ . ___

2. ___ . ___   4. ___ . ___

22. MEDICAID RESUBMISSION CODE | ORIGINAL REF. NO.

23. PRIOR AUTHORIZATION NUMBER

24. A. DATE(S) OF SERVICE From MM DD YY To MM DD YY	B. PLACE OF SERVICE	C. EMG	D. PROCEDURES, SERVICES, OR SUPPLIES (Explain Unusual Circumstances) CPT/HCPCS MODIFIER	E. DIAGNOSIS POINTER	F. $ CHARGES	G. DAYS OR UNITS	H. EPSDT Family Plan	I. ID. QUAL.	J. RENDERING PROVIDER ID. #
1								NPI	
2								NPI	
3								NPI	
4								NPI	
5								NPI	
6								NPI	

25. FEDERAL TAX I.D. NUMBER SSN EIN

26. PATIENT'S ACCOUNT NO.

27. ACCEPT ASSIGNMENT? (For govt. claims, see back) YES NO

28. TOTAL CHARGE $

29. AMOUNT PAID $

30. BALANCE DUE $

31. SIGNATURE OF PHYSICIAN OR SUPPLIER INCLUDING DEGREES OR CREDENTIALS (I certify that the statements on the reverse apply to this bill and are made a part thereof.)

SIGNED DATE

32. SERVICE FACILITY LOCATION INFORMATION

a. NPI b.

33. BILLING PROVIDER INFO & PH # ( )

a. NPI b.

NUCC Instruction Manual available at: www.nucc.org

PLEASE PRINT OR TYPE

APPROVED OMB-0938-0999 FORM CMS-1500 (08-05)

CARRIER

PATIENT AND INSURED INFORMATION

PHYSICIAN OR SUPPLIER INFORMATION

SAMPLE

▶ **Figure 7.7** CMS 1500.

Reprinted from Centers for Medicare and Medicaid Services. Available: www.cms.gov/cmsforms/downloads/CMS1500805.pdf

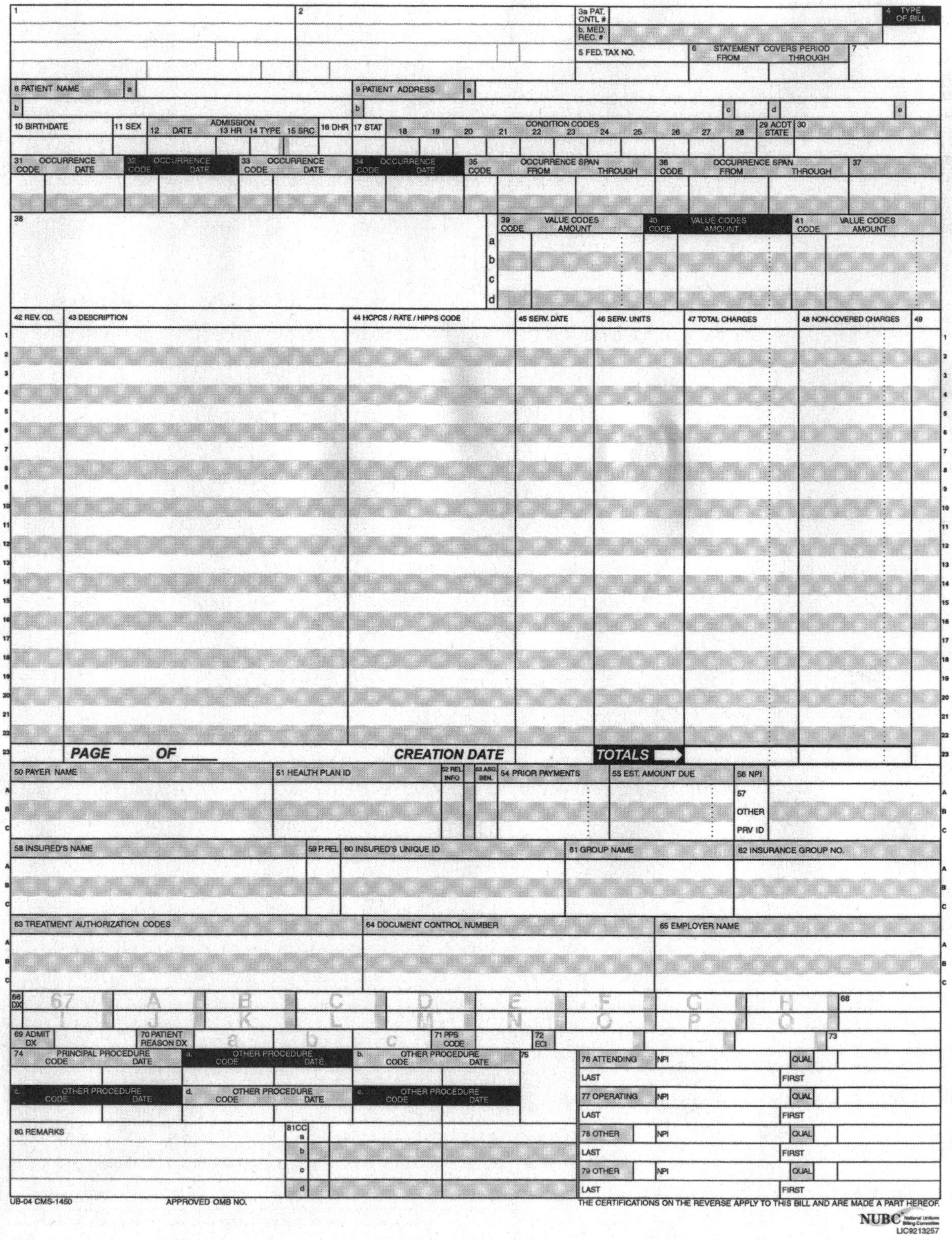
1
2
3a PAT. CNTL #
b. MED. REC. #
4 TYPE OF BILL
5 FED. TAX NO.
6 STATEMENT COVERS PERIOD FROM THROUGH
7
8 PATIENT NAME a b
9 PATIENT ADDRESS a b c d e
10 BIRTHDATE | 11 SEX | ADMISSION 12 DATE 13 HR 14 TYPE 15 SRC | 16 DHR | 17 STAT | CONDITION CODES 18 19 20 21 22 23 24 25 26 27 28 | 29 ACDT STATE | 30
31 OCCURRENCE CODE DATE | 32 OCCURRENCE CODE DATE | 33 OCCURRENCE CODE DATE | 34 OCCURRENCE CODE DATE | 35 CODE OCCURRENCE SPAN FROM THROUGH | 36 CODE OCCURRENCE SPAN FROM THROUGH | 37
38 | 39 VALUE CODES CODE AMOUNT | 40 VALUE CODES CODE AMOUNT | 41 VALUE CODES CODE AMOUNT (a b c d)
42 REV. CD. | 43 DESCRIPTION | 44 HCPCS / RATE / HIPPS CODE | 45 SERV. DATE | 46 SERV. UNITS | 47 TOTAL CHARGES | 48 NON-COVERED CHARGES | 49
1–23
PAGE ____ OF ____ CREATION DATE TOTALS
50 PAYER NAME | 51 HEALTH PLAN ID | 52 REL. INFO | 53 ASG. BEN. | 54 PRIOR PAYMENTS | 55 EST. AMOUNT DUE | 56 NPI | 57 OTHER PRV ID (A B C)
58 INSURED'S NAME | 59 P. REL | 60 INSURED'S UNIQUE ID | 61 GROUP NAME | 62 INSURANCE GROUP NO. (A B C)
63 TREATMENT AUTHORIZATION CODES | 64 DOCUMENT CONTROL NUMBER | 65 EMPLOYER NAME (A B C)
66 DX | 67 A B C D E F G H | I J K L M N O P Q | 68
69 ADMIT DX | 70 PATIENT REASON DX a b c | 71 PPS CODE | 72 ECI | 73
74 PRINCIPAL PROCEDURE CODE DATE | a. OTHER PROCEDURE CODE DATE | b. OTHER PROCEDURE CODE DATE | 75
c. OTHER PROCEDURE CODE DATE | d. OTHER PROCEDURE CODE DATE | e. OTHER PROCEDURE CODE DATE
76 ATTENDING NPI QUAL LAST FIRST
77 OPERATING NPI QUAL LAST FIRST
78 OTHER NPI QUAL LAST FIRST
79 OTHER NPI QUAL LAST FIRST
80 REMARKS | 81CC a b c d
UB-04 CMS-1450 APPROVED OMB NO. THE CERTIFICATIONS ON THE REVERSE APPLY TO THIS BILL AND ARE MADE A PART HEREOF.
NUBC National Uniform Billing Committee LIC9213257

▶ **Figure 7.8** UB-04 (also CMS 1450).

Reprinted from Centers for Medicare and Medicaid Services. Available: www.cms.gov/Transmittals/downloads/R1104CP.pdf

Athletic trainers should work with an insurance agent to purchase insurance services. Although athletic trainers can buy insurance directly or by bidding, those pursuing this option should always be sure to determine the layers and limits of the coverage, deductibles and copayments that might be required, and exclusions to the policy.

PURCHASING INSURANCE SERVICES

An athletic trainer might have the responsibility for evaluating and buying an athletic accident policy for a school sports medicine program. A variety of persons, including athletic directors, business office personnel, and risk managers, often share this function. Even if athletic trainers are not directly involved in evaluating and selecting insurance, they should not hesitate to offer their input, especially if they will be responsible for implementing the system.

Insurance is usually purchased through an agent. The U.S. Small Business Administration (1981) suggests that well-qualified **insurance agents** should be able to

- provide advice on the type and amount of insurance required,
- provide suggestions on the specific details of insurance policies, and
- provide timely service in the event of a claim.

Like sports medicine supplies and equipment, athletic accident insurance can be purchased in a variety of ways. One method is simply to contact a local insurance agency and ask the agent to write a policy covering the elements that the institution desires. This method requires the least time and effort on the part of the athletic trainer, but it is without question the least desirable. Investigating the wide range of insurance products and their prices is the surest method of obtaining the best protection for the lowest cost.

Another method that educational institutions commonly use is a formal bidding process to purchase insurance services. The advantage to the bidding method is that it allows institutions to obtain athletic accident insurance at the lowest possible cost. But this system has disadvantages too. First, every insurance plan has hidden costs, the most significant of which is usually the time the institution's employees spend learning the system and filing the claims. If an institution awards athletic accident contracts to the lowest bidder annually, employees will spend a great deal of time learning new insurance systems—time that they could spend on more productive work. Another disadvantage of the bidding system, especially for institutions that bid for multiyear contracts, is that the initial low price of the premium may rise as the institution establishes a claims history with the company, which may raise rates to ensure that it makes a profit.

Bidding for insurance coverage can be a stressful and often frustrating process. The inexperienced athletic trainer may be involved in making a decision that affects tens of thousands of dollars for an institution yet possess no formal training or experience regarding the process. One method of improving leverage during bidding and negotiations is to consider collaborating with institutions that may be in your conference, in your geographical region, or of like size in terms of the number of participating student-athletes. This can also help inexperienced athletic trainers. Regardless of how the process is managed, an athletic trainer should be prepared to provide the past three to five years of a claims history to present to potential insurance providers so that they can analyze the trends of the injury claims in an effort to provide a fair bid for services.

An alternative to both the bidding and direct purchasing systems just described is for the athletic trainer and other institutional representatives to interview several insurance companies and carefully evaluate their products and prices. This process allows for easy clarification of questions and provides an opportunity to determine the procedures for processing claims.

No matter which purchasing method is used, each proposal should be evaluated with the following points in mind:

- What are the monetary limits of the coverage? What are the time limits of the coverage? Does the policy offer **layered coverage**? If so, what are the limits for each layer of coverage? Is there a layer of catastrophic coverage?
- What specific exclusions to the coverage are listed? What riders are available to cover these exclusions?

- Does the policy provide primary coverage or secondary (excess) coverage? If secondary, how does it interface with personal insurance? How does it handle student-athletes whose parents are covered by HMOs or PPOs?

- What deductibles, if any, apply to the policy? Who will be responsible for paying the deductible?

- What **copayments**, if any, does the policy require? Who is responsible for the copayments?

- Whom does the policy cover? Does it cover ancillary and support personnel, such as athletic trainers, coaches, student managers, and cheerleaders?

- Under what circumstances are covered individuals protected? How does the policy handle out-of-season injury?

- What is the annual premium? If a multiyear contract, how and under what circumstances will the annual premium change?

- What specific steps must the institution take to file claims? How much staff time and effort will be required to do so?

APPLICATIONS TO ATHLETIC TRAINING: THEORY INTO PRACTICE

Apply the concepts discussed in this chapter to the following two case studies to prepare for situations you might face in actual practice. The questions at the end of the studies are open-ended—many solutions may be correct. The case studies may be used for homework, exam questions, or class discussion.

■ Case Study 1

Barbara Cummings, ATC/PT, was beginning to have second thoughts about her decision four months earlier to sell her private sports medicine and physical therapy practice to Universal Health Care Services. She had thought that by selling the practice to Universal, a huge medical practice conglomerate operating in 47 states, she would be able to improve her bottom line while the parent company assumed the risk of adding the new, expensive equipment she desperately needed to remain competitive with the local hospital's sports medicine clinic. Unfortunately, she soon discovered that Universal put so much pressure on her to increase revenue that patient care was beginning to suffer. Still, she thought that she had to do something to meet Universal's expectations or she would have to leave the practice she had worked so long to establish.

Bob Thaxton, Universal's manager of clinic operations for 10 northern states, visited Barbara's clinic and told her she would have to institute the following billing and insurance practices immediately:

- All new patients were to be discharged immediately when they met their insurance limits.
- No patients were to be discharged until their insurance expired.

- Every patient was to be billed for a minimum of 1 hour of therapy to cover expenses associated with overhead at the home office.
- Patients without insurance were not to be accepted.

Although Barbara was upset with the new regulations, she thought she had no choice but to conform to the standards established by the company. The day after Bob Thaxton's visit, she implemented the new regulations.

QUESTIONS FOR ANALYSIS

1. What potential legal pitfalls do the new billing and insurance regulations pose for Barbara and her staff? What ethical dilemmas, if any, do these regulations pose?

2. How could Barbara implement the regulations without violating the law? Would these actions serve her patients well? Why or why not?

3. What other revenue-enhancing procedures, besides those mandated by Universal, could Barbara implement? How would they serve her patients more efficiently and effectively than the procedures required by Universal?

■ Case Study 2

Libby Wilson, Northwest State University's head athletic trainer, was called into the athletic director's office and told that a new university policy required all service contracts to be awarded to the lowest bidder. The new rule was to take effect beginning with the next fiscal year, which was only two months away. Libby would have to put together a bidding package for the university's athletic accident insurance, the ambulance service, and the team physician's contract. The athletic director gave her one month to secure the bids. This schedule would give him enough time, he thought, to evaluate the bids, award the contracts, and have the services in place by the time the new fiscal year began.

Although Libby was not happy about having to put these services out for bid, she went to work right away. She knew that the insurance bid would be the most complicated, so she decided to tackle that part of the project first. She put together a bidding document that requested cost quotations based on the following requirements:

■ Excess coverage for 500 student-athletes in 18 sports, including football and gymnastics

■ Excess coverage for all ancillary and support personnel

■ Coverage limits up to $50,000 with lifetime catastrophic coverage for amounts above $50,000

Libby included a copy of the university's claims history for the previous five years (an average of 75 claims per year) and sent the bidding package to three insurance companies that specialized in athletic accident insurance. Two weeks later she received the bids. She developed table 7.3 to help the athletic director understand the bids.

QUESTIONS FOR ANALYSIS

1. What advantages and disadvantages are likely to accompany the university's new policy regarding the athletic accident insurance program?

2. If you were in Libby's position, would you have followed the same process in securing bids for insurance? Why or why not? What would you have done differently?

3. Based on the information in table 7.3, which company's insurance policy represents the best value? Do you need any other information to reach this conclusion?

4. The Good Insurance Company will write a policy only with a maximum of $25,000 per claim. The university's catastrophic insurance coverage does not take effect until $50,000 in medical bills has been paid. If the university decided to purchase the Good Insurance Company's policy, what options should it investigate to decrease its risk between $25,000 and $50,000?

TABLE 7.3 NSU Athletic Accident Insurance Bid Summary

| Company | Coverage | PREMIUM DEDUCTIBLE PER CLAIM | | |
		$0	$100	$250
Professional Underwriters	$50,000	$20,000	$17,500	$15,000
Best Insurance Company	$50,000	$18,000	$16,000	$14,000
Good Insurance Company	$25,000	$12,000	$10,000	$8,000

SUMMARY

Reimbursement provides an opportunity to receive equitable remuneration for professionally delivered health care services. While reimbursement for services and involvement with various forms of insurance did not play a role in the early days of athletic training, they have become more commonplace in the practice of athletic training today. Various types of insurance exist, including (but not limited to) health, accident, medical, and liability. For student-athletes, medical, health, and accident insurance exist to support injuries and illnesses that occur as a result of sport participation. The athletic trainer is often involved with the data collection and claims processing associated with these types of insurance plans. A series of steps are taken to ensure proper filing of an insurance claim, and the types of services provided will often be dictated by the specific type of plan an individual or the individual's affiliation (or both) has contracted with. All policies and plans have advantages and disadvantages, and each person should take the time to understand the specific type of insurance plan that he maintains. The entire process associated with insurance and reimbursement can be time sensitive and complicated, requiring the athletic trainer to be competent and remain current regarding industry standards.

KEY CONCEPTS AND REVIEW

1. Understand the difference between medical, health, and accident insurance.

As the cost of medical care continues to rise and the quality of insurance continues to fall, it is becoming increasingly important for athletic trainers to understand insurance systems. Insurance not only protects the assets of educational institutions that sponsor athletic programs but also safeguards the income and livelihood of athletic trainers employed by sports medicine clinics. Most athletic accident policies cover only acute injuries with no connection to preexisting conditions and do not pay for illnesses or overuse conditions. Medical and health insurance policies are generally more comprehensive and are usually designed to help cover a percentage of an insured person's medical bills or to provide coverage for activities designed to maintain good health.

2. Understand the advantages and disadvantages of self-insurance, primary coverage, and secondary coverage.

The three choices available to most educational institutions when buying insurance services are self-insurance, primary coverage, and secondary, or excess, coverage. Secondary coverage is the most common type of insurance plan, because it uses the patient's personal health insurance as a first layer of coverage. Primary insurance is expensive; it pays all covered expenses from the first dollar. Some institutions choose to self-insure, gambling that they will not incur large claims that would drain institutional coffers.

3. Define the types of injuries covered by most athletic accident policies.

Most athletic accident policies cover only acute injuries that occur in officially sanctioned practices or games. These policies usually do not cover chronic injuries, illnesses, or degenerative conditions.

4. Understand the basic legal responsibilities associated with third-party reimbursement.

Athletic trainers reimbursed for services through third-party insurance plans should maintain patient–practitioner confidentiality. They should never release medical records to third-party payers unless the patient has provided written authorization. Athletic trainers commit fraud when altering the date of an injury, treatment, or assessment or when failing to record payments from an insurance company on a patient's bill. Claiming reimbursement for services not provided is also illegal and is punishable by substantial fines.

5. Understand the role of procedural coding in the third-party reimbursement system.

CPT coding lists procedures on insurance claim forms in the form of a code. Diagnostic coding provides third-party payers with a standardized system for determining the kinds of medical conditions that health care providers are treating when they seek reimbursement.

6. Organize a claims-processing system for a sports medicine program in an educational setting.

Claims processing in educational settings is different from claims processing in a sports medicine clinic. In each case, patients enrolled in some managed care plans must receive authorization from primary care providers before services are rendered. Athletic trainers in educational settings should communicate the limits of the school's athletic accident insurance policy to parents. Each athlete who submits an insurance claim needs a separate file, and bills should not be submitted to the school's insurance company until the athletic trainer has received an explanation of benefits report from the athlete's personal health insurance company.

7. Understand the steps required to file a claim for reimbursement from a third-party payer.

All diagnoses and procedures must be converted to coded form using the ICD-10-CM and the CPT list of codes. Claims can be submitted on the standard CMS 1500 form for private practice settings, the UB-04 (CMS 1450) form for hospitals, on a scannable form, or electronically using a computer. Athletic trainers responsible for this process must keep meticulous records of all procedures, charges, and payments.

8. Evaluate and purchase an athletic accident insurance policy for an educational institution.

Athletic trainers are frequently responsible for purchasing or recommending the purchase of athletic accident insurance. Price, policy exclusions, limits of coverage, deductibles, and claims-processing workload should all be considered when the policies offered by various insurance companies are being evaluated.

CHAPTER 8

Legal Considerations in Sports Medicine

OBJECTIVES

After reading this chapter, you should be able to do the following:

1. Define and discuss the legal principles most applicable to athletic training settings.

2. Identify the types of situations most likely to hold liability concerns for athletic trainers.

3. Understand the different types of credentialing laws that affect the practice of athletic training.

4. Understand the elements required to prove negligence on the part of an athletic trainer.

5. Be aware of the various legal defenses available to athletic trainers against charges of malpractice.

6. Identify the most important elements of providing effective legal testimony.

7. Identify and put into practice methods that avoid legal liability while improving the quality of athletic training care.

► As the only certified athletic trainer for a large metropolitan high school, Todd Russell has over 500 student-athletes to care for. One Thursday, as Todd was in the athletic training room packing for a Friday night football game on the other side of the state, the assistant soccer coach and one of his players carried in Enrique Vasquez, the team's backup goalkeeper, and laid him on a treatment table. Todd examined Enrique's injured left ankle. Enrique explained that he had been involved in a collision in front of the goal, but he wasn't sure how he had injured the ankle. Most of his pain was located over the medial malleolus. Mild swelling was present. Active range of motion was painful in inversion and eversion, but not too bad in plantar- and dorsiflexion. Todd told Enrique that he had probably sprained the deltoid ligament on the medial aspect of his ankle. He applied ice with an elastic bandage and elevated the injured foot. Because the team physician usually stopped in on Thursdays, Todd decided to keep Enrique in the athletic training room and have the physician examine the ankle. Todd returned to his packing while Enrique iced the ankle.

Todd removed the ice after 30 minutes, and the team physician arrived 10 minutes later. After evaluating the problem, the physician told Enrique that Todd's assessment was probably correct but that he wanted Enrique's family doctor to see him the next day to get an X ray. Todd, who was present when the team physician gave the instructions, made sure that Enrique understood what he needed to do. He gave Enrique a pair of crutches and returned to his preparation for the football game.

Because the football team would be playing their game nearly 300 miles away, Todd was not in school on Friday. Enrique, whose parents had no medical insurance, decided not to see his family physician or get an X ray. He used the crutches only sparingly, thinking that walking on the injured ankle would decrease the stiffness he felt. When he woke up on Saturday, however, his ankle was so swollen and painful that his mother took him to the emergency room, where a displaced fracture of the tibial malleolus was diagnosed.

Enrique underwent surgery later that day to stabilize the fracture. Unfortunately, he developed an infection and was hospitalized for the next two weeks. The infection caused scarring of the articular surfaces of the joint, leaving Enrique with a permanently stiff, sore ankle.

Several months later, both Todd and the team physician were surprised to learn that Enrique's family was suing them, along with the school board.

The law is sort of hocus-pocus science
that smiles in yer face while it picks yer pocket.

—CHARLES MACKLIN

Todd Russell faces the same pressures as many athletic trainers: too many athletes to care for and not enough time to provide that care. Yet the expectations he faces from coaches, physicians, parents, and administrators are substantial. They expect him to be caring, thorough, tireless, and wise every day (and night and weekend) he comes to work. If he makes a mistake, it is typically overlooked. But if he were to make the wrong mistake with the wrong person, his professional standing, his personal assets, and his self-respect could be seriously jeopardized.

Athletic trainers have been aware for some time that they need a general understanding of certain legal principles to protect themselves and the institutions that employ them from the risk of lawsuits (Gieck, Lowe, and Kenna 1984). Wise athletic trainers, however, also realize that basic knowledge of legal principles, when applied thoughtfully and consistently, helps inform and improve their professional practice. These legal standards often provide extra incentive for athletic trainers to do what they ought to be doing routinely in their professional practice, whether they will be sued or not (Danzon 1985).

Of course, this chapter cannot provide definitive, comprehensive coverage of all the law related to the practice of athletic training. But it does present to athletic training students the legal issues they are likely to encounter in their professional practice. If an athletic trainer confronts a specific legal issue or problem, the best source of information is an attorney who is experienced in handling similar cases (Horsley and Carlova 1983). Effective policies and procedures, formed by consultation with both attorneys and insurance companies, also help guide athletic trainers through the minefield of legal perils they face daily.

LEGAL PRINCIPLES

The common threat that confronts all athletic trainers who provide sports medicine services to patients is **malpractice**. Scott (1990, p. 6) defines health care malpractice as "liability-generating conduct associated with the adverse outcome of patient treatment. Liability may be based on

Athletic trainers can be subject to judicial claims based on a variety of legal theories, and those in different settings must be aware of the legal concepts specific to their setting.

- negligent patient care,
- failure to obtain informed consent,
- intentional conduct,
- breach of a contract,
- use/transfer of a defective product, or
- abnormally dangerous treatment."

Torts

Although athletic trainers may enter patient–practitioner relationships that are implied contracts, unhappy patients are less likely to bring a legal action based on **breach of contract** than on an accusation that the athletic trainer committed a **tort** (Wadlington, Waltz, and Dworkin 1980). A tort is a legal wrong other than breach of contract for which a remedy will be provided, usually in the form of monetary damages. Actions based on tort law are pressed by plaintiffs in civil legal proceedings, whereas criminal cases are initiated by the government. All the legal grounds for malpractice, other than breach of contract, are based on tort law. Of the three types of tort—intentional tort, negligent tort, and strict liability tort—negligence, which focuses on the conduct of the practitioner, is the most common basis for most malpractice actions.

Negligence

Athletic trainers are usually sued under a negligent tort theory (Leverenz and Helms 1990a). **Negligence** is a type of tort in which an athletic trainer fails to act as a reasonably prudent athletic trainer would under the circumstances (Drowatzky 1985). Athletic trainers can demonstrate that their actions have been both reasonable and prudent by adhering to certain standards in the performance of their duties. Standards emerge from several sources, including individual, societal, institutional, and professional values (Leiske 1985). Standards derived from individual and societal values are often implicit (for example, patients should be treated with respect). Standards derived from institutional and professional values are typically more explicit. Policies and procedures usually codify these standards. Position statements of professional associations also include them. For example, the American College of Sports Medicine's position statement on exercise and fluid replacement and the Inter-Association Task Force on Exertional Heat Illnesses Consensus Statement create a professional standard that athletic trainers and others involved in the health care of physically active patients should adhere to during hot, humid weather. (You can go to a search engine and look up these two statements.) Similarly, the American Heart Association's statement on cardiovascular preparticipation screening of competitive athletes creates a standard to which team physicians and athletic trainers should adhere when organizing and conducting preseason physical exams. Finally, the National Collegiate Athletic Association (NCAA) has established a comprehensive set of standards to which athletic trainers in college athletics should adhere (see the *NCAA Sports Medicine Handbook,* www.ncaa.org/).

Athletic trainers can be negligent through either omission or commission. **Omission** is the failure to do something that one should have done under the circumstances. **Commission** occurs when an athletic trainer performs an act that she should not have performed. To prove that an athletic trainer was negligent, the aggrieved patient must be able to substantiate the following five components (Ciccolella 1991):

- Conduct by the athletic trainer
- Existence of duty
- Breach of duty
- Causation
- Damage

Conduct

To substantiate a charge of negligence, the plaintiff must be able to prove that the athletic trainer, by either commission or omission, did something that links him to the case. Nonactions, such as thoughts, attitudes, or intentions, cannot render the athletic trainer negligent. Only when athletic trainers take an action (or fail to take an action) can the plaintiff successfully accuse them of negligence. In the opening case, Todd Russell's failure to contact Enrique's parents might constitute proof of the conduct portion of a negligence claim.

Duty

When does an athletic trainer owe a duty to an injured athlete or other physically active patient? Generally, athletic trainers employed by educational institutions have a duty to provide athletic training services to student-athletes actively engaged in those institutions' athletic programs. Athletic trainers employed by professional sport teams have the same duty toward team members. This duty has its legal origin in the athletic trainer's contract, in which he or she agrees to provide these services in return for payment. Whether a high school or university athletic trainer owes a duty to the student who is injured in an intramural basketball game or a physical education class is less clear—it depends on the responsibilities defined by the employment contract. In many athletic training settings, coaches, coaches' families, athletic department staff, and other personnel often ask the athletic trainer for a consult and assume that such interaction is a courtesy. While this courtesy is often extended without question, it remains unclear from contract to contract whether or not it is considered an appropriate part of the job description of the athletic trainer. For that reason, athletic trainers should have an employment contract with a clearly written position description delineating their specific responsibilities.

Athletic trainers employed by sports medicine clinics have greater leeway in deciding whom they will accept as patients. Consequently, the injured athletes and other physically active patients they owe a duty to should, in theory, be only those patients they choose to treat in their clinics. Enough exceptions to this general rule exist, however, that sports medicine clinic owners should consult with their attorneys to find out whom they might owe a duty to and under what circumstances. For example, sports medicine clinics that have a contract to provide services to a health maintenance organization might have a duty to provide services to the HMO's subscribers.

Abandonment is another issue related to duty that affects athletic trainers. Once an athletic trainer chooses to provide services to an injured athlete or other physically active patient, whether a duty originally existed or not, the athletic trainer does not have the legal freedom simply to walk away from the case except under certain circumstances. An athletic trainer cannot forsake even patients who do not cooperate or who fail to pay their bills—unless she provides adequate warning and enough time for the patient to find alternative care.

If the physically active patient recovers and the athletic trainer and the patient agree that further treatment is no longer necessary, they can jointly terminate the relationship. If the patient has been referred, the athletic trainer has a duty to inform the referring agent, usually a physician, that treatment is being discontinued.

An athletic trainer can also discontinue services without fear of being charged with abandonment if the patient voluntarily terminates the relationship. The athletic trainer should make sure (and should be able to prove), however, that the patient understands the consequences of discontinuing the therapy. If the patient simply stops coming for treatment, the athletic trainer should be sure to document his attempts to make contact. If the athletic trainer is away from the sports medicine center and leaves the patient's care in the hands of another practitioner, abandonment might also be charged. If the practitioner substituting for the athletic trainer commits a negligent act, the athletic trainer might be found negligent as well. Athletic trainers can avoid this problem by informing patients when they plan to be gone and making sure that patients agree to be treated by the substitute practitioner. The athletic trainer owes a duty to the patient to make sure that the substitute is competent and is capable of providing the same standard of care.

In general, the duties owed by an athletic trainer to athletes and other physically active patients are those described in the Board of Certification (BOC) *Role Delineation Study*. The courts have identified several specific duties:

- Provide or obtain reasonable medical assistance for injured patients as soon as possible under the circumstances in such a way as to avoid aggravation of the injury (a probable breach of this duty occurred in the opening case). This implies having an effective emergency action plan, complete with necessary first aid supplies and communications with ambulance services.
- Maintain the confidentiality of the patient's medical records.
- Provide adequate and proper supervision and instruction.
- Provide safe facilities and equipment.
- Fully disclose information about the patient's medical condition to the patient.

Breach of Duty

The next step in proving negligence against an athletic trainer requires the aggrieved athlete or other physically active patient to establish by a preponderance of the evidence that the athletic trainer actually breached a duty owed the patient. The issue here is whether the athletic trainer exercised the **standard of care** that other reasonably prudent athletic trainers would have exercised under the circumstances. The athletic trainer can consult the standards of practice of various medical and athletic professional organizations to determine a standard of care if questions arise. Note that the standard of care does not require an athletic trainer to be the *most* knowledgeable or competent athletic trainer in the profession. If this were the case, nobody could meet the standard. Instead, the standard requires athletic trainers to perform their duties as other competent athletic trainers would under similar circumstances. In determining whether athletic trainers have met the standard of care, the laws of various states require that their actions be compared with those of other athletic trainers in one of the following three settings (Scott 1990):

- The same locality
- Similar communities
- The same or similar circumstances

For a useful guide to standards in sports medicine, see D.L. Herbert, 1992, *The Sports Medicine Standards Book* (Canton, OH: Professional Reports Corporation).

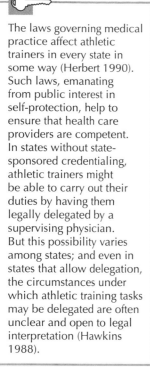

The laws governing medical practice affect athletic trainers in every state in some way (Herbert 1990). Such laws, emanating from public interest in self-protection, help to ensure that health care providers are competent. In states without state-sponsored credentialing, athletic trainers might be able to carry out their duties by having them legally delegated by a supervising physician. But this possibility varies among states; and even in states that allow delegation, the circumstances under which athletic training tasks may be delegated are often unclear and open to legal interpretation (Hawkins 1988).

The standard of care expected of athletic trainers in fulfilling their duties to their patients can depend on whether the state has credentialed the profession. Herbert (1990) posits that in those states without statutory credentialing, the athletic trainer might be held to the standard of care of other regulated health professionals, including physicians. Indeed, in *Gillespie v. Southern Utah State College* (669 P.2d. 861 [Ut. 1983]), an athletic training student was held to the standard of care of a physician in the treatment of a sprained ankle that later developed serious complications (Leverenz and Helms 1990b).

Causation

After an aggrieved athlete or other physically active patient has demonstrated that an athletic trainer breached a duty to exercise reasonable care, the patient must prove that the breach was in fact the legal cause of the injury (or made the original injury worse). The courts use two tests to determine causation. First, the plaintiff must prove **actual cause**. Actual cause is established if the patient can demonstrate that the athletic trainer's actions were a considerable determining factor in the damage claimed. The athletic trainer might be found only partially responsible for causing or aggravating the injury. Team physicians, coaches, and institutions might be named as codefendants in negligence cases, because all of them might have contributed to the injury. If more than one defendant was responsible for causing or aggravating the injury, those defendants will be found jointly and severally liable for the negligence, which means that each might end up paying a portion of the damages, consistent with her percentage of fault as determined by the court.

The second causation test is the requirement to demonstrate the existence of **proximate (legal) cause**. Proximate cause exists when an athletic trainer acts in a way that leads to harm or injury to another or to an event that injures another. Inherent in the notion of proximate cause is the **foreseeability** of the harm allegedly precipitated by the athletic trainer. The requirement that harm must be foreseeable is positive for athletic trainers—it doesn't penalize them for results that were improbable or unlikely. One of the problems in the opening case is that the team physician and athletic trainer did not ensure that an X ray of Enrique's injured ankle was obtained, although they should have known that if a fracture was present it could have been aggravated by delayed or improper treatment. In short, they should have foreseen serious consequences.

Damage

The final element in establishing negligence is to determine whether the aggrieved patient actually suffered damages. If an athletic trainer breached a duty without causing any harm, no negligence occurred. The athletic trainer who oversteps his level of training by suturing a wound, for example, cannot be found negligent unless the plaintiff can prove that she suffered harm as a result (but a charge of practicing medicine without a license would probably have merit). Although physical damage is the most common and easily proved, the law recognizes other forms of damage as well. Emotional distress and loss of consortium (injury to the marital relationship) are just two examples (Herbert 1990).

REDUCING THE RISK OF LEGAL LIABILITY

In addition to the certification requirements of the BOC, most states regulate the practice of athletic trainers. This state credentialing is important for the protection of the public and the advancement of the profession.

Credentialing

Athletic trainers must become familiar with the practice acts that regulate the profession. Both practicing athletic trainers and students should have such understanding, because the law is likely to define different roles and responsibilities for these two groups. Athletic training practice acts vary a great deal among states. The acts define *athlete* and *athletic trainer* differently. Some limit the scope and setting in which an athletic trainer may practice. Some limit the types of therapeutic modalities athletic trainers can use. Most have specific educational requirements that might or might not correspond to those required for certification by the BOC. Most state laws require physician supervision. Some states also allow other health professionals, such as physical therapists, chiropractors, and dentists, to supervise an athletic trainer under certain circumstances. In states without specific credentialing for athletic training, an athletic trainer should obtain a copy of the state's **medical practice act** to determine the scope and setting of practice that the law permits athletic trainers and other health care providers.

Four types of credentialing laws regulate the practice of athletic training: **licensure, certification, registration**, and **exemption**. Athletic trainers practicing in states with athletic training practice acts should review the state law to determine what type of credentialing they require—each type has different implications. In addition, the definitions and level of restrictiveness of each type of credentialing vary from state to state.

> As of May 1, 2011, athletic trainers had established a legal basis for their practice in 49 states. For the most current list, visit www. nata.org and click on the link for "Government Affairs/Advocacy."

■ **Licensure.** Licensure is the most restrictive form of governmental credentialing. The intent of licensure is to protect the public by limiting the practice of athletic training to those who have met the requirements of a licensing board established under the law. Licensure laws generally prohibit unlicensed individuals from calling themselves athletic trainers. More importantly, they prohibit unlicensed persons from performing the tasks reserved for athletic trainers under the law. States that license athletic trainers usually require a specific educational background that comprises both course work and experience, in addition to passing a licensing examination administered by the board. Some states that license athletic trainers accept the equivalent of the BOC standards, but many have different requirements as well. Licensing boards are powerful legal entities because they are usually authorized to set the rules, in accordance with the law, that govern who may practice and who may not. They also set the fee required for license applications and renewals. Because licensure is the most restrictive form of state credentialing, athletic trainers commonly view it as the most desirable of the four regulatory options.

■ Athletic Training: State Regulation

STATES THAT LICENSE ATHLETIC TRAINERS

Alabama	Nebraska
Arizona	Nevada
Arkansas	New Hampshire
Connecticut	New Jersey
Delaware	New Mexico
Florida	New York
Georgia	North Carolina
Idaho	North Dakota
Illinois	Ohio
Indiana	Oklahoma
Iowa	Rhode Island
Kansas	South Dakota
Maine	Tennessee
Massachusetts	Texas
Michigan	Vermont
Mississippi	Virginia
Missouri	Wisconsin

STATES THAT CERTIFY ATHLETIC TRAINERS

Kentucky
Louisiana
Pennsylvania
South Carolina

STATES THAT REGISTER ATHLETIC TRAINERS

Minnesota
Oregon
West Virginia

STATES THAT EXEMPT ATHLETIC TRAINERS FROM OTHER HEALTH PROFESSIONS' PRACTICE ACTS

Hawaii

STATES THAT HAVE NO REGULATION FOR CERTIFIED ATHLETIC TRAINERS

Alaska
California

■ **Certification.** Certification is a less stringent form of professional regulation than licensure. A person who is certified is generally recognized to have the basic knowledge and skills required of practitioners in the profession. Both states and professional associations can certify health care practitioners. The National Athletic Trainers' Association Board of Certification (NATABOC), for example, is the recognized certifying agency for ensuring that athletic trainers have the basic knowledge and skills to carry out their duties as defined by the *Role Delineation Study*. Athletic trainers who meet the requirements for NATABOC certification and maintain their certification are entitled to use the board's credential. Some states also certify athletic trainers. States get the authority to certify athletic trainers from a credentialing law passed by the state legislature and signed by the governor, the same process that gives them the authority for licensure. Unlike licensure, however, state certification usually protects only an athletic trainer's title, not the specific tasks that he performs. Noncertified persons could not call themselves athletic trainers, but they could perform the duties of an athletic trainer.

■ **Registration.** Registration is another form of professional regulation that is less restrictive than licensure. In states that have registration laws, athletic trainers are required to register with the state before practicing. Some states allow a grace period during which athletic trainers may practice without being registered as long as they begin their application for registration within the period established by the state's board. Because the registration law prohibits unregistered persons from practicing, it becomes a form of title protection for an athletic trainer. States that require registration might or might not require screening devices such as examinations, although most prescribe the educational requirements necessary to register as an athletic trainer.

■ **Exemption.** Some states have provided the legal basis for athletic trainers to practice by exempting them from complying with the practice acts of other professions, typically the physical therapy, physician assistant, medical, and masseuse practice acts. Although exemption is often viewed as the least restrictive form of professional regulation, athletic trainers might still be required to meet a variety of standards, usually related to educational background or certification by the NATABOC, to qualify. In addition, athletic trainers are required to act according to the standards of the profession and the boundaries of their training.

Risk Management

Athletic trainers have been concerned with issues of legal liability for many years. As larger numbers of athletic trainers moved into management positions or took on management responsibilities along with their clinical duties, the broader construct of **risk management** became more important. Although athletic trainers are still concerned with the basics of avoiding legal liability in their clinical practices, they are increasingly called on to help their schools, professional teams, clinics, and companies manage the risks that form the foundation for this liability.

What Is Risk Management?

At its most fundamental level, risk management is a process intended to prevent financial loss for an organization. In a broader sense, however, the goal of risk management is to prevent losses of all kinds (financial, physical, property, activity, time) for everyone associated with an organization, including its directors, administrators, employees, and clients (Culp, Goemaere, and Miller 1985). This broader application is warranted, because losses experienced at one level of an organization are usually felt at other levels. For example, if Enrique from the opening case is successful in his lawsuit against the school district, the board of education will have fewer dollars to spend on all programs, including Todd's athletic training program. Controlling the risks that led up to Enrique's injury and the subsequent difficulties he experienced is in everyone's best interests.

As van der Smissen (2001) appropriately points out, risk management is more than the act of developing safety checklists. A comprehensive risk management program involves careful analysis of the risks facing the program or organization and development of a plan for addressing those risks. She recommends using four general strategies for managing risk:

- **Avoidance.** When an activity, procedure, or event is so risky that dire consequences are likely, the organization may simply choose to avoid the activity. Avoidance is an especially appropriate risk management approach when the negative consequences of a particular activity have high costs.

- **Transference.** When activities are associated with high financial risk but low frequency (for example, catastrophic sport injury) or lower financial risk but high frequency (for example, fractures, joint injuries requiring surgery), a common method to reduce the risk of these activities is to transfer all or part of the risk to another entity. The organization usually accomplishes this by purchasing insurance designed to cover the financial loss associated with certain well-defined risks. Exculpatory clauses in waivers signed by athletes and their parents are another example of a method to transfer the risk associated with sport participation to the participants and away from the organization, although this method has many flaws.

- **Retention.** Every organization—including organizations in which athletic trainers work—has activities or sponsors programs that have a level of risk deemed acceptable in light of the organization's mission. These risks are viewed as part of the cost of doing business. To eliminate the activities associated with these risks would fundamentally change the nature of the organization. The organization accepts and retains risks like these. These risks are still associated with a predictable level of financial cost, however, and the organization must account for it in the organization or program budget. Ideally, the organization should establish a reserve fund to cover costs that rise above predicted levels.

- **Reduction.** Careful development, implementation, monitoring, and evaluation of policies and procedures can reduce risks. Ideally, every risk that an organization knowingly retains should be accompanied by one or more policies and procedures designed to reduce the frequency and financial effect of that risk. For guidance on reducing risk in athletic programs, see the later section "Specific Risk Reduction Strategies."

How Are Risks Identified?

Risk identification is rarely as easy as it seems. Some risks are obvious to anyone. If you begin to administer an ultrasound treatment to an athlete or other physically active patient and notice that the power cord is frayed and the wire is exposed, you have identified a rather obvious risk factor. You could even quantify the risk in this case, because you could safely assume that 100% of the people who contact the exposed wire will receive an injury ranging from a minor burn to an electrical shock that induces cardiac arrest. Most risks in athletics are more difficult to identify and quantify. For example, how would you answer an athletic director who wanted to know if the rubberized gym floor was the cause of the high rate of anterior cruciate ligament (ACL) injuries among your school's female basketball players? What evidence could you provide to support your answer? Could you calculate the risk of ACL injury with any accuracy? Assessing this risk is obviously difficult, because not every female basketball player at your school will suffer an ACL injury. Of those who do, not all will suffer the injury while playing in the gym at school. Two ways to identify and assess risk in athletics are real-world observation and inference from controlled experiments (Graham and Rhomberg 1996).

Real-World Observation   Observation of real-world events is the most rudimentary form of risk assessment. This method involves making inferences regarding the risk of certain activities based on clinical practice and experience. Real-world observation is usually the first step in the discovery of cause-and-effect relationships between hazardous practices and their results.

Athletic trainers can help prevent losses (physical and financial) for their employers and patients by instituting a risk management plan. Both real-world observations and controlled experiments can identify risks. Preparing properly for activity, conducting safe activities, managing injuries properly, and maintaining appropriate records are all part of a risk management plan.

For example, athletic trainers in the 1960s observed many cases of heat illness among athletes who had been denied access to fluids during heavy exercise in hot weather. The athletic trainers surmised that this practice led to dehydration and all its negative side effects. Their observations led to an accurate assessment of a risk that was later validated in laboratory studies. Unfortunately, however, real-world observation can often lead to spurious conclusions. In the case of the gym floor previously mentioned, all the women's sport coaches who used that gym were so convinced that the floor was the cause of the high incidence of ACL injuries that they lobbied the administration to tear out the rubberized floor and replace it with a wooden floor. The project cost more than $1 million. Two years later, the rate of ACL injuries was just as high on the new wooden floor as it had been on the rubberized floor. In this case, factors other than the playing surface must have caused the high incidence of ACL injuries. The coaches' observations were incorrect and led to an expensive "solution" that solved nothing.

Controlled Experiments Another way to identify and assess risks is to engage in data-driven controlled studies. This method is more difficult to implement because it is time intensive, costly, and frequently impractical. Using the preceding example, the people involved would probably have received better information regarding the effect of playing surface on ACL injuries if they had replaced one court with wood and left another with the original rubberized surface. If they had then randomly assigned players to practice on each of the courts and tracked the incidence of ACL injury as a function of player exposures, they would have gotten a much better answer (but not a perfect one) to the question of whether they should replace the rubberized floor.

This type of controlled study—the kind used to establish the safety and efficacy of prescription drugs—is rarely practical for athletic or physical activity settings. One method that is practical, however, involves using an epidemiological approach to identifying risks. Epidemiology can help athletic trainers draw inferences regarding potential risks by tracking the incidence of injuries and all their associated factors, including athlete characteristics, playing surface, weather, and type of activity. Most commercially available injury-tracking database software programs allow athletic trainers to do this.

When the school administration asked the athletic trainer in the gym floor case for an opinion regarding the advisability of switching to a wooden floor, he did an analysis of knee injuries in women's basketball and volleyball using 10 years of data from the school's injury-tracking database and the NCAA Injury Surveillance Study, in which his school was a participating member. The results indicated that the rate of injury was the same for wooden and rubberized gym floors. In addition, twice as many knee injuries occurred during away contests (where the teams usually played on wood surfaces) as occurred on the rubberized floor during home games. His conclusion was that there was no basis to recommend the commitment of $1 million to switch to a wood floor. The money was spent anyway. Knee injury rates continued as before.

Planning for Risk

Even the most prepared and conscientious organizations will, despite their best efforts, experience unwanted events from time to time—including life-threatening emergencies. One of the most important roles that athletic trainers can play in helping the organization prepare for these events is by taking the lead in developing emergency action plans. An **emergency action plan (EAP)** is a blueprint for handling emergencies that helps establish accountability for their management (Andersen, Courson, Kleiner, and McLoda 2002). Every organization that sponsors an athletic or physical activity program should have a written EAP. Indeed, the failure to have such a plan could constitute a breach of the institution's legal responsibility to conduct safe programs. The plan should cover every aspect of the program—including practices, games, and conditioning sessions. A variety of people, including every person or classification of person who will have a role in implementing the plan, should contribute to the EAP. These people typically include athletic trainers, athletic training students, team physicians, coaches, athletic administrators, campus safety officers, campus health center personnel, local law enforcement personnel, firefighters, EMS personnel, athletic venue managers, and hospital personnel. The plan should be reviewed annually at a minimum, with all vested parties taking part in the review. In addition, it is helpful to test the plan from time to time by conducting a dry run involving the people who will be responsible for implementing the plan in an actual emergency. This includes the emergency response team who would be summoned by a call in an emergency situation. Dry runs can often identify components that may be overlooked despite significant planning and attention to detail during the plan's development and revisions. Athletic trainers who frequently visit facilities should become familiar with the respective emergency action plans during each visit. Each EAP should contain the following elements:

- A list of personnel involved in implementing the plan, including their roles, responsibilities, contact information, and a chain of command for decision making. Each person involved in implementing the EAP should have current training and certification in CPR (including use of an automatic external defibrillator), first aid, and bloodborne pathogen transmission prevention.

- The procedures to be followed in the event of an emergency, including communication and transportation procedures.

- Venue-specific directions that instruct personnel in the specific steps to be taken for each activity area. A map of each activity area indicating driveways, doors, gates, and telephone locations is critical. The plan should also include a list of the emergency equipment on hand at each venue, posted in an easily visible location.

- Instructions on which emergency care facility will serve as the location to which injured athletes will be taken. Hospital staff should be notified in advance of all contests and events that could result in emergencies requiring their services.

- A system for documenting the actions taken during an emergency and evaluating those actions to improve the emergency plan.

- A plan for directing athletic personnel during inclement weather, including a lightning safety plan (Walsh et al. 2000).

- A plan to communicate with an injured athlete's caretaker, parents, or other responsible individuals who will provide appropriate support and levels of follow-up supervision. Generally, parents should be contacted prior to treatment of a minor. However, since this is not always possible, legislatures and courts have articulated the emergency medicine doctrine for minors (Martin 1994). In part, this doctrine states that medical treatment may be initiated in emergency situations "when delaying treatment to first secure parental consent would endanger the life or health of a minor." Most state laws require parental notification as soon as possible, even in states that allow emergency treatment of minors without such parental approval.

For the complete text of the NATA's position statement on emergency planning and lightning safety, as well as its position statement for emergency planning in athletics, visit www.nata.org and click on "Statements" and then "Position Statements."

Specific Risk Reduction Strategies

Besides considering van der Smissen's (2001) general risk reduction strategies, outlined earlier, athletic trainers should think about implementing Rankin and Ingersoll's (2000) four-part strategy to help control risk in athletic programs:

1. Preparation for the activity
   - Administer preparticipation physical exams
   - Monitor fitness levels
   - Assess activity areas
   - Monitor environmental conditions

2. Conduct of the activity

- Maintain equipment
- Use proper instructional techniques
- Provide adequate work–rest intervals

3. Injury management

- Have a physician supervise all medical aspects of the program
- Evaluate and treat injuries correctly and promptly
- Supervise student athletic trainers

4. Records management

- Document physician orders
- Document the treatment plan
- Document the treatment record
- Document the patient's progress

Mulder (2003) recommends implementing a computer-aided planned maintenance system for medical equipment monitoring, as it is a relatively simple and straightforward task for most settings. The main purpose of such a system is to monitor and administer preventive maintenance activities. Though the cost of these systems may be more expensive in larger settings, such as hospitals, these types of settings often require a more formal tracking system to ensure compliance.

Medications, Legal Liability, and Athletic Trainers

The medical management of athletes' health with pharmaceutical agents is one of the areas of sports medicine that has great potential for legal liability for the athletic trainer. Research conducted by the NCAA reveals that many college and university athletic programs improperly—and illegally—administer and dispense both prescription and nonprescription medications (Laster-Bradley and Berger 1991). Most do so in an effort to provide injured or ill athletes with a comprehensive regimen of therapeutic tools to encourage their full and speedy recovery. Providing medications in the athletic training facility is generally thought to improve physician and athlete convenience. But poorly organized and delivered pharmaceutical management of athletic injuries and illnesses can both compromise an athlete's health and subject the athletic trainer and her employer to significant legal liability.

The sections that follow pertain to prescription and nonprescription medication policies in colleges and universities with adult populations. Medication policies for K through 12 schools are much more restrictive. Generally, neither prescription nor nonprescription medications can be provided to a minor, except in single doses as authorized in writing by the child's parent or guardian. The National Federation of State High School Associations' 1998 position statement on drugs, medications, and supplements for participants in interscholastic sports specifies that "school personnel, including coaches should not dispense any drug, medication or supplement except with extreme caution and in accordance with state regulations and school district policy. School district policies should be developed in consultation with health care professionals, senior administrative staff of the school district and parents." Athletic trainers in high school settings should avoid administering or dispensing medications of any kind to their student-athletes except under the most tightly controlled, parent-authorized circumstances consistent with school board policy.

Athletic trainers should understand the difference between drug administration and drug dispensing. Different laws regulate each; see table 8.1 (Huff 1998). **Drug administration** occurs when a legally authorized and licensed health care practitioner administers a single dose of a medication to a patient. Only certain health care professionals (in most states, physicians, pharmacists, physician assistants, and nurses) may legally administer prescription medications, and then only on the direct order of a physician. **Drug dispensing** is the act of preparing and packaging medications for subsequent use by a patient. Physicians cannot legally delegate the responsibility to dispense prescription medications to a person who is not authorized by law to dispense, including athletic trainers, unless they possess a legal dispensing license in the state that they practice in.

Prescription Medications

The simplest and surest way to ensure that athletic trainers comply with state and federal laws governing the administration and dispensing of prescription medications is to enact policies and procedures that forbid the storage or dispensing of such pharmaceuticals in the athletic training facility. When team physicians provide written prescriptions to student-athletes that are taken to and filled by local or campus health center pharmacies, the athletic trainer and the university are in a much safer legal position. If athletic trainers choose to keep prescription medications in the athletic training facility, however, they must be aware of and strictly enforce the practices that may make this permissible under certain circumstances (Nickell 2006):

TABLE 8.1 Agencies and Regulations Governing Provision of Pharmaceutical Care

Regulation	Enforced/administrated by	Purpose
Federal Food, Drug and Cosmetic Act (FDCA) of 1938	Food and Drug Administration	Regulates the quality, strength, bioequivalence, and labeling of prescription and nonprescription drugs
Durham-Humphrey Amendment of 1951	Food and Drug Administration	Separates prescription from nonprescription drugs
Current Good Manufacturing Practice Regulations of 1962	Food and Drug Administration	Mandates standards for repackaging of medications
Federal Controlled Substances Act of 1970	Drug Enforcement Authority	Regulates controlled substances (drugs that have potential for abuse)
Poison Prevention Packaging Act (PPPA) of 1970	Food and Drug Administration	Regulates packaging of prescription and nonprescription drugs in child-resistant safety containers
Medical Device Act of 1976	Food and Drug Administration	Regulates classification and performance standards of medical devices
Federal Anti-Tampering Act of 1983	Food and Drug Administration	Mandates tamper-resistant packaging on all nonprescription drugs
Fair Packaging and Labeling Act	Food and Drug Administration	Mandates labeling of the contents of nonprescription drugs to assist consumers in identifying similar products
Prescription Drug Marketing Act of 1987	Food and Drug Administration	Mandates accountability of sample drugs from receiving through administering or dispensing
Anti-Drug Abuse Act of 1987	Drug Enforcement Authority	Regulates anabolic steroids as controlled substances
Omnibus Reconciliation Act of 1990 (OBRA '90)	Food and Drug Administration	Mandates drug review, patient medication records, and verbal patient education as part of dispensing of prescription medications
State Pharmacy Practice Acts	Individual State Boards of Pharmacy	Regulates the provision of pharmaceutical care within each state; laws and regulations may vary considerably between states
State Medical Acts	Individual State Boards of Medicine	Regulates the practice of medicine within each state

- Formal, written policies and procedures must be in place to govern the administration and dispensing of prescription medications. These policies and procedures must comply with local, state, and federal law. Huff (1998) recommends that the university or college ask state regulatory agencies (such as the state board of pharmacy) to review and evaluate such policies and procedures because submitting to review can demonstrate intent to abide by all pertinent laws.

- Only the minimum amount and variety of medications necessary to treat the most common injuries and illnesses should be maintained in the athletic training facility. A pharmacist should check the stock regularly to ensure security, proper labeling, and compliance with expiration dates. Drug reference materials should be maintained near the medication storage area.

- Prescription medications must be kept in a locked cabinet that keeps the drugs cool and dry. To ensure compliance with laws regulating administration and dispensing of these medications, only the team physician should have a key to the cabinet, and persons who are not licensed for those activities, including athletic trainers, should not have access to the cabinet.

- Prescription medications—including samples—must be packaged and labeled according to state and federal regulations.

- The drug storage cabinet and the physician's field kits containing prescription medications (athletic trainers are not allowed to carry prescription medications in their field kits) are extensions of the pharmacy that issued the medication. A pharmacist must regularly inspect and inventory the drug cabinet and physician's field kits.

- Controlled substances (drugs with a high potential for abuse) must never be maintained in or dispensed from the athletic training facility.

- A comprehensive record-keeping system must be maintained that includes a properly formatted, written prescription for each medication administration or dispensation, an inventory of all drug stocks, a log book that documents when medications are provided to an athlete, and a record of the patient education provided to each athlete when he receives a medication.

- Athletic trainers who wish to carry inhaled asthma medications or EpiPens in their kits must seek permission from the state board of pharmacy.

- All prescriptions should be scripted to a person's name. Commonly used medications (such as prescription hydrocortisone) should not be labeled "training room" and used as a community medication.

Nonprescription Medications

Although nonprescription medications do not require the same level of control or carry the same level of risk that prescription medications do, their administration or dispensation by athletic trainers is still an activity that requires careful, consistent compliance with well-crafted policies and procedures. Improper use of nonprescription medications, also known as **over-the-counter (OTC) medications**, can have serious adverse health consequences. Athletic trainers who wish to provide their athletes with OTC medications for the treatment of minor injuries and illnesses should comply with the following guidelines:

For the most recent version of the NCAA's guidelines regarding prescription medications, visit www.ncaa.org and search "banned drugs."

- Because providing an OTC medication to an athlete may be considered a medical act in some jurisdictions, policies and procedures governing the administration of OTCs should be developed by the team physician and reviewed by legal counsel.

- OTC medications should be administered only in compliance with the team physician's instructions.

- OTC medications should be stored in a locked, dry, cool (59 to 86 degrees Fahrenheit) environment and should be checked regularly to ensure that they are not expired or in poor condition (NCAA 2002).

- OTC medication stored in field kits should be inventoried and replaced regularly to avoid environmental deterioration.
- OTC medications should be administered only in single doses.
- OTC medications must be packaged and labeled in compliance with the federal seven-point label requirement (see table 8.2).
- Athletes must be provided with appropriate oral and written education regarding the OTC medication, including indications, contraindications, dosing, adverse effects, and drug interaction warnings.
- OTC medications should be administered to athletes only after a review of their medical history and condition, other drugs they may be taking, and drug allergies.
- Records of OTC administration must be maintained and should include the athlete's name, name of the medication, date of administration, dosage, and signature of the person administering the medication.

TABLE 8.2 Federal Seven-Point Label Requirements

The label of a nonprescription drug is required to contain the following information:
1. The name of the product
2. The name and address of the manufacturer, packer, or distributor
3. The net contents of the package
4. The established name of all active ingredients and the quantity of certain other ingredients, whether active or not
5. The name of any habit-forming drug contained in the preparation
6. Cautions and warnings needed to protect the consumer
7. Adequate directions for safe and effective use

Reprinted from *Clinics in Sports Medicine,* Vol. 17, P. Huff, "Drug distribution in the training room," pgs. 211-228. Copyright 1998, with permission from Elsevier.

Product Liability

Injured athletes and other physically active patients can sue equipment manufacturers based on any of three legal theories. First, the manufacturer can be sued for negligence. If the risk of injury from the use of its product was foreseeable and the company did not exercise due care in reducing or eliminating the risk, the company may be found negligent. A second approach involves suing a manufacturer for breach of an implied warranty. If a product is found by the court to be unfit for the purpose for which it was intended, then the plaintiff might be able to collect damages because the equipment includes an implied warranty that it works the way it is supposed to work. Finally, an injured patient might be able to argue that an equipment manufacturer is strictly liable. Under this legal theory, a company can be found liable if a patient using its product is injured, regardless of the foreseeability of risk or the care the manufacturer took to prevent an injury.

Athletic trainers can help prevent lawsuits that have components of product liability by instituting the following practices:

- Read the warning labels and instruction manuals for every piece of equipment you use.
- Insist that athletes read the warning labels on all equipment they use.

Equipment Liability

Athletic trainers must understand that the improper design, manufacture, or use of products can result in legal liability for the company that made the equipment and, in some cases, for the athletic trainer who issued or used the equipment. A product can be found defective in one of four ways (Settle and Spigelmyer 1984):

- Faulty design
- Faulty construction
- Failure to provide adequate warning
- Failure to conform to an express warranty

Athletic trainers can protect themselves against the threat of legal liability in many ways. Wise athletic trainers will take care to implement each of these strategies in their practice.

- Make sure that athletes understand the information in the warning label. Ask them if they have any questions (this is especially important if their primary language is different from the language used on the label). Ask them to sign a statement indicating that they have read and understand the warning label.

- Never modify, alter, or otherwise reconfigure a piece of equipment. Doing so might invalidate its express warranty and might shift a sizable percentage of the legal liability away from the manufacturer and toward the athletic trainer.

- Inspect and maintain equipment according to the schedule recommended by the manufacturer. Keep records of all such maintenance.

- Obtain, read, and disseminate to staff all of the documentation for equipment, and provide training in the equipment's proper use. Document this training for verification and offer retraining as needed (Cohn et al. 1998).

Additional Strategies

At the beginning of this chapter, it was suggested that knowledge of legal liability would help improve the quality of care offered by an athletic trainer. To place that sweeping statement into context, consider the following suggestions as part of a strategy to avoid the threat of legal liability (Graham 1985).

- **Build relationships.** Develop and maintain good relations with athletes and other physically active patients, parents, coworkers, subordinates, and other health care professionals with whom you work or to whom you commonly refer patients. You should build trust relationships and promote a constant flow of two-way communication with these groups.

- **Insist on a written contract.** Have a written contract supported by a detailed position description that clearly delineates the athletic trainer's job functions. This document is one of the most important defenses you can offer against a charge of negligence, because it helps establish those to whom you might owe a legal duty.

- **Obtain informed consent.** Obtain informed consent for the services you perform. In the case of minors, obtain informed consent from their parents (see figure 6.8 on p. 201). Warn athletes and parents of the dangers, including permanent disability and death, inherent in their particular sport. Repeat such warnings annually.

- **Provide physical examinations.** Be certain that every athlete undergoes a physical examination by a state-licensed medical practitioner. Make certain that the content of the physical examination is consistent with nationally recognized standards in terms of both content and frequency.

- **Know the profession and its standards.** Develop and maintain a database of information about injuries and illnesses that are most common to each sport you work with. This documentation will enhance your qualifications as an expert in your field. Practice your profession unafraid, but keep in mind the standards of practice embraced by the profession. Regularly refer to professional position and consensus statements for current acceptable approaches to the standard of care.

- **Document hazards.** Make a documented attempt to reduce injuries by recommending or personally taking action to remove or modify potential hazards. Consider establishing a safety committee charged with conducting an ongoing program of risk assessment and reduction. Be aware, however, that a paper trail documenting safety hazards can also be used against you or your institution, especially if the hazards are not corrected or the corrections go undocumented.

■ **Establish policies.** Adopt and scrupulously adhere to policies and procedures designed to reduce the incidence of injury and to guide the actions of sports medicine personnel when injuries do occur. Keep all emergency first aid equipment in working order and available to those who might need to use it.

■ **Document activities.** Document the details of all injuries, treatments, and rehabilitative procedures so that a chronology of events can easily be determined after the fact. Maintain medical records until well after the statute of limitations for malpractice liability has expired (this will vary from state to state).

■ **Maintain confidentiality.** Maintain the confidentiality of the patient's medical record. When you wish to share the information with others, obtain written permission of the patient first.

■ **Provide proper instruction.** When interacting with athletes and other physically active patients, be certain that the instruction you provide allows for safe participation. If you give instructions to a patient in a rehabilitation program, for example, make sure that the patient understands how to progress and knows the warning signs associated with reinjury. If you are instructing athletes in an off-season conditioning program, make sure that they can perform the exercises properly and that they use commonly accepted safety techniques such as spotting each other when using free weights.

■ **Supervise your staff.** Insist that every staff member adhere to prescribed programmatic procedures. Make sure that supervisees understand your requests. Check to make sure that they are carrying out your requests as required by the procedures specified in the program's handbook. When deviations occur, be sure to correct the supervisee's behavior.

■ **Participate in continuing education.** Take part in continuing athletic training education by attending seminars and symposia and reading sports medicine literature. Alter your techniques as technology and knowledge advance. Document your continuing education activities and the changes that result.

■ **Recognize your qualifications.** Practice only within the limitations of the laws of your state and the boundaries of your training. Be consistent with the standard of care expected of other reasonably prudent athletic trainers. Be quick to refer injured athletes and other physically active patients to physicians and be sure to follow their instructions carefully. Avoid the distribution of prescription medications and be cautious in your use of over-the-counter medications.

■ **Maintain insurance coverage.** All athletic trainers, certified and student alike, should have malpractice and liability insurance to safeguard their personal assets in the event of a legal action. Even if a malpractice suit is frivolous and eventually dismissed, the costs associated with defense are usually beyond the means of most athletic trainers. In some cases, the employer's general liability policy will adequately protect you. In many cases, however, institutional liability insurance policies specifically exclude health care activities. In addition, the maximum benefit of institutional policies might not cover the fantastic costs associated with medical litigation. Athletic trainers who do not have adequate protection through their employer's liability insurance policy should seriously consider buying their own policies. Athletic trainers must evaluate the limits of coverage of both their employer's malpractice insurance policies and their personal malpractice insurance policies. The limits of these policies often determine what kinds of activities the athletic trainer can engage in. Some policies, for example, cover job-related duties but exclude volunteer activities. Under these circumstances, an athletic trainer who provides medical services at summer sports camps would probably want to have her employer write these activities into her job description so that the policy would cover them. Activities that an athletic trainer undertakes with malicious intent or gross negligence are frequently not covered.

Informed consent is a process whereby patients are educated about the risks and benefits of a medical procedure and give their permission for enactment of the procedure. For informed consent to be valid, the patient must (1) be of legal age and be mentally competent, (2) be fully informed and demonstrate a full understanding of the risks and benefits, and (3) voluntarily offer consent without duress or pressure (Herbert 1990).

The National Athletic Trainers' Association offers malpractice and liability insurance to its members through Marsh Affinity Group Services. Visit www. personal-plans.com/ nata/welcome.do for more information.

STRATEGIES FOR DEALING WITH LEGAL CHALLENGES

Despite the best efforts of athletic trainers to practice within the law, some will inevitably face legal challenges at some point in their careers. When facing a lawsuit or other legal challenge, well-informed athletic trainers should be aware of both the defenses available to them and the do's and don'ts of providing testimony.

Legal Defenses

Athletic trainers accused of malpractice have several possible legal defenses. None of these, however, provides ironclad protection against a lawsuit; each defense has exceptions that could leave the athletic trainer liable even though the general principle might be valid. The best defense, of course, is to provide high-quality athletic training services consistent with the standard of care expected in the profession and by the statutory regulations of the state. The statute of limitations, sovereign immunity, assumption of risk, Good Samaritan immunity, and comparative negligence are legal defenses that might apply to claims of athletic trainer malpractice.

■ **Statutes of limitations. Statutes of limitations** are state laws that fix a certain length of time during which an aggrieved patient may sue a health care provider. The statute of limitations applies in most states to health care providers who have been statutorily recognized by the state. States that regulate athletic training practice, therefore, probably extend the statutes of limitations to cover athletic trainers, but other states might not. Athletic trainers who are employed by physicians, hospitals, or physical therapists in states that don't provide credentials might also be protected because their employers are regulated. Although the statute of limitations usually specifies the period, many exceptions can lengthen the period during which an athlete or other physically active patient can bring suit.

■ **Sovereign immunity. Sovereign (governmental) immunity** is a legal doctrine that holds that neither governments nor their agents can be held liable for negligent torts (Baley and Matthews 1984). In theory, athletic trainers employed in public schools, colleges, and universities are immune from legal liability because they are agents of governmental entities. In fact, however, many governmental units, including the federal government, have substantially lowered this traditional shield against legal liability (Herbert and Herbert 1989). Athletic trainers employed in public institutions should not proceed as if they are immune by virtue of their positions, even though Leverenz and Helms (1990b) have identified three cases in which athletic trainers avoided liability based on a claim of governmental immunity (*Garza v. Edinburg Consolidated Independent School District,* 576 S.W.2d. 916 [Tx. 1979]; *Lowe v. Texas Tech University,* 540 S.W.2d. 297 [Tx. 1976]; and *Sorey v. Kellett,* 849 F.2d. 429 [5th Cir. 1988]).

■ **Assumption of risk.** One of the oldest and most common defenses that educational institutions and their employees have used against legal liability in athletic injury cases is **assumption of risk**. In this defense, the athletic trainer asserts that the injured athlete or other physically active patient was aware of the risks involved and decided to proceed anyway, thereby absolving the institution and the athletic trainer from any liability for damages. Scott (1990) points out that this defense is valid only when two conditions are met. The athlete must "fully appreciate" the type and magnitude of the risk involved in participating in the activity. The athlete must also "knowingly, voluntarily, and unequivocally" choose to participate in the activity in the face of the inherent risks. Skillful attorneys usually have little trouble defeating this defense, especially when the injured party is a minor. To protect against legal liability and improve their chances of being able to use this defense should the need arise, many schools and colleges provide educational sessions, complete with videos and printed materials, that warn student-athletes and their parents of the specific dangers inherent in their sports. Fol-

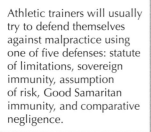

Athletic trainers will usually try to defend themselves against malpractice using one of five defenses: statute of limitations, sovereign immunity, assumption of risk, Good Samaritan immunity, and comparative negligence.

lowing these sessions, participants are asked to sign a statement affirming that they have been warned of the dangers associated with the sport (including permanent disability and death), that they understand these risks, that they have been offered the opportunity to ask questions regarding the risks, and that they voluntarily choose to participate regardless of the risks.

■ **Good Samaritan immunity.** A defense that athletic trainers can use in a limited number of settings is immunity by virtue of a **Good Samaritan law**. Good Samaritan laws enacted in some states protect health care providers who voluntarily come to the aid of injured persons. These statutes might or might not cover athletic trainers, although about two-thirds of the states with Good Samaritan laws protect everyone who comes to the aid of an injured person, and the rest specify the classes of people who are protected under the law (Gallup 1995). Specific Good Samaritan laws in some states protect volunteer team physicians from legal liability (Benda 1991). If the physician receives compensation of any kind, the immunity from liability does not apply. Because athletic trainers are increasingly volunteering to serve at state games and charitable athletic events, this defense might become more popular. The injured person, of course, must consent to be treated. The statutes do not protect an athletic trainer from willful or wanton misconduct or from gross or intentional negligence.

■ **Comparative negligence.** As was true in the opening case, physically active patients sometimes ignore the prescriptions of their health care providers, a disregard that can lead to injury or aggravate an injury. The courts often use the doctrine of **comparative negligence** to determine if the liability for these injuries should be divided between the plaintiff and the defendant. Comparative negligence determines the degree of fault an athletic trainer and a patient have for causing an injury. The athletic trainer's financial liability depends on the formula used in the state in which the case is tried. In most states, patients can collect damages only if their comparative culpability is less than half the total. In some states, however, plaintiffs can be awarded financial restitution equal to the athletic trainer's percentage of fault. For instance, if Enrique's negligence accounted for 25% of the total fault for the aggravation of his injury, Todd Russell and his team physician might have to pay 75% of the damage claim.

Providing Testimony at a Deposition or Trial

As a fact witness, the athletic trainer either had responsibility for treating an injured patient or has knowledge of the facts of the case. The athletic trainer has few choices about appearing in court under this circumstance, because the court will probably issue a **subpoena** ordering appearance.

An attorney might retain an athletic trainer as an expert to testify on behalf of a client. Expert witnesses are paid to provide testimony that educates the judge and jury about the standard of care that should be applied in a particular case. As an expert witness, the athletic trainer should agree with the positions that the attorney will ask her to take at trial. She should also be sure the attorney who hired her has the facts to support the case. Otherwise, she will appear ignorant and foolish on the witness stand. In many cases, the expert opinion of an athletic trainer is considered during pretrial phases, and the case itself may be settled or dismissed without a trial. The opinion of the athletic trainer is deemed very valuable during these times as it may sway a plaintiff or defendant's case in one direction or another, possibly leaning toward the determination of an outcome if a trial were to occur.

Whether athletic trainers are subpoenaed or appear as expert witnesses, they should observe the following guidelines to safeguard their credibility (Horsley and Carlova 1983):

■ Avoid memorizing the testimony.

■ Never guess. If you're unsure of the answer to a question, admit lack of knowledge on that point.

■ Testify only on issues about which you are an expert. Do not testify beyond the boundaries of your experience.

Although athletic trainers are sued infrequently, they might be called on to provide **testimony** in a court. An athletic trainer might give testimony either at a deposition, which is an informal series of questions posed under oath before a trial, or at the trial itself. He might be called as either a fact witness or an expert witness.

- Prepare for your testimony by carefully studying the records of the case before entering the courtroom. If you need to refer to the medical records while on the stand, understand that the records will be considered evidence that the opposing attorney will be able to access.

- Discuss your testimony with your attorney or the attorney retaining you as a witness before giving it in the courtroom.

- Use common language. Whenever you use medical language, attempt to interpret it for the judge and jury.

- Be sure that your testimony in court is consistent with any depositions you might have made before the beginning of the trial. Always review the deposition before taking the stand.

- Ask the judge for guidance if you feel the need to expand on a yes-or-no question posed by an attorney.

- Ask the judge for guidance if you think that answering a question would violate the athletic trainer–patient relationship.

- Use illustrations (charts, drawings, slides, photographs, and so on) to help make your point when appropriate.

- If you are charged with malpractice and your malpractice insurance company has provided a lawyer you feel uncomfortable with, hire your own attorney.

- Maintain a professional, dignified demeanor at all times. Dress neatly; answer in a normal tone of voice at an even rate; and be respectful of the judge, jury, and attorneys.

- Remain composed at all times.

- Be prepared to be subjected to hostile questioning.

- Avoid responding to hypothetically posed questions. These are not based on facts and merely serve as speculation.

APPLICATIONS TO ATHLETIC TRAINING: THEORY INTO PRACTICE

Apply the concepts discussed in this chapter to the following two case studies to help you prepare for similar situations in actual practice. The questions at the end of the studies have many possible correct solutions. The case studies can be used for homework, for exam questions, or to spur class discussion.

Case Study 1

Larry Donelson was pleased when the management of the professional football team that employed him allowed him to hire an additional athletic training student for the preseason training camp. The preseason was a hectic time, and he was grateful for the help that students were able to provide. One of the students whom he had decided to hire this year, Rich Hayes, was only a sophomore. Larry usually hired only students who had completed their junior year, but Rich had come highly recommended by his supervising athletic trainer, an old friend of Larry's, so Larry had decided to take a chance on Rich.

James Star was a 10th-round draft choice trying to make the team that summer. James had played college football at the university that Rich was attending. Although James felt good about his performance in the first two weeks, a knee injury suffered in the first scrimmage had kept him out of practice since then. Fortunately, the knee was starting to feel better, and James hoped that he could return to limited practice within a couple of days.

One day the head coach surprised everybody by announcing that the team would have the next morning off. The athletic training students, knowing they wouldn't have to wake up at 5:30 A.M. as usual, decided to visit a local pub that night. The bar was the only one in the small college town where the team had its training camp, so most of the players went there as well.

Rich saw James at the pub and joined him. Three beers later, the topic of James' knee injury came up. When James told Rich that he was feeling better and would probably be back in a couple of days, Rich confided that while he was cleaning a whirlpool a couple of days earlier, he had heard Larry Donelson, the team physician, and the head coach talking about James. When James asked what they had said, Rich told him they were simply discussing the details of James' knee injury and his prospects for full recovery. After two more beers, James had the whole story.

When the team released him the next week, James immediately contacted his agent, an attorney, who filed a lawsuit on his behalf alleging that the team had concealed the true nature of James' injury, which resulted in his termination and subsequent unemployment.

QUESTIONS FOR ANALYSIS

1. What legal principles are involved in this case? How do they apply? Does James have a strong case? Why or why not?

2. How could this situation have been avoided? What policies and procedures should Larry Donelson institute to prevent this kind of problem?

3. Who, if anyone, is at fault in this case? If more than one person is at fault, how is a judge or jury likely to determine the percentage of each person's liability?

4. What records could Larry use to defend himself and the team?

Case Study 2

Christine Campbell, the assistant athletic trainer for Northwest State University, was off the bench like a shot when she saw the basketball team's star center fall to the floor holding her knee. After conducting an examination on the floor, Christine decided to take the player to the athletic training room for a complete examination by the team physician. She and the student manager, who were both at least 10 inches shorter than the player, helped her hobble off the court toward the athletic training room. As they were passing the locker room, the student manager slipped on a wet spot, causing the player to put her full weight on the injured knee. She cried out in pain and told Christine that she felt a "pop."

After the team physician, a general practitioner employed by the student health service, completed his examination, he informed the player that she had torn the anterior cruciate and medial collateral ligaments in her knee and would need surgery to correct the problem. He instructed Christine to do the following things, all of which he recorded in his postevaluation dictation for the athlete's medical record:

1. Apply an elastic wrap from the toes to midthigh.

2. Apply a knee immobilizer.

3. Fit the athlete with crutches.

4. Arrange an orthopedic consultation for the next day.

5. Give enough 800-milligram ibuprofen for three days.

Later that night, a phone call from the athlete's roommate woke Christine, who found out that the athlete had become violently ill and had been rushed to the hospital by ambulance after suffering a reaction to the medication that Christine had given her.

QUESTIONS FOR ANALYSIS

1. What legal principles are involved in this case? What liability concerns should be addressed? What policies and procedures should be implemented to address these concerns?

2. What would you have done differently, if anything, if you had been in Christine's position?

3. Who, if anyone, is at fault in this case? If more than one person is at fault, how should a judge or jury determine the degree to which each person is liable?

SUMMARY

Athletic trainers are challenged every day with legal considerations. It is expected that all athletic trainers will practice within a standard of care, performing duties that other reasonably prudent athletic trainers would have performed under similar circumstances. Negligence occurs when an athletic trainer fails to act as a reasonably prudent athletic trainer would act under such circumstances. Malpractice refers to liability-generating conduct associated with the adverse outcome of a patient's treatment. To provide protection to the public, athletic trainers are regulated on a state-wide basis (licensure, registration, certification, exemption). In addition to adverse treatment outcomes, liability also rests with adverse conditions arising from poor facility management, faulty equipment, and improper dispensing of medication, to name a few examples. Risk management is the process intended to prevent losses of all kinds (financial, physical, property, activity, time) for everyone associated with an organization, including its directors, administrators, employees, and clients. Ongoing evaluation of one's practice and practice setting helps to reduce the risk of adverse outcomes.

KEY CONCEPTS AND REVIEW

1. Define and discuss the legal principles most applicable to athletic training settings.

Although the thought of legal action against an athletic trainer is unsettling, prudent athletic trainers will take advantage of their legal knowledge to improve the quality of the service they provide to their physically active patients. The best and most important source of legal advice, of course, is an attorney experienced in dealing with health care malpractice issues.

2. Identify the types of situations most likely to hold liability concerns for athletic trainers.

Risk management is a process designed to prevent losses of all types for everyone associated with an athletic program. The two ways to identify and assess risks are real-world observation and inference from controlled studies. The best risk management programs use both methods. The athletic trainer can reduce risk in four areas: preparation for the activity, conduct of the activity, management of injuries, and proper records management.

3. Understand the different types of credentialing laws that affect the practice of athletic training.

Credentialing laws, including licensure, certification, registration, and exemption, are designed to ensure basic competencies to protect the public. All athletic trainers should become familiar with the laws in their state to determine their legal basis for practice. Athletic trainers who practice in states without credentialing laws, although they might be protected by the delegatory clause of the medical practice act, might be held to the standard of care of a physician in a malpractice case.

4. Understand the elements required to prove negligence on the part of an athletic trainer.

Torts are legal wrongs, other than breach of contract, for which a court will determine a remedy, usually in the form of monetary damages. Negligence is the kind of tort most commonly charged against athletic trainers. To prove negligence, the aggrieved person must demonstrate conduct by the athletic trainer, existence of duty, breach of duty, causation (including actual and proximate cause), and damage. Athletic trainers will be held to the same standard of care as other reasonably prudent athletic trainers in the same or similar circumstances.

5. Be aware of the various legal defenses available to athletic trainers against charges of malpractice.

Although several defenses against charges of malpractice exist, including statutes of limitations, sovereign immunity, assumption of risk, Good Samaritan immunity, and comparative negligence, the athletic trainer's best defense is to practice in a manner consistent with the standards of the profession.

6. Identify the most important elements of providing effective legal testimony.

Should an athletic trainer be called to provide testimony, either as a fact witness or as an expert witness, he should prepare by reviewing the records of the case, consulting with the attorney, and speaking only to the facts of the case within the limits of his experience and training.

7. Identify and put into practice methods that avoid legal liability while improving the quality of athletic training care.

Athletic trainers will improve their practice while simultaneously protecting themselves from liability if they build relationships with their patients, insist on written employment contracts, obtain informed consent, screen all athletes during a physical exam, and abide by the standards of the profession. They should also document hazards, establish and adhere to written policies, document patient care activities, maintain confidentiality, and provide proper instruction to injured patients. Finally, athletic trainers must also supervise their staffs, participate in continuing education, practice within the boundaries of their qualifications, and maintain a liability insurance policy.

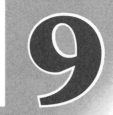

Ethics in Sports Medicine

OBJECTIVES

After reading this chapter, you should be able to do the following:

1. Understand the definition and purpose of ethical standards and their relevance for the athletic trainer.

2. Define what the term "professional" means as it relates to an athletic trainer.

3. Identify the appropriate code of ethics that applies generally to the profession of athletic training, along with codes that might apply to specific settings within the profession.

4. Identify the situations and circumstances in which ethical concerns are most frequent.

5. Develop strategies for avoiding ethical problems and for dealing with them if they occur.

6. Recognize elements of cultural competence as they relate to athletic training.

7. Recognize the ethical challenges and overall issues associated with whistle-blowing.

Portions of this chapter are reprinted or adapted from R.R. Ray and D. Wiese-Bjornstal, 1999, *Ethical perspectives in counseling* (Champaign, IL: Human Kinetics), 161-175. By permission of Richard Ray.

▶ Tammy Johnson is the certified athletic trainer at a National Collegiate Athletic Association (NCAA) Division III college. As the school's first athletic trainer, Tammy was instrumental in developing and building support for a drug and alcohol program that included both educational and athlete code of conduct components. Included in the athlete's code of conduct was a zero-tolerance clause that prohibited all athletes from consuming alcoholic beverages during their seasons. Athletes caught violating this rule would be forced to miss two games.

One night Tammy received a call at home from a student who had taken a class from her a couple of years before. The student was a waiter at a local restaurant and had observed one of the school's basketball players drinking in the restaurant's bar two nights earlier. He had been reluctant to tell anyone about the incident because he knew the athlete would have to miss the first round of the NCAA tournament later in the week if he was turned in. The student finally decided that he had to do something to ease his conscience, however, so he called Tammy in the hope that she would be willing to report the violation. Tammy spent 45 minutes on the phone gathering all the details of the event, including the names of other students who had been with the basketball player. She even got the name of the waitress who had served the basketball player and his friends. She also informed the student who had called her that if he insisted on going forward with the allegations he could expect some questions from the basketball coach and the athletic director. He said that would be OK as long as justice was served.

The next day, Tammy went to the basketball coach and informed him of the allegations. The coach, who was trying to prepare for the biggest game of the year, was upset but said that he would talk to the player and try to reach resolution on the matter as soon as possible. Later that afternoon, the coach pulled Tammy aside in the hallway and told her that he and all of his assistants had confronted the player with the allegation that he had been drinking. The coach told Tammy that the athlete denied consuming any alcohol, although he did admit to being in the bar. The basketball coach told Tammy that he believed his player, and that as far as he was concerned the matter was closed. When Tammy asked the coach if he had informed the athletic director as required by the school's drug and alcohol policy, the coach simply said that he didn't think the case merited any further investigation and he didn't want to take any of the AD's time with such a trivial matter.

Fame is vapor, popularity an accident, riches take wing. . . .
The only thing that endures is character.

—HORACE GREELEY

As Tammy's case demonstrates, athletic training is a profession that places many pressures on its practitioners. Athletic trainers face pressure from coaches, whose security needs are met through winning games; from athletes and other physically active patients, who are often willing to sacrifice their health for short-term glory; and from a variety of other sources. One common by-product of this pressure is the temptation to make decisions or perform acts that, although seemingly innocent, are not in the best interests of patients or of the profession.

All athletic trainers have a responsibility to act in an ethical manner. Unfortunately, fulfilling this responsibility is not always easy. Ethical decision making requires both the knowledge of ethical responsibilities and the willpower to endure the inevitable hardships that accompany ethically correct decisions. The purpose of this chapter is to introduce the topic of ethics as it applies to athletic trainers. In the chapter we will identify some of the most common situations in which ethical breaches can occur, and we will consider steps that the athletic trainer can take to minimize their occurrence.

Ethical practice is not limited to the managerial roles assumed by athletic trainers; ethical dilemmas arise in other domains of the profession as well. An athletic trainer's injury management, rehabilitation, education, and counseling roles are particularly rich with potential ethical problems. Although not all ethical problems are related to the managerial role, many are. All require some degree of decision making. Decision making is the single most common element among all managerial functions, and the ability to make good decisions is one of an athletic trainer's most important managerial skills.

DEFINING ETHICS

Ethics is the study of the rules, standards, and principles that dictate **right conduct** among members of a society. Such rules are based on moral values. Principles of ethics have developed from a long, rich history of philosophical debate. They are deeply embedded in our choices of how we govern and conduct ourselves as a civilized society and serve as the basis for many of our norms for social interaction. Ethics also reflect many of the tenets of a variety of religions and have been influenced by religious philosophies from around the world. All of these influences and history have led us to depend on the principles of ethics to form the moral backbone of the most important things that we do as contributors to a conscientious society. In the professions, ethics provide a perspective from which to judge the rightness or wrongness of a professional's actions; they are a reflection of the conscience of the profession (Appelbaum and Lawton 1990).

> Ethics help define acceptable behavior among members of a group. Professions establish codes of ethics to provide behavioral guidelines for their members and to help protect the public from the actions of unethical practitioners.

Why Professions Establish Ethical Standards

Professions are defined by a commitment to certain characteristics that set them apart from nonprofessional groups within our society. One of the most important of these characteristics is a commitment to high standards of ethical behavior by the members of the profession. The professional organization of each of the professions that provide health care services to athletes and other physically active patients writes a **code of ethics** to establish its ethical standards. The purposes of these codes are to provide a guide to appropriate conduct for members, to provide a reference by which to judge members when their conduct comes into question, and to provide assurance and protection to the public served by members of the profession.

Ethical Standards Relevant to Athletic Training

Sports health care professionals should comply with the code of ethics of the national professional organization for their primary profession. Athletic trainers must adhere to several sets of professional standards. The *NATA Code of Ethics* (National Athletic Trainers' Association 1995) is intended to guide the actions of every member of the NATA in the practice of athletic training (see appendix B). The code consists of four general principles, each with its own substatements. A breach of the principles embodied in this document would be viewed seriously and could result in suspension or revocation of certification. Athletic trainers who hold dual credentialing as physical therapists must adhere to the American Physical Therapy Association *Code of Ethics* (American Physical Therapy Association 2010). Similarly, athletic trainers who hold other certifications or credentials, such as nurses, occupational therapists, physicians, physician assistants, or emergency medical technicians, are bound by the codes of ethics of the organizations that represent those professions. Code of ethics documents provide guidelines for ethical conduct within the respective professions and apply to the entire range of practice patterns and settings applicable to those professions. Their standards are enforceable for the members of each organization but should also be considered applicable to nonmembers within the profession.

Despite variations in how different professions view their own ethical conduct, the foundation for forming guidelines for each can be based on six underlying principles (Rubin 2002):

Go online to find the code of ethics for the following organizations: American Counseling Association, American Psychological Association, American Association of University Professors *(Statement on Professional Ethics)*, the International Federation of Sports Medicine (FIMS), and the American Physical Therapy Association (APTA).

1. Autonomy: A patient's right to be fully informed, to make his or her own health care decisions, and to have his inherent dignity respected
2. Beneficence: Commitment to do good, to try to do the best for each patient
3. Nonmaleficence: Commitment to avoid doing bad things, to do no harm
4. Fidelity: Subordination of one's needs to those of the patient
5. Veracity: Truth telling and honesty
6. Justice: Concept that all patients should be treated fairly without regard to race, religion, and so on

Unfortunately, becoming informed about the NATA's code of ethics is often not enough, even for athletic trainers without dual credentials. The various practice domains force athletic trainers to examine the ethical codes of other disciplines to make sure that they do not stray from accepted practice in those disciplines. For example, when providing counseling to student-athletes, athletic trainers should be sure to adhere to the *Code of Ethics* of the American Counseling Association (1995) or to the *Ethical Principles of Psychologists and Code of Conduct* of the American Psychological Association (1992). Athletic trainers who are also teachers might be bound by the ethical codes of professional educators' societies, such as the American Association of University Professors (1995). Finally, ethical standards exist that are specific to particular employment settings.

Efforts to implore members of professions and professional associations to adhere to an ethical code of conduct are necessary to establish public trust that in the eyes of some has been waning in recent years (Cohen 2006). Public trust is based on altruism, respect, honesty, integrity, dutifulness, honor, excellence, and accountability. While the overwhelming majority of health care providers abide by their professional ethical guidelines, some are faced with a unique set of challenges related to these principles. This is seen in cases in which individuals hold dual certifications and credentials, such as a certified athletic trainer who is also a physical therapist, or a physical therapist who is also a chiropractor. In these circumstances, the professional who attempts to follow ethical principles of both professionally affiliated organizations may find that the organizations are at odds with one another. Position statements and other organizational initiatives may conflict between the two organizations, placing the health care professional in a difficult predicament. Professional organizations are focused on supporting, endorsing, and protecting their professional members; thus they may not be very sympathetic toward health care professionals who hold dual memberships.

Medical Ethics

While professionals in different disciplines define their own set of ethical standards, those in health care typically follow a set of guidelines referred to as **medical ethics**. Campbell and colleagues (2001) defined medical ethics as a moral philosophy that helps practitioners and others discern if and under what circumstances various health care practices are right or

---

■ Five Principles of the NATA Code of Ethics

1. Members shall respect the rights, welfare, and dignity of all.
2. Members shall comply with the laws and regulations governing the practice of athletic training.
3. Members shall accept responsibility for the exercise of sound judgment.
4. Members shall maintain and promote high standards in their provision of services.
5. Members shall not engage in conduct that could be construed as a conflict of interest or that reflects negatively on the profession.

wrong. For physicians, the foundation for ethical practice has been established by the Hippocratic Oath:

I swear to fulfill, to the best of my ability and judgment, this covenant:

I will respect the hard-won scientific gains of those physicians in whose steps I walk, and gladly share such knowledge as is mine with those who are to follow.

I will apply, for the benefit of the sick, all measures [that] are required, avoiding those twin traps of overtreatment and therapeutic nihilism.

I will remember that there is art to medicine as well as science, and that warmth, sympathy, and understanding may outweigh the surgeon's knife or the chemist's drug.

I will not be ashamed to say "I know not," nor will I fail to call on my colleagues when the skills of another are needed for a patient's recovery.

I will respect the privacy of my patients, for their problems are not disclosed to me that the world may know. Most especially must I tread with care in matters of life and death. If it is given me to save a life, all thanks. But it may also be within my power to take a life; this awesome responsibility must be faced with great humbleness and awareness of my own frailty. Above all, I must not play at God.

I will remember that I do not treat a fever chart, or a cancerous growth, but a sick human being, whose illness may affect the person's family and economic stability. My responsibility includes these related problems, if I am to care adequately for the sick.

I will prevent disease whenever I can, for prevention is preferable to cure.

I will remember that I remain a member of society, with special obligations to all my fellow human beings, those sound of mind and body as well as the infirm.

If I do not violate this oath, may I enjoy life and art, respected while I live and remembered with affection thereafter. May I always act so as to preserve the finest traditions of my calling and may I long experience the joy of healing those who seek my help.

The Hippocratic Oath is believed to have been written by Hippocrates, who is considered the father of Western medicine, around the late fifth century B.C. The oath is taken by new physicians and other new health care practitioners to swear in the presence of others that they will uphold their professional ethical standards. Today, the Hippocratic Oath has been translated from its original format to both classic and modern versions (the modern version is presented here).

Medical ethics goes beyond the relationship between a single practitioner and a patient. All health care professionals must work collaboratively despite their variance of training in an effort to offer maximum benefits for all patients involved in the health care system (Davidoff 2000; Gibson 2002). A group of interdisciplinary health care providers consisting of physicians, nurses, health care administrators, academics, ethicists, lawyers, economists, and philosophers met to develop ethical principles that might be useful for all individuals involved in the health care delivery system. This group has since become known as the Tavistock (named after a square in London where the meeting took place) group, and the set of principles derived from their discussions is referred to as the Tavistock Principles. The principles were all-encompassing, designed to benefit those who are responsible for the health care system, those who work in it, and those who use it.

The following are the seven principles defined by the Tavistock group (Magee 2010):

1. **A Human Right:** Health care is a human right.

2. **Balance Patient Centered With Population Sensitive:** The care of individual is at the center of health care delivery but must be viewed and practiced within the overall context of continuing work to generate the greatest possible health gains for groups and populations.

Medical ethics is a moral philosophy that helps practitioners and others discern if and under what circumstances various health care practices are right or wrong.

Athletic trainers can usually act in an ethical manner by acting within the law. They can become involved in ethical dilemmas as either a primary party or a third party.

3. Comprehensively Manage Disease Burden and Promote Prevention: The responsibilities of the health care delivery system include the prevention of illness and the alleviation of disability.

4. Professional Collaboration: Cooperation with each other and those served is imperative for those working within the health care delivery system.

5. Quality Improvement: All individuals and groups involved in health care, whether providing access or services, have the continuing responsibility to help improve its quality.

6. Safety: Initially there was anxiety over "do no harm" because it is so strongly associated with doctors. But this principle seemed important to include because there is increasing recognition of just how much harm health care systems produce and of how policies with benign intentions can create harm.

7. Openness: This last principle might be both the most banal and the most profound. Nobody could argue against being open, honest, and trustworthy; yet every day in every health care system, people fail on all three counts.

RELATIONSHIP BETWEEN LEGAL AND ETHICAL CONSIDERATIONS

Ethical considerations often overlap with, contradict, or otherwise interact with issues of **law**. In convenient circumstances, difficult ethical decisions are consistent with the law, but an athletic trainer must recognize that in some situations what is ethical might not be legal and what is legal might not be ethical. This issue is especially difficult for those in health care roles who must consider issues of confidentiality and protection of individual **rights** to privacy. The right of an athlete to privacy might well conflict with the law when the law dictates that a specific type of information be reported. The multiple roles served by athletic trainers make the issue even more difficult because of the many different types of information for which they are responsible. The most recent large-scale issue of this kind is the reporting of human immunodeficiency virus (HIV) status required by some health departments. Ideas regarding how an athletic trainer might deal with such conflicts are included later in this chapter. What is clear is that professional codes of ethics usually dictate that it is unethical to engage in any practice activity that is illegal (Makarowski and Rickell 1993).

Defining a Professional

As simple as the term may sound, "professionalism" is not clearly defined and agreed on among those in all health care disciplines (Swick 2000). Concepts of professionalism have been reported to change according to age, experience level, educational rank, and gender (Nath et al. 2006). Nath and colleagues found that younger health care professionals in training were more likely than their older peers or faculty to view certain behaviors as unprofessional. Isear (1997) defined three elements of professionalism:

1. Clinician–patient relationship (trust, confidence)

2. Collegial relationships (with other health care professionals, including professional growth)

3. Attire and hygiene (personal intangibles, such as punctuality, adhering to commitments, understanding role limitations)

Isear's elements are similar to those of Chambers (2004), who incorporates more of a community-based approach toward the characteristics of a professional:

1. Be a community of practitioners who simultaneously work for themselves, customers, and peers.

2. Help patients and clients who are individuals making their own personal choices.

3. Serve private and personal needs of customers seeking wholeness.

4. Work as agents on behalf of customers instead of transacting services.

5. Function in a relationship of trust.

Implementing these elements does not appear to be an overwhelming task to request of a health care professional. Why, then, are they not adhered to regularly by all? Even though most health care professionals place a high value on the components of professionalism, not all believe that they are easy to incorporate into daily practice. The three most common barriers to professionalism as reported by medical residents are time constraints (51.5%), high workloads (21.9%), and having to work with challenging or difficult patients (16%) (Ratanawongsa et al. 2006).

Professionalism is not just an expectation for practicing clinicians, educators, and administrators. The process of developing skills and characteristics to become a competent professional must be nurtured while students engage in their formal academic preparation. Professionalism is one of the six core competencies of both the Accreditation Council for Graduate Medical Education (ACGME) and the American Board of Medical Specialties (ABMS) (DeRosa 2006). Professionalism is taught at the medical school level and in residency programs, as well as in all athletic training education programs. A fact that merits discussion is that after one completes all academic requirements and becomes farther removed from formal education, less emphasis is placed on grade point average and more attention is paid to interpersonal skills and professional behaviors. Physical therapy educators have also attempted to define professionalism in an effort to promote such behavior as a part of student preparation (Jette 2003). Similar to what Isear (1997) suggested for athletic trainers, surveys of physical therapy students identified the following attributes associated with professionalism: self-presentation, accountability, integrity, and values.

The Athletic Trainer as a Primary Party

An athletic trainer may face ethical issues in many different forms. The most menacing will be those in which the athletic trainer is a **primary party** to the ethical concern. To be a primary party means that the athletic trainer is directly involved in the situation as a person who has behaved in an ethically questionable manner or who is the victim of an unethical act committed by another person. Of primary concern in this chapter is the former situation, in which the athletic trainer is the **perpetrator** of an unethical act.

The next few paragraphs address three types of situations in which an athletic trainer might become entangled as a primary party in an ethical dilemma. Although this set of situations is not exhaustive, these are the scenarios that occur most often or that have the greatest potential to harm the individuals involved. By adhering to codes of ethics, the athletic trainer will do much to protect both the patient and himself.

Breach of Confidentiality

One of the most frequently recurring ethical situations faced by athletic trainers involves **breach of confidentiality**. This situation is especially difficult for several reasons. First, an athletic trainer often serves in many roles that relate to an athlete. The athletic trainer often needs to share information with the team organization, with coaches, or with colleagues who are also responsible for some aspect of the athlete's care. Those needs, legitimate or not, sometimes conflict with what is in the best interest of athletes and

■ Types of Unethical Conduct

The following are the most common or serious situations in which an athletic trainer might become a primary party:

- Breach of confidentiality
- Conflict of interest
- Exploitation

with the responsibilities that the athletic trainer has for their health care. Consider Tammy's case in the opening scenario. If the basketball player who violated the school's alcohol policy had come to Tammy, admitted the violation, asked Tammy for help in treating his dependency, and asked her not to tell the coach, Tammy would have found herself in a difficult ethical position. On one hand, she has a responsibility to maintain the confidentiality of the athletes under her care. On the other hand, she might have a contractual obligation to uphold the policies of the institution that employs her and turn in the athlete for appropriate discipline under the rules of the alcohol policy.

Confidential information obtained as part of the professional relationship that an athletic trainer has with an athlete or other physically active patient might be personal, private, and sensitive. The athletic trainer should handle such information carefully to avoid ethical as well as legal breaches of confidentiality. In some situations, the most appropriate ethical behavior might even jeopardize an athletic trainer's job.

The second reason it might be difficult for an athletic trainer to maintain confidentiality is that many people are often involved in the care of an athlete or other physically active patient. This situation is especially common when student and intern practitioners who might not be fully cognizant of concerns for confidentiality are involved. When an athletic trainer is responsible for the supervision of students and interns, she will also be held responsible for student or intern actions. The athletic trainer can become a primary party in a breach of confidentiality even if she was not the immediate perpetrator of the breach.

The final concern relative to confidentiality is the high profile of athletes and of the athletic industry in our society. The pressures of the press and the public's desire to know everything possible about a high-profile athlete can be significant threats to an athlete's right to privacy and to the confidentiality of information that an athletic trainer is privy to. To avoid breaches of confidentiality, athletic trainers should take proactive and diligent measures to protect information and communications. Several suggestions for such measures are offered in the following sidebar.

The codes of ethics note three exceptions to the rule of confidentiality. No reason for a breach of confidentiality other than those listed next serves as an excuse for its occurrence. A professional should recognize the difference between a **reason** and an **excuse** and should accept a reason as an excuse only when it is both unavoidable and justifiable. These reasons would be considered excusable; any other reason would be inexcusable.

■ Measures to Protect the Confidentiality of Information and Communications

- Publish established policies regarding communication with coaches, administrators, media, and so on.
- Establish and follow responsible procedures for documentation, and store records in a secure environment.
- Allow access to the records only to persons with a legitimate role in providing health care to the patient.
- Release information only with written permission of the patient involved.
- Designate a specific person to handle all requests for health-related information; train all persons in the organization and remind them regularly to refer all inquiries to that person.
- Never discuss the health status of an athlete or other physically active patient in public, and never in private, unless all persons present have a legitimate need and have authorization to access the information.

Exceptions to the Rule of Confidentiality

- When the client is in clear and imminent danger
- When other persons are in clear and imminent danger
- When legal requirements demand the release of confidential information

Conflict of Interest

Athletic trainers are also susceptible to ethical breaches based on **conflicts of interest**. Here again, the particular threat to ethical practice is a result of the multiple roles that an athletic trainer might fill. The responsibilities that an athletic trainer has to a team organization, to the coaching staff, and to himself will often conflict with his responsibilities to an athlete or other physically active patient. The temptation to act or to advise an athlete or other patient in a manner that serves the team or protects the job or other interests of the athletic trainer might go unrecognized.

In Tammy's case, the threat to confidentiality of information comes about because she has a conflict of interest. Her personal concern for her job conflicts with the best interests of the athlete to keep the information confidential. These can be particularly difficult conflicts of interest to resolve, because the coach and organization might have a legitimate need to know the information and might threaten to fire the athletic trainer.

A nearly universal component in most codes of ethics for health care professionals is the responsibility to place the best interests of the patient above all other concerns. This standard applies to every role assumed by an athletic trainer. Athletic trainers who receive payment to use a particular product might have a conflict of interest when treating patients with that product. An athletic trainer's role is particularly sensitive because the athletic trainer and the patient must develop a high degree of trust in one another. If the athletic trainer breaches this trust through a conflict of interest, rebuilding it might be impossible and the relationship might disintegrate. For that reason, among others, athletes with sensitive counseling or psychological concerns might be better off if they are referred to a counselor not affiliated with the institution or the team. The athletic trainer's role as administrator is also subject to conflicts of interest. When decisions regarding allocation of resources, including time, money, and personnel, clash with the health care needs of the athletic patient population, a conflict of interest might be present that could lead to an ethical breach.

Avoiding conflicts of interest is not enough. Athletic trainers should be careful to avoid even the appearance of a conflict. People interpret ethical standards in different ways. Sometimes a well-considered action will appear unethical to those who don't know why the decision was made or why the action was taken. Unfortunately, if the action appears to involve a conflict of interest and is therefore considered unethical, the trust required to maintain a reputation of high integrity will be damaged.

Exploitation

Exploitation of an athlete or other physically active patient by an athletic trainer is a particularly manipulative and self-interested form of conflict of interest. Exploitation involves the intentional use of another person or group of persons to achieve a selfish objective. When patients confide in an athletic trainer, they become particularly vulnerable to exploitation because they might reveal things about themselves that would otherwise be unknown. Under such circumstances, patients are vulnerable to exploitation for money, information, sex, self-endangerment (for example, manipulating an athlete to play while injured), goods, or any number of other reasons. For an athletic trainer to perpetrate such a situation would be clearly unethical.

The Athletic Trainer as a Third Party

An athletic trainer might also be involved in ethical dilemmas as a **third party**. To be a third party means that the athletic trainer is not personally involved in the dilemma but has professional responsibilities because of her knowledge of the situation. An athletic trainer has the responsibility not only to intervene in the best interest of the client but to also protect others from harm whenever there is apparent risk of harm occurring. Tammy's situation in the opening case is a good example of how an athletic trainer can become embroiled in an ethical dilemma as a third party.

One of the primary differences between being involved in a situation of ethical concern as a third party and being involved as a primary participant is that as a third party, an athletic trainer can act more appropriately to help find a resolution. When an athletic trainer's involvement is as a primary participant, especially in the presence of a conflict of interest or exploitation, he must often remove himself from the situation and request that someone else intervene to help resolve it. If he is involved in an ethical concern as a third party, the circumstance is much different. In this case the athletic trainer is often in a good position to orchestrate a solution. The solution will often entail providing information and perspectives to the patient or managing other people and information to resolve the ethical dilemma.

An athletic trainer can become a third party to an ethical dilemma because of what she learns directly from a patient or because knowledge comes to her attention from other sources. Such knowledge can create difficult circumstances, because conflicts often occur between the professional's responsibility to maintain confidentiality, her responsibility to protect the patient from harm, her responsibility to protect others from harm, and other loyalties she might have that affect the patient.

Five categories of knowledge are most likely to render an athletic trainer a third party to an ethical dilemma.

Breach of Confidentiality, Conflict of Interest, or Exploitation of a Patient

As in situations when the athletic trainer is directly involved, breach of confidentiality, conflict of interest, or exploitation of a patient by a third party can be harmful to patients. Knowledge of such situations makes it incumbent upon the athletic trainer to intervene on behalf of the patient. Intervention usually does not mean that the athletic trainer has responsibility for correcting the situation. Bringing the situation to the patient's attention is usually sufficient because the patient can then take responsibility for the circumstance from a fully informed perspective. In the case of patients who are **minors** or who might otherwise be unable to protect themselves in such a situation, the athletic trainer should inform the parents or **guardians**, refer the situation to the appropriate authorities (particularly when there are legal concerns), or intervene directly.

■ Categories of Knowledge That Make an Athletic Trainer a Third Party to an Ethical Dilemma

- Knowledge of the occurrence of a breach of confidentiality, conflict of interest, or exploitation involving a patient
- Forbidden knowledge
- Knowledge of high-risk behaviors
- Knowledge of illegal activities
- Knowledge of situations in which the welfare of the patient conflicts with the welfare of another individual or group of individuals

Imagine, for example, that a college women's softball player goes to her athletic trainer for advice because she is frustrated about not getting enough playing time. She states that she thinks the woman playing ahead of her is getting all the playing time not because she is a better player but because she has a romantic relationship with the coach. The athletic trainer, as a third party having knowledge of this exploitation, would be ethically bound to intervene on behalf of both athletes.

Forbidden Knowledge

Forbidden knowledge is information about a situation that an athletic trainer is forbidden to act on. Such information might come from athletes or other physically active patients (about themselves or others), or it might come from another person. Typically, the person prefaces the sharing of information with a phrase such as "If I tell you this, you must promise not to share it with anyone" (Makarowski and Rickell 1993).

An athletic trainer should be wary of anyone who wants to share information but refuses to allow it to be acted on. To agree to such terms might preclude the athletic trainer from taking necessary actions that would otherwise supersede the promise, including the reasons cited earlier. An athletic trainer who receives forbidden information should insist that the patient offering it trust him to act in the patient's best interests. The patient should be assured that the athletic trainer will maintain the confidentiality of the information (provided that there is no threat of harm to the patient or to other persons affected by the information, and provided that the athletic trainer is not legally required to release the information). If a patient is unable to agree to those terms, the athletic trainer should offer him a referral to someone with whom he can trust the information, and the athletic trainer should strongly encourage the patient to follow through with it.

When someone other than the patient involved offers forbidden information, an athletic trainer must clarify that she is obligated to act in the best interest of the patients under her care. Offering to use the information in an anonymous fashion might be appropriate, but an athletic trainer must not forfeit the right to use it when necessary.

A word of caution regarding the use of knowledge is in order, particularly in the context of forbidden knowledge. To take action on knowledge that is inaccurate or untrue can be harmful to athletic trainers, to the athletes or other physically active patients they are responsible for, or to others. The offer of forbidden knowledge by a patient or by others is a common avenue by which an athletic trainer is at risk for being **manipulated**. The athletic trainer should use any information cautiously, particularly when the accuracy of the information is in doubt. In some circumstances, delaying action on a piece of information until it can be verified might be appropriate. For example, if the student who informed on the basketball player in the opening case is known to carry a grudge against the athlete or the program, Tammy would be wise to try to obtain independent confirmation of his allegations before acting.

Knowledge of High-Risk Behaviors

Knowledge of **high-risk behaviors** is another area of potential ethical concern for an athletic trainer. This knowledge might come to you from your own observation, from a report from an athlete or other physically active patient under your care, or from others. This particular concern extends to situations in which a patient is at risk for harm because of his high-risk behaviors or the high-risk behaviors of others. It also includes situations in which the high-risk behavior of the patient puts others at risk.

When an athletic trainer has knowledge that a patient is engaging in potentially harmful high-risk behaviors that put only the patient at risk, the ethical responsibility is not to prevent the behaviors as much as it is to be sure that the individual involved is aware of the associated risks. The athletic trainer may also wish to help the person find alternatives to the high-risk behaviors. The athletic trainer's responsibilities in a case like this, therefore, are to provide the patient with information, education, and counseling so that she can make an informed choice regarding her participation in the behaviors.

When the high-risk behavior of an athlete puts others at risk, the athletic trainer has the responsibility to intervene, if only to make the other individuals aware of the risk so that they can protect themselves. For example, if an athletic trainer becomes aware that one of the athletes in her care is engaging in unprotected sexual activity with multiple partners, she might have an ethical duty to confront the athlete in a private setting and warn him of the consequences of such behavior. Another example is often seen in a college or university setting when a student-athlete tests positive following a drug screen. While established guidelines of confidentiality may exist regarding which individuals within an organization need to know of the positive test results, these guidelines may cover only the communication methods with administrators and coaches. However, others, such as strength and conditioning coaches, may have a justified need to be informed since they are working with student-athletes in a potentially risky environment—one in which a lack of judgment in thought processes could certainly lead to serious injury.

Knowledge of Illegal Activities

Knowledge of illegal activities related to an athlete or other physically active patient can also create a difficult ethical situation. An athlete might admit to illegal activities as part of an advising session, or the information might come to the attention of the athletic trainer from an outside source, as it did in Tammy's case. That case would have been even more complicated had Tammy known, for example, that the athlete had used a false ID to obtain alcohol in the bar. In that scenario, Tammy would have an ethical responsibility to the bar and the police, in addition to her responsibility to uphold the college's policy.

One of the difficulties of having knowledge of illegal activities is that legal authorities might be aware of those activities and seek information from the athletic trainer. The other difficulty occurs when legal authorities are unaware of the illegal activities. Both of these circumstances demand that the athletic trainer be familiar with her legal obligations as a professional and also demand careful consideration of the specific situation. Legal concerns become entangled with issues of confidentiality, responsibility to the client, privileged communication status, legal reporting requirements, and many others. Athletic trainers who have knowledge of a patient's illegal activities should consider seeking legal counsel to protect their own status and that of the patient.

Knowledge of Conflicting Interests

A central concept in ethics is that individuals have a right to **self-determination** (Appelbaum and Lawton 1990). This right, however, can come into conflict with the rights and welfare of other individuals or groups in society. For example, suppose an athletic trainer knows that a wrestler has a contagious skin disease that is difficult to see. In this example, the right of a capable and otherwise healthy athlete to compete would conflict with the right of other athletes to be protected from the skin disease.

Knowledge of situations in which the welfare of a patient conflicts with the welfare of another individual or group of individuals can present challenging ethical questions for the athletic trainer. Social conventions or law governs many of these types of situations, but some areas are not clearly defined. The athletic trainer might have the opportunity to remediate some of these difficult ethical situations. It is possible to resolve many of them by seeking permission to take action or disclose information, or by bringing the involved parties together to develop a mutually acceptable solution to the problem. Indeed, most situations in which the rights and welfare of individuals conflict can be resolved by providing an opportunity for the affected parties to become familiar with the perspectives of the other parties. Most people are reasonable and willing to compromise when they understand the concerns of others who might be affected by their actions.

THREE APPROACHES TO ETHICAL DECISION MAKING

Mangus and Ingersoll (1990) describe three approaches to ethical decision making in athletic training: ethical egoism, utilitarianism, and formalism. All these approaches are valid. Some would be best for certain situations whereas others would only compound the ethical concern. The wise athletic trainer will weigh the benefits and drawbacks of each approach on a case-by-case basis.

- **Ethical egoism.** The ethical egoism approach to ethical decision making involves athletic trainers' making decisions that result in the greatest benefit to themselves. Using Tammy as an example, she would be employing the ethical egoism approach if she simply dropped the issue as the coach suggested. One could argue that she did her duty by bringing the allegations to the proper authorities as specified in the school's policy. By making the decision to drop the case, Tammy is removing herself from any potential conflict that might develop were she to pursue it further. Her life gets easier. She benefits.

- **Utilitarianism.** The utilitarian approach to ethical decision making involves choosing a course of action that benefits the greatest number of people. The utilitarian approach is not easily demonstrated through Tammy's case. One could argue that by dropping the case as the coach suggested, Tammy would be serving the basketball team well because it would be able to keep the star player for the upcoming tournament. One could also argue that Tammy would be serving a potentially much larger group—all the athletes in the school's program—by aggressively pursuing the charges against the wishes of the coach. If the player is "brought to justice" under the terms of the school's alcohol policy, the other members of the athletic program will receive a clear message that such behaviors will not be tolerated.

- **Formalism.** The formalistic approach to ethical decision making is most likely to be followed by athletic trainers who see a clear professional duty that they believe should be implemented universally. If Tammy were a formalist, it is quite likely that she would not accept the coach's self-serving excuse for dropping the case, especially in light of the fact that the coach never informed the athletic director as required by the policy. She would probably go to the athletic director in an effort to satisfy herself that she had fulfilled her ethical responsibility to the school, its athletic program, and ultimately the athlete in question.

THE ACT OF "WHISTLE-BLOWING"

A professional athletic trainer who feels obligated to abide by established policies might view Tammy's initial actions of informing the basketball coach about his player's misconduct as completely appropriate; others may think Tammy could have handled the matter in a "softer" way, intending no formal inquiry beyond a "friendly" discussion between the coach and the player.

Even though reporting of people who are perceived to have violated rules follows a set of rules in an attempt to "do the right thing," it is often referred to as "whistle-blowing." Whistle-blowers are typically employees or former employees who report misconduct to persons who have the power to take action (Miethe 1999). Though the reporting in some cases can be done anonymously, the act is still considered whistle-blowing. Individuals may initiate or participate in whistle-blowing for a number of reasons. It is believed that the typical whistle-blower is motivated by a sense of altruism and egoism while possessing strong moral convictions and a sense of responsibility to act appropriately. Whistle-blowers often think that the consequences of not bringing the truth to light may be too great to bear and therefore must act (Alford 2001). Some whistle-blowers feel that double standards exist within their employment setting and are uncomfortable not bringing issues to superiors; they may even feel ashamed of their work setting for allowing wrongdoings to go on.

The three approaches to ethical decision making are ethical egoism, utilitarianism, and formalism. The approach you use depends on the situation at hand.

The reporting of possible wrongdoings would appear on the surface to be the appropriate form of action in any workplace setting. As previously discussed in this chapter, this is an ethical decision that people must make on their own, since there may be significant adverse consequences for the whistle-blower. As Bok (2004) said of the whistle-blower's situation,

> "The whistle blower hopes to stop the game; but since he is neither the referee nor the coach, and since he blows the whistle on his own team, his act is seen as a violation of loyalty."

Laws designed to protect the whistle-blower do not work very well. Even if the whistle-blower has disclosed an obvious wrongdoing, there are a host of procedural and technical legalities that can fail to protect him (Alford 2001). All health care organizations should establish procedures for employees to report wrongdoing without fear of reprisal. These should include a range of actions such as anonymous reporting. A few years ago, the corporate world faced a financial scandal in which numerous employees of the company known as Enron sensed a betrayal of financial responsibility on the part of their superiors, when their initial actions were not responded to. The end result was federal criminal charges against the leaders of the organization and a significant amount of lost life earnings for the employees. This outcome led to the passing of the Sarbanes-Oxley Act, written to prohibit retaliation against whistle-blowers in publicly traded companies. This act also encouraged a standard for other industries to follow, including profit and not-for-profit health care organizations (Griffin 2005). Laws that have been enacted have not completely addressed the repercussions seen with whistle-blowing. Alford (2001) reported that two-thirds of whistle-blowers he had worked with ended up losing their jobs. Most never got their jobs back or even ended up working in the same field again. Some lost significant wages leading to bankruptcy, loss of their homes, and even loss of their families. Many of these individuals at the time of their reporting felt strongly that they were doing the correct thing. However, after dealing with the consequences, they regretted their actions and would advise others against whistle-blowing.

At the time of decision making, judgment as to whether or not one should report another person for a possible wrongdoing is not always clear. Why is judgment unclear in the heat of the moment, with the right decision becoming more apparent to a whistle-blower only as time passes? This thinking process and ultimate learning from a particular situation is not unique to whistle-blowing. Many decisions in life are difficult and confusing to make at the most critical time. However, after time has passed and we have the opportunity to assess the outcomes, we learn from our experiences and apply the learned knowledge toward future situations.

Specifically in relation to whistle-blowing, Miethe (1999) recommends a series of questions for potential whistle-blowers to consider prior to taking action:

1. Do you have documented evidence of wrongdoing? Is the evidence specific as to time and place? Can the evidence be corroborated through other sources of evidence?

2. Are other coworkers aware of the problem and are they willing to come forward?

3. Have you consulted family, close friends, and an attorney to get their advice before proceeding?

4. Do you have the financial resources to be able to defend yourself in the event you lose your job or need to pay for an attorney?

5. Will your disclosures make a difference in organizational practices?

PRACTICING ETHICALLY AS AN ATHLETIC TRAINER: SPECIFIC RECOMMENDATIONS

The following recommendations are intended to serve as a functional guide to ethical practice in athletic training. The guidelines in this list should minimize the occurrence of ethical conflicts and facilitate the resolution of those that do occur.

■ **Study the relevant professional codes of ethics.** Begin with the code of ethics of the NATA and then review the codes of ethics of organizations that apply to your specific employment setting and the roles you play in that setting.

■ **Learn to recognize situations in which ethical concerns are present or might appear to be present.** This undertaking requires careful consideration of how all your personal and professional relationships might affect the athletes or other physically active patients whom you treat.

■ **Increase your sensitivity to situations in which ethical concerns are present.** Remember that ethics are relative and that the athletic trainer needs to be aware of how a situation may appear to persons viewing it from their own social or cultural perspective. Sensitivity requires that you be able to appreciate a situation from the point of view of others who are affected, particularly the patients under your care. Beyond that, you should treat every ethical concern seriously, or you will be perceived as insensitive and uncaring—and there is no better formula for professional trouble than that.

■ **Consult with others whenever there are questions, especially when the answers are not clear or when they are not clearly defensible.** Good consultation serves to protect the athletic trainer as well as the patient because it provides an outside, objective perspective on the situation of concern. In addition, a small group often has more wisdom than any individual does.

■ **Refer when the concern is beyond your legal scope of practice or your competence.** Everyone's best interests are served when athletic trainers make prudent use of referrals in critical, complicated, and difficult cases. To do this, however, athletic trainers must be acutely aware of their own limitations and must be sure to follow prescribed protocols for referral.

■ **Refer when you become a primary party in an ethical dilemma or when you might be perceived by a patient or outside observers to be a primary party.** When an athletic trainer becomes a primary party in a situation of ethical concern, both the professional and the patient are at risk and the situation might become worse. In addition, even the perception of such a situation can be destructive. Referral to a health care professional not involved in the conflict is generally considered necessary and prudent in such situations.

■ **Document carefully and often.** As in all areas of practice, careful, accurate documentation is essential. This includes documentation of all policies and procedures that have been read and agreed to by all those that the guidelines pertain to.

■ **Follow your conscience.** Good conscience requires knowledge and awareness. For the athletic trainer, good conscience requires knowledge of the moral and ethical standards applicable to the profession, and it requires awareness of the individual circumstances that each patient faces. Athletic trainers most often fail to be conscientious not so much because they lack knowledge but because they lack awareness. To be aware, they must be reflective and considerate, which takes time and effort. As athletic trainers, we must guard against becoming too busy or too routinized to allow ourselves the time and energy to be reflective and considerate. Otherwise we risk failing to be conscientious.

■ **Fully disclose to a patient all your roles.** More than anything else, disclosure is an ethically critical component for informed consent in an athletic trainer's relationship with an athlete or other physically active patient. Identify all the roles you assume that might involve the athlete directly or indirectly. Avoid circumstances in which you are responsible for roles that have conflicting interests regarding the patient. Examples of the types of situations that warrant disclosure include, but are not limited to, the following:

1. You should be sure that athletes understand that you also have responsibility for other athletes on a team and that you might be obligated to use or act on information that affects their health or safety.

Most athletic trainers are committed to practicing ethically, but they are not interested in becoming ethicists to do so. Fortunately, ethical practice doesn't require becoming an ethicist, but it does require an understanding of the meaning and intent of the relevant codes of ethics, reflection on the situations and actions that occur in practice, and the development of professional habits and awareness that are consistent with ethical practice.

2. The organization that an athlete plays for often employs the athletic trainer. The athlete needs to understand this potential conflict of interest, because the practitioner might be required or might have strong incentives to act in the best interest of the organization rather than of the athlete.

3. Athletic trainers often make available services, referrals, or goods in which they have a financial interest. The athletic trainer should disclose this conflict of interest to the athlete or other physically active patient and provide alternatives.

4. Patients should be informed that an athletic trainer also has social and legal obligations that might require her to divulge information that could be in conflict with the patient's own best interest. If a patient tells you about certain illegal activities, the law might require you to report that information. Furthermore, the patient should be informed that information might be divulged when it indicates that the patient or others are in imminent danger.

■ **Consider possible courses of action carefully.** When confronting an ethical dilemma, (1) identify the greatest variety of choices possible, including those that might seem extreme; (2) investigate each of the possible choices identified; and (3) judge your choices from an other-centered perspective rather than from a self-centered or egocentric perspective.

■ **Allow patients to make their own fully informed choices rather than imposing solutions on them.** An informed perspective requires exploration of the positive and negative implications of every conceivable choice. Having relevant information allows athletes or other physically active patients to judge which course of action is in their best interest and is a necessary prerequisite to self-determination. Allowing patients to make their own choices helps them take responsibility for their destiny.

These actions, when combined, dramatically reduce the occurrence of ethical conundrums.

CULTURAL COMPETENCE

Diversity is observed each day in all facets of life. Health care providers are diverse both as individuals and as practitioners. Similarly, athletes and patients are diverse. They are diverse in their thinking, in their values, and in their actions. The cultural background of individuals is recognized as a major contributor toward their actions and expressed beliefs. Tammy's cultural background likely played a role in her thought process while she developed her college's drug and alcohol program. She chose to bring the allegations about the student-athlete to the basketball coach because it was a policy issue and an ethical concern, and in all likelihood she felt the need to address the issue based on her established cultural values and beliefs.

It is not uncommon for health care providers to make decisions for patients taking into account their own values. While a provider may mean well, this approach may not be optimal if his values differ from those of the patient (Campbell et al. 2001). What part of one's cultural background leads to the development of values and beliefs? There is no one simple component. Numerous elements integrate with one another to formulate cultural beliefs.

Campinha-Bacote (2003) has identified all of the following as indicators of one's cultural makeup: race, ethnicity, religious affiliation, language, physical size, gender, sexual orientation, age, disability, political orientation, socioeconomic status, occupational status, and geographic location. Despite whatever indicators compose one's makeup, all individuals should be provided health care services on an equitable basis (Campbell et al. 2001). In athletics, such indicators may also include type of sport (revenue generating versus nonrevenue generating) and level of participation (varsity versus junior varsity, travel team versus recreation team, division I versus division III).

Cultural competence has taken on a greater role over the last two decades in the United States as the result of a rapidly changing population demographic. The Census Bureau estimates that by 2050, diverse racial/ethnic groups will constitute approximately 48% of the U.S. population (Bigby 2003b; Callister 2005).

Defining Cultural Awareness and Cultural Competence

Schlabach and Peer (2008) define **culture** as the shared values, beliefs, traditions, and customs of a particular group. A group can be identified by similar race, religion, ethnicity, or any of the previously mentioned indicators. And while there is really no single acceptable definition of "culture," it consists of a sum of social characteristics of a given group of people (Spector 2004). Coaches fall under this definition of culture; and to a certain extent, subgroups of coaches exist who form cultural views related to their own sport and its idiosyncrasies. Athletic trainers have become accustomed to working with some coaches who truly believe that an athlete's health and well-being come first above all other aspects of sport and life, with equal health care afforded to all. Some coaches, unfortunately, seek preferential treatment for athletes who play more significant roles on the team. While this lends itself to an ethical dilemma, the example demonstrates the ongoing relationship between cultural competence and ethical decision making.

As a health care professional, the athletic trainer will cross the paths of individuals on a daily basis who represent different cultures. While it is unrealistic to assume that an athletic trainer can become aware of all of the potential cultural differences, cultural awareness in and of itself is a critical first step toward becoming a competent health care provider. As one becomes aware, one becomes more competent. **Cultural awareness** represents a set of behaviors that an individual or group of individuals (organizations, businesses) possesses and implements through consistent actions that demonstrate appropriate awareness of diverse cultures. As there are numerous versions of the definition for culture, there are also several components of cultural competence (Bigby 2003b). Within health care, being culturally competent equates to being sensitive to issues of culture, race, gender, sexual orientation, social class, language, and economic situation (Lipson 1996). Callister (2005) explained cultural competence nicely by relating areas of culture to a particular domain:

- cultural awareness and knowledge (cognitive domain)
- cultural skills (behavior domain)
- cultural sensitivity (affective domain)
- cultural encounter (environmental domain)

With the growing cultural shift in the United States, cultural competence has taken on an increasingly important role in an effort to eliminate health care disparities (Callister 2005). However, cultural awareness and cultural competence are not simply talked about and learned in a meeting. Athletic trainers should strive to systematically incorporate culturally competent principles into policies, the administrative structure, and clinical service delivery models in their athletic training settings (Bigby 2003b; Taylor and Lurie 2004; Varricchio 1997). To put it simply, cultural awareness reflects on the process of an individual self-reflecting, while cultural competence is the process of applying one's cultural awareness toward one's actions and the actions of others.

Challenges Associated With Establishing Cultural Competence

Reading and learning about different cultures is helpful for any practitioner. Most athletic trainers are confronted with issues of race, class, sex, and cultural diversity on a daily basis (Geisler 2003). Equally important is understanding how certain cultures perceive how they are treated within the health care system. For example, blacks and Latinos perceive that they receive a lower quality of health care as compared to whites. Blacks, Hispanics, and Asian Americans are more likely to report difficulty in accessing health care, paying for medications, and identifying a regular physician than whites; they are also more likely to rate the quality of care they receive from health care providers and the health care system in general more negatively (Bigby 2003a; Johnson et al. 2004). How does knowing this type of information help an athletic trainer become more culturally competent? This is part of becoming culturally sensitive, a component of the affective domain as defined by Callister (2005).

Culturally sensitive challenges may also be prevalent and may be exacerbated by the behaviors of health care practitioners who knowingly or unknowingly provide differential treatment, lack a sense of awareness of cultural issues, and perhaps even choose to spend less time spent with certain patients (Bigby 2003a). Ethnocentrism, the conviction that one's own culture is superior, can also hinder effective cross-cultural care (Juckett 2005).

National Standards for Cultural Competence

The profession of athletic training does not have set guidelines related to cultural competence. While the guidelines for accreditation for entry-level athletic training education programs refer to ethical behaviors, learning styles, and other related indicators, the words "cultural" and "diversity" do not appear in the guidelines administered by the Commission on Accreditation for Athletic Training Education (CAATE). However, the NATA established the Ethnic Diversity Advisory Committee, defining its purposes as follows: "Identify and address issues relevant to American Indian/Alaskan Natives, Asian/Pacific Islanders, Black, non-Hispanic and Hispanic members. Additionally, address health care concerns affecting physically active individuals in these ethnic groups. Advocate sensitivity and understanding toward ethnic and cultural diversity throughout the profession and the association." The profession of athletic training would benefit from strategies designed to incorporate cultural awareness and competence into the formal didactic and clinical curriculums (Geisler 2003). The NATA educational competencies that do refer to cultural competence state that cultural competence should be incorporated into all aspects of professional practice as a foundational behavior.

In 2000, the Office of Minority Health of the U.S. government published the *National Standards on Culturally and Linguistically Appropriate Services in Health Care (CLAS Standards)*. These standards (presented in the sidebar on p. 279) provide a framework for building the cultural and linguistic competence of home health care agencies and can be integrated into athletic training practice settings (Narayan 2001).

Cultural awareness and competence can be as simple as respecting others' beliefs and interest in receiving alternative or complementary therapies. Nontraditional athletic training treatment interventions, such as aromatherapy, reflexology, or hypnotherapy, may be the treatment of choice for some patients. While disagreeing with such forms of care and perhaps even being able to cite a lack of evidence to support such treatments, an athletic trainer should respectfully acknowledge the wishes of a patient and perhaps take the time to learn more about why the patient prefers such a form of care (Spector 2004).

Athletic training curriculums and clinical education experiences teach us formal and informal methods of what we perceive to be appropriate health care delivery services. However, some elements of our health care delivery approach may seem strange to people from different cultures. For example, preventive medicine is not practiced in all cultures, and in some countries patients must wait months just to see a physician regardless of the severity of the symptoms. Additionally, we have been taught to expose the body part that needs to be examined for proper skin inspection. Some cultures find it offensive to remove portions of clothing even for medical purposes (Campinha-Bacote 2003). As an athletic trainer, being aware of such concerns prior to performing an assessment or treatment intervention will likely lead to an improved patient–practitioner interaction.

Cultural awareness and competence can also take the form of recognizing certain medical conditions that are associated with a specific race, gender, or ethnicity. For example, the sickling of red blood cells is a genetically inherited trait that occurs only in blacks and causes normally shaped red blood cells to assume a "sickle" shape. This can ultimately result in hemolysis and thrombosis of the red blood cells since the abnormally shaped cells do not move easily through the blood vessels. Proper screening and recognition of individuals who carry the sickle cell trait and who are involved with competitive and contact or collision types

CLAS Standards

CULTURALLY COMPETENT CARE

Standard 1

Health care organizations should ensure that patients/ consumers receive from all staff member's effective, understandable, and respectful care that is provided in a manner compatible with their cultural health beliefs and practices and preferred language.

Standard 2

Health care organizations should implement strategies to recruit, retain, and promote at all levels of the organization a diverse staff and leadership that are representative of the demographic characteristics of the service area.

Standard 3

Health care organizations should ensure that staff at all levels and across all disciplines receive ongoing education and training in culturally and linguistically appropriate service delivery.

LANGUAGE ACCESS SERVICES

Standard 4

Health care organizations must offer and provide language assistance services, including bilingual staff and interpreter services, at no cost to each patient/consumer with limited English proficiency at all points of contact, in a timely manner during all hours of operation.

Standard 5

Health care organizations must provide to patients/consumers in their preferred language both verbal offers and written notices informing them of their right to receive language assistance services.

Standard 6

Health care organizations must assure the competence of language assistance provided to limited English proficient patients/consumers by interpreters and bilingual staff. Family and friends should not be used to provide interpretation services (except on request by the patient/consumer).

Standard 7

Health care organizations must make available easily understood patient-related materials and post signage in the languages of the commonly encountered groups and/ or groups represented in the service area.

ORGANIZATIONAL SUPPORTS FOR CULTURAL COMPETENCE

Standard 8

Health care organizations should develop, implement, and promote a written strategic plan that outlines clear goals, policies, operational plans, and management accountability/oversight mechanisms to provide culturally and linguistically appropriate services.

Standard 9

Health care organizations should conduct initial and ongoing organizational self-assessments of CLAS-related activities and are encouraged to integrate cultural and linguistic competence-related measures into their internal audits, performance improvement programs, patient satisfaction assessments, and outcomes-based evaluations.

Standard 10

Health care organizations should ensure that data on the individual patient's/consumer's race, ethnicity, and spoken and written language are collected in health records, integrated into the organization's management information systems, and periodically updated.

Standard 11

Health care organizations should maintain a current demographic, cultural, and epidemiological profile of the community as well as a needs assessment to accurately plan for and implement services that respond to the cultural and linguistic characteristics of the service area.

Standard 12

Health care organizations should develop participatory, collaborative partnerships with communities and utilize a variety of formal and informal mechanisms to facilitate community and patient/consumer involvement in designing and implementing CLAS-related activities.

Standard 13

Health care organizations should ensure that conflict and grievance resolution processes are culturally and linguistically sensitive and capable of identifying, preventing, and resolving cross-cultural conflicts or complaints by patients/ consumers.

Standard 14

Health care organizations are encouraged to regularly make available to the public information about their progress and successful innovations in implementing the CLAS standards and to provide public notice in their communities about the availability of this information.

Reprinted from Office of Minority Health of the US Government. 2000.

of sports are essential. This demonstrates not only competent health care delivery but also cultural competence.

The process of becoming culturally competent must be differentiated from what can be referred to as stereotyping. Salimbene (2005) offers the following tips for avoiding a stereotypical approach to patients:

1. Find out where the patient is on the continuum of health beliefs and practices often associated with his or her population group.

2. Refrain from judging any of the beliefs or practices the patient reveals during the interview.

3. Honor the patient's decision-making process.

4. Negotiate, don't dictate, your treatment plans.

5. Modify both your personal and your medical approach according to where the patient is on the continuum of health beliefs and practices.

APPLICATIONS TO ATHLETIC TRAINING: THEORY INTO PRACTICE

Use the following two case studies to help apply the concepts in this chapter to real-life situations. The questions at the end of the studies have many possible correct solutions. The case studies can be used in class discussion or for homework or test questions.

■ Case Study 1

Gerry Cramer is an athletic trainer at a large university with a successful athletic program. One morning Gerry made a routine trip to the student health service to pick up lab reports and X rays. As he gathered his materials, a secretary asked him if Sean O'Connor (a star basketball player) had been dating a student named Mary Johnson (a nonathlete on campus). When Gerry responded that Sean had dated Mary a few months ago, the secretary proceeded to say how unfortunate it was that Mary had recently tested positive for HIV. Gerry was startled to hear this news. Although Mary wasn't under the care of the athletic training staff and Gerry didn't really know her, he was concerned about how this circumstance might affect Sean O'Connor, who was under the care of the athletic training staff.

QUESTIONS FOR ANALYSIS

1. What are the major ethical issues Gerry should be concerned about following this exchange? Should Gerry pursue additional details and information from the secretary? If so, what?

2. To whom is Gerry primarily responsible in this situation? What responsibilities does Gerry have toward Sean, and what responsibilities does Gerry have toward Mary? What other persons might be involved and warrant consideration?

3. What should Gerry do with the information about Mary's HIV status? Should Gerry use the information as a basis for counseling Sean? Under what conditions should Gerry use the information? What alternatives should Gerry be investigating?

4. What is the worst mistake Gerry could make in trying to fulfill the responsibilities of an athletic trainer to an athlete in this situation? What would be the ideal resolution to this ethical situation? What alternatives fall between the two extremes? How should Gerry proceed?

5. If it is determined at some time that Sean O'Connor is HIV positive, how should the athletic training staff handle that outcome? Who needs to know? What permission is necessary for the staff to relay the information? Who is responsible for the safety of other athletes, for coaches, for the athletic training staff, and for officials with regard to their risk of exposure?

6. What risks does Gerry face because he has this information? What steps should Gerry take to avoid becoming another victim in this ethical dilemma?

7. What elements of professionalism are involved in Gerry's decision-making process?

Case Study 2

Shawna Jackson, an athletic training student at Big Hills University, was assigned to work with the cross country team this fall. As was their custom, the team always spent the first week of the season at a mountain lodge to facilitate both intense training and a sense of team unity. During the first day at the lodge, a runner approached Shawna complaining of pain in his left great toe. Shawna examined the toe and noted that it was red, warm, and tender around the margin of the nail. "You're probably just developing a small blister from all the running you've been doing," Shawna informed the athlete. "Let's try padding and lubrication and see if that makes it feel better." Shawna applied a felt "doughnut" and some lubricant, and the runner told her that the toe felt better. Shawna didn't see the athlete for this or any other injuries the rest of the week.

A few days after the team returned from their trip, the same runner who had seen Shawna nearly 10 days earlier limped into the athletic training room and told Mary Ricard, the staff certified athletic trainer, that he had pulled his left groin. When Mary asked him when this happened, the athlete shrugged his shoulders and told her that it had started hurting a little the day before but that it was much worse today. When Mary examined the athlete, she observed several cracked calluses and blisters on his left foot. The left great toe was swollen, red, and warm. A faint red streak ran from the ankle to the posterior aspect of the knee. The left inguinal lymph nodes were swollen to

golf-ball size. Mary told the runner that he had a serious infection in his left leg and made an immediate appointment for him to be seen by the team physician.

When Mary returned from taking the cross country runner to the hospital for IV antibiotic therapy, she checked his file and found the note that Shawna had entered describing her physical exam and treatment for the runner's "blister." Mary immediately picked up the phone and dialed Shawna's room.

QUESTIONS FOR ANALYSIS

1. What are Mary's ethical responsibilities in this case? What ethical responsibilities does Shawna have? Are they the same? Are they different? Why or why not?

2. Should Mary tell the athlete that Shawna might have mishandled his toe injury? Does the athlete have a right to know this? Why or why not?

3. Which, if any, of the five principles of the NATA Code of Ethics apply (applies) to this case?

4. How do ethics and the law interface in this case? Where do the athletic trainer's ethical responsibilities end and the athlete's legal rights begin?

5. Does the concept of whistle-blowing come into play in this case? If so, how?

SUMMARY

Being a professional is part of being an athletic trainer. Professionalism has been defined in many different ways, though it encompasses one's level of trust, appearance, communication, and interpersonal relationships with colleagues and patients, among other characteristics. Being a professional also involves following a set of ethical principles. The NATA has established a code of ethics, and states that enforce regulatory status also abide by a set of ethics. Athletic trainers should follow a strategic process designed to avoid unethical behaviors and also be familiar with the steps one should take when making ethical decisions. Whistle-blowing is a process whereby an employee reports a colleague for unethical behavior, and the individual who makes the report or complaint is sometimes faced with retaliation. Despite an effort to do the right thing, the whistle-blower must decide if the act of reporting is worth the potential consequences. As the population of the world in general changes around us, we continue to note changes in cultures: in our communities, in our professions, in the sporting world, and in the health care delivery system. Becoming culturally aware of one's own values and beliefs is a component of becoming culturally competent overall.

KEY CONCEPTS AND REVIEW

1. Understand the definition and purpose of ethical standards and their relevance for the athletic trainer.

Ethics is the study of the rules, standards, and principles that dictate right conduct among members of a society. Ethical standards are useful for athletic trainers because they provide a framework for decision making that helps the athletic trainer place the needs of the patient above all other considerations. Athletic trainers who practice unethically are at risk of failing to meet the needs of their patients.

2. Define what the term "professional" means as it relates to an athletic trainer.

Professionalism is not clearly defined and agreed upon among those in all health care disciplines. However, most agree that certain elements compose professional behaviors. These include, but are not limited to, trust, confidence, professional growth, punctuality, and service-oriented behaviors.

3. Identify the appropriate code of ethics that applies generally to the profession of athletic training, along with codes that might apply to specific settings within the profession.

Athletic trainers are often called upon to serve in many roles while working with athletes and other physically active patients. To carry out each role well, it is essential that they be familiar with the ethical standards that are customarily applied to these roles. Athletic trainers should review the code of ethics of the NATA as well as those of other professional groups that might credential them.

4. Identify the situations and circumstances in which ethical concerns are most frequent.

The most common types of ethical problems that directly involve an athletic trainer are breach of confidentiality, conflict of interest, and exploitation. Athletic trainers might also have ethical responsibilities when they have knowledge of such situations; when they are privy to forbidden knowledge; or when they have knowledge of high-risk behaviors, illegal activities, or conflicts between the welfare of different parties involved in a situation.

5. Develop strategies for avoiding ethical problems and for dealing with them if they occur.

Athletic trainers can reduce the occurrence of ethical dilemmas by studying the appropriate codes of ethics and learning to recognize and be sensitive to situations in which ethical concerns are present. Prudent practice includes obtaining consultation with an uninvolved professional whenever there are questions about an ethical situation and referring patients when their problems are beyond the legal scope of practice or competence of the athletic trainer. Athletic trainers should present patients seeking their services with the conditions of the activity, including disclosure of potential conflicts between roles, and the circumstances that affect the confidentiality of information transmitted in their professional relationship. They should document all professional activities prudently and make referrals whenever they become involved as a primary party in an ethical dilemma. Whenever possible, athletic trainers should encourage athletes and other physically active patients to make their own fully informed choices regarding their care.

6. Recognize elements of cultural competence as they relate to athletic training.

Cultural competence is the ability to act with sensitivity to issues of culture, race, gender, sexual orientation, social class, language, and economic situations.

7. Recognize the ethical challenges and overall issues associated with whistle-blowing.

Whistle-blowing poses ethical challenges as to how an individual chooses to report perceived or known wrong-doing within one's own organization. Formal versus informal reporting mechanisms are considered, and challenges such as retaliation and workplace humiliation may result following whistle-blowing episodes.

Preparticipation Physical Exams and Drug-Testing Programs

OBJECTIVES

After reading this chapter, you should be able to do the following:

1. Understand and support the rationale for administrating preparticipation physical examinations.

2. Understand the strengths and weaknesses of the various preparticipation physical examination models.

3. Organize and implement a comprehensive preparticipation physical examination program in a variety of settings.

4. Understand and support the rationale for administrating drug-testing programs in athletics.

5. Understand the legal ramifications of drug testing in athletic programs.

6. Organize and implement a comprehensive drug-testing program.

> ▶ Randall Tate, ATC, smelled trouble when he walked into the athletic director's office to begin his first day on the job as the new athletic trainer at Eastmont Prep School. "Randy," the AD began, "we've had a few problems since you interviewed for the job last spring. I'm embarrassed to have to tell you this, but we had a big drug scandal among an influential group of our student-athletes just before graduation. I've personally always suspected that the drug problem here was bigger than most people were willing to admit, and the problems we had last year just confirmed my suspicions. I had a long meeting with the administration and the board of trustees about a month ago, and they have agreed to allow us to drug test our student-athletes beginning this fall. I know it may not seem fair to dump all this on you when you haven't been on the job for even five minutes, but you're going to be my point man on this. You are the only one with the medical expertise we need to make sure this is done right. I told the board that we would conduct our first round of testing during the fall sports physicals next month." "Are the physical examinations all arranged?" asked Randall. "I've got the date and the doctors all lined up," the AD responded. "All the other details are up to you."

A high-grade athlete will seldom bother the trainer with his own ills.
The trainer will be forced to draw him out.

—DR. FORREST "PHOG" ALLEN

Few duties consume more of an athletic trainer's administrative time and energy than the organization and administration of preparticipation physical examinations (PPEs) and drug-testing programs. Seasoned athletic trainers have experience to guide them through the many potential pitfalls involved, but new athletic trainers may require guidance in planning these two important activities. Although drug testing is a managerial task required of a relatively small segment of our profession, the consequences associated with poor planning in this area are significant, for both the athlete and the institution or team. PPEs, on the other hand, are an activity long associated with sports medicine and engaged in by most athletic trainers. Even athletic trainers employed in sports medicine clinics frequently organize, conduct, or otherwise assist in the provision of PPEs to local high school athletes.

This chapter will help you understand and be able to apply the principles associated with efficient organization of PPEs and drug-testing programs. Although the chapter includes some discussion of the medical justification for the content of the PPE and drug-testing programs, the primary focus is how to plan, organize, and otherwise manage this aspect of your professional responsibilities. A basic knowledge of the medical aspects of these two activities is assumed.

ORGANIZING PREPARTICIPATION PHYSICAL EXAMINATIONS

The PPE is arguably the first step in injury prevention in school, college, and professional sports. Athletic trainers play an important role in helping to organize this aspect of the injury-prevention program. For the PPE to be effective, it must (1) identify disease or processes that will affect the athlete, (2) be sensitive and accurate, and (3) be practical and affordable (American Academy of Family Physicians 2005).

Few administrative tasks are viewed as more fundamental to an athletic trainer's role than the planning, organization, and execution of the **preparticipation physical examination (PPE)**. As the people to whom coaches, athletic directors, school administrators, and parents look for leadership in all things medical, athletic trainers are in a unique position to suggest and implement policy regarding injury prevention as it may be achieved through the information identified and learned with the effective administration of the PPE.

Why PPEs Are Performed

Anyone with any degree of experience in sport as a participant, coach, athletic trainer, or administrator has probably asked, "Why do we have to do these physicals every year? It just seems like a formality." This is a legitimate question. PPEs take a lot of time and energy to organize. They can be expensive to administer, despite the fact that many of the providers who participate serve in a volunteer role. They require significant effort on the part of many people, all of whom could be doing other things. Finally, athletes and coaches, who would rather spend the time practicing, often view them as no more than a necessary evil. So why are PPEs so important? PPEs are important for at least four reasons.

Injury and Illness Prevention

The most compelling reason to perform PPEs is that, properly performed and with data that are subsequently acted on, the PPE can provide information that allows an athlete to participate in sport activities with reduced risk of injury or illness. This justification for the PPE is valid, of course, only if the medical team conducting the PPE uses the data generated by the exam. If seemingly minor findings are discovered during the PPE and are not followed up with appropriate treatment, then the PPE is more than a waste of time; it becomes a potential source of liability for the medical staff.

One of the functions of the PPE is to determine an athlete's readiness for participation in her chosen sport (National Collegiate Athletic Association 2002). On rare occasions, this may involve using the information generated by the PPE to disqualify an athlete from participation. This action should be taken only when participation in the given sport would foreseeably lead to an exacerbation of the athlete's medical condition or would cause harm to other participants. As the medical director of an institution's sports medicine program, the team physician should have the final authority to approve for or disqualify prospective athletes from participation (Herbert 1997). The wise team physician will consider the input of the athlete's personal physician, parents (especially in the case of a minor), and specialists involved in the case. The final authority, however, rests with the team physician (Herbert 1996). See table 10.1 for a list of **disqualifying conditions**. The team physician has six options for determining medical qualification to participate (American Academy of Orthopaedic Surgeons 2000):

1. **Passed.** The athlete is cleared for participation in all sports with no reservations or contraindications.
2. **Passed with conditions.** The athlete has a medical condition that requires follow-up. The athlete may participate in some activities. The athlete may resume full activity pending satisfactory follow-up.
3. **Passed with reservations.** The athlete may not participate in contact or collision sports (whichever is appropriate).
4. **Failed with reservations.** The athlete is not cleared for his or her requested sport. Other sports may be considered. Contact or collision is not permitted.
5. **Failed with conditions.** The athlete must be reevaluated for participation after his or her medical condition is addressed and resolved.
6. **Failed.** The athlete may not participate in any sport at any level of exertion or competition.

Compliance With Association Rules

Most school- and college-based athletic programs are subject to the rules of the athletic associations of which they voluntarily choose to be members. At the high school level, the National Federation of State High School Athletic Associations (NFHS) defers on the issue of required PPEs to the various state associations. The guidelines published by these state organizations vary considerably. Some require the completion of a standard form signed by

TABLE 10.1 Disqualifying Conditions

Condition	Contact/ collision[1]	Limited contact/ impact[2]	NONCONTACT Strenuous[3]	NONCONTACT Moderately strenuous[4]	NONCONTACT Nonstrenuous[5]
Atlantoaxial instability	No	No	Yes[6]	Yes	Yes
Acute illnesses	[7]	[7]	[7]	[7]	[7]
Cardiovascular					
Carditis	No	No	No	No	No
Hypertension					
• Mild	Yes	Yes	Yes	Yes	Yes
• Moderate	[8]	[8]	[8]	[8]	[8]
• Severe	[8]	[8]	[8]	[8]	[8]
Congenital heart disease	[9]	[9]	[9]	[9]	[9]
Eyes					
Absence or loss of function of one eye	[10]	[10]	[10]	[10]	[10]
Detached retina	[11]	[11]	[11]	[11]	[11]
Inguinal hernia	Yes	Yes	Yes	Yes	Yes
Kidney: absence of one	No	Yes	Yes	Yes	Yes
Liver: enlarged	No	No	Yes	Yes	Yes
Musculoskeletal disorders	[8]	[8]	[8]	[8]	[8]
Neurologic					
History of serious head or spine trauma, repeated concussions, or craniotomy	[8]	[8]	Yes	Yes	Yes
Convulsive disorder					
• Well controlled	No	Yes	Yes	Yes	Yes
• Poorly controlled	No	No	Yes[12]	Yes	Yes[13]
Ovary: absence of one	Yes	Yes	Yes	Yes	Yes
Respiratory					
Pulmonary insufficiency	[14]	[14]	[14]	[14]	[14]
Asthma	Yes	Yes	Yes	Yes	Yes
Sickle cell trait	Yes	Yes	Yes	Yes	Yes
Skin: boils, herpes, impetigo, scabies	[15]	[15]	Yes	Yes	Yes
Spleen: enlarged	No	No	No	Yes	Yes
Testicle: absence of or undescended	Yes[16]	Yes[16]	Yes	Yes	Yes

[1]Boxing, field hockey, football, ice hockey, lacrosse, martial arts, rodeo, soccer, wrestling.
[2]Baseball, basketball, bicycling, diving, high jump, pole vault, gymnastics, equestrian, skating, softball, squash, handball, volleyball.
[3]Aerobic dance, crew, fencing, discus, javelin, shot put, running, swimming, tennis, track, weightlifting.
[4]Badminton, curling, table tennis.
[5]Archery, golf, riflery.
[6]Swimming: no butterfly, breaststroke, or diving starts.
[7]Needs individual assessment (e.g., contagiousness to others, risk of worsening illness).
[8]Needs individual assessment.
[9]Patients with mild forms can be allowed a full range of physical activities; patients with moderate or severe forms, or who are postoperative, should be evaluated by a cardiologist before athletic participation.
[10]Availability of American Society for Testing Materials (ASTM)-approved eye guards may allow competitor to participate in most sports, but this must be judged on an individual basis.
[11]Consult ophthalmologist.
[12]No swimming or weightlifting.
[13]No archery or riflery.
[14]May be allowed to compete if oxygenation remains satisfactory during a graded exercise test.
[15]No gymnastics with mats, martial arts, wrestling, or contact sports until not contagious.
[16]Certain sports may require a protective cup.

a physician, whereas others have rules that are much more relaxed. Athletic trainers working in high school settings should check with their state's athletic association to become familiar with the rules specific to that state.

The National Collegiate Athletic Association (NCAA 2010) also publishes guidelines for the conduct of the PPE. The NCAA instructs its member colleges to provide every student-athlete with a comprehensive PPE, complete with cardiovascular screening, upon entry to the athletic program. Updated histories and blood pressure screening should be performed annually thereafter, with additional PPEs only as warranted by these histories. This guideline reflects the modified recommendations of the American Heart Association (1996, 1998).

Education and Counseling of Athletes

Because the PPE is frequently the only opportunity that many adolescent athletes have to interact with a physician, some have suggested that the focus of the PPE be redirected toward counseling and educating young athletes on a variety of health-related issues (Goldberg et al. 1980; Koester 1995). Koester's HEADS topics (Home life, Education, Activities, Drugs, Sex, Suicide) provide a useful guide to initiating conversations with young athletes in an effort to prevent the kinds of health problems that they are most likely to experience (see tables 10.2 and 10.3). Some institutions also use the PPE as an opportunity to educate athletes about the benefits of hepatitis B vaccination. Additional areas of education that can be addressed during the PPE may include nutrition; alcohol, tobacco, and drug use; and sexually transmitted diseases.

The ability of a health care professional to elicit high-quality information and to provide meaningful feedback regarding an adolescent's potential health risks depends on several factors. The typical **mass screening** in the gym or locker room is a poor setting for this kind

TABLE 10.2 HEADS Topics and Sample Questions for the Mature Adolescent

Topic	Sample Questions
Home life	Problems with parents or siblings, living arrangements, parents' drug use?
Education	Grade level, grades, enjoy school, future plans?
Activities	What do you do for fun, extracurricular activities, who are your friends, what are weekends like?
Drugs	Do you or your friends drink alcohol, how much, how often, do you drink until you are drunk, use marijuana, cocaine, inhalants, other drugs?
Sex	Are you sexually active, use birth control, condoms, sexual preference, number of partners, do you know about risks (pregnancy, STDs, HIV)?
Suicide	Have you ever been depressed, do you feel like you are under too much pressure, thought of or attempted suicide?

Reprinted, by permission, from M.C. Koester, 1995, "Refocusing the adolescent preparticipation physical evaluation toward preventive health care," *Journal of Athletic Training* 30: 352-360.

TABLE 10.3 HEADS Topics and Sample Questions for the Younger Adolescent

Topic	Sample Questions
Home life	Problems with siblings or parents, living arrangements, adequate diet?
Education	Grade level, grades, enjoy school, future plans?
Activities	What do you do for fun, extracurricular activities, who are your friends, what are weekends like?
Depression	Ever stressed out or depressed, how do you handle it?
Safety	Seat belts, helmets, guns in the house or at a friend's house?

Reprinted, by permission, from M.C. Koester, 1995, "Refocusing the adolescent preparticipation physical evaluation toward preventive health care," *Journal of Athletic Training* 30: 352-360.

of activity. The level of training and comfort of the examiner are important. Finally, young athletes are likely to open up only to those they know and trust, so it is important to use health care professionals who are familiar with this sample of athletes for this portion of the PPE.

Compliance With Standards of Practice

Although not codified in federal or state statutes, both the athletic and medical communities understand and accept the requirement to provide a PPE that at least meets minimal standards. Failure to provide such a PPE is a gross violation of the standards of practice for anyone charged with safeguarding the health of athletes. No fewer than six explicit national standards, not counting all those promulgated by individual state associations, have been published (Herbert 1992). See the following sidebar for a list of organizations that either or endorse or actually provide recommended standards for the administration of PPEs.

When PPEs Should Be Conducted

The ideal time to conduct PPEs is six to eight weeks before athletes intend to begin vigorous training for their sports (Anderson and Hall 1995). This schedule allows adequate time for remediation of most problems that the PPEs are likely to detect. An option common in many school and college settings is to conduct PPEs one season before athletes intend to participate in their sports. For example, screening of football players would occur just before the summer recess. Basketball players would be screened in early fall at the beginning of the school year. Screening for spring sport athletes would occur around the end of December. Although this system works well for high schools and small colleges that conduct sport seasons exclusively during specific times of the year, larger schools that sponsor nontraditional seasons may have to screen all their athletes in either late spring or summer because even spring sports jump into full gear as soon as school begins in fall.

As discussed earlier, the frequency with which PPEs should be conducted is a matter of some debate. The least rigorous standard requires a complete and comprehensive PPE when an athlete enters an athletic program, with annual **health history updates** thereafter (see figure 10.1). Most high school programs require a PPE every year, although a few states require only one PPE every three years (Kibler 1990). Although athletic trainers are obligated to comply with the standards for their particular settings, the fact remains that the frequency of the PPE relates closely to its content. The more comprehensive and detailed the PPE, the less frequently it needs to be repeated. The less comprehensive and detailed the PPE, the more frequently it needs to be repeated. The nature of the sport is another factor that should influence the frequency with which PPEs should be repeated. Contact and collision sports

---

■ Organizations That Endorse or Provide Recommended Standards For PPEs

American Academy of Family Physicians (AAFP)

American Academy of Pediatrics (AAP)

American College of Cardiology (ACC)

American College of Sports Medicine (ACSM)

American Heart Association (AHA)

American Medical Society for Sports Medicine (AMSSM)

American Orthopaedic Society for Sports Medicine (AOSSM)

American Osteopathic Academy of Sports Medicine (AOASM)

National Collegiate Athletic Association (NCAA)

National Federation of State High School Athletic Associations (NFHS)

HOPE COLLEGE HEALTH CLINIC
ATHLETIC PHYSICAL UPDATE

Name _____ (M or F)____ Age_____ Date _____

S.S. # _____   Year in school   Fr   So   Jr   Sr

Sport _____

1. List any significant illnesses, injuries, or surgery you have had since your last Hope College physical exam (mono, pneumonia, knee or joint injury, etc.).

2. What past or present medical problems (injuries, illnesses, etc.) do you feel we should check?

3. Are you now suffering from any medical problems?

Signature _____

White copy to Health Center, yellow copy to Athletic Dept.

▶ **Figure 10.1**   Sample annual health history update form.

with high injury rates may warrant more frequent repetition of the PPE than sports for which injuries are less frequent and serious.

A common method of administering PPEs that is not necessarily ideal is to perform the service on the day the athletes return to their first team or individual organized practice. This day often coincides with reviewing compliance-related issues, issuing sport equipment, and finally holding the first practice, all within the same day. The benefit of this timing to the school and team is that all of the activities are managed within a well-organized, compact time period. However, this format can lead to some challenges for the sports medicine team. Primarily, findings of concern identified through the process will require some additional review, possible scheduling of further tests, and follow-up prior to granting clearance for participation. Any deficiencies identified at this time would not benefit from a period of rehabilitation before the start of the formal practice schedule as they would if the PPE was performed six to eight weeks in advance. Perhaps of greatest concern is the "carte blanche" attitude that a coaching staff may take toward the PPE if it is performed just prior to the first practice. In this circumstance, the coaching staff is likely very excited to see the athletes perform for the first time at practice after a long period away from formal competition; and any delay in this opportunity can lead to disappointment, irrational bargaining, and in some cases adverse behaviors toward the medical staff for simply doing their job appropriately.

Where and How PPEs Should Be Conducted

Much debate exists regarding the optimal setting for the PPE. Before attempting to decide where and how to conduct PPEs, athletic trainers should try to answer the following questions:

1. What kind of information do we need to get from the PPEs?
2. How many people will we be able to recruit to help conduct the PPEs?
3. How many of the people we recruit will be trained medical personnel with an interest and experience in sport health care?
4. What options do we have in terms of physical facilities for the PPEs?
5. Do the facilities to which we have access have adequate provisions for privacy?
6. How much time do we have for conducting PPEs?
7. What expenses will we incur?
8. Will the people conducting the PPEs be volunteers, or will they expect to be paid?
9. Will the individuals performing the physical examinations require background checks according to state laws?
10. How many athletes will we need to service?
11. What are the characteristics of the athletes to be screened? Adults? Children? Male? Female?
12. Do the planned dates conflict with any holidays or major local, school-related, or other events?
13. Do the facilities have ample parking if large numbers of participants are expected?

Office-Based PPEs

Determining the methods to employ in conducting PPEs involves consideration of many important issues (see table 10.4). All other factors being equal—which they never are—the privacy of a physician's office is probably the ideal place. This setting allows the physician to examine and counsel the athlete with a minimum of interruption and to focus on the athlete and his problems. In addition, physicians who conduct PPEs in their offices have the advantage of being able to call more easily on the wide range of medical equipment and services they may need to provide the comprehensive care the athlete requires. Accessing specialized equipment and services can be difficult in a mass screening in a gymnasium.

If an office-based PPE is the technique of choice, the next issue is to identify the appropriate physician to conduct the examination. Should all athletes be examined in the team physician's office, or should their personal physicians screen them? Many people disagree about this issue as well.

On one hand, the team physician is presumably more versed in sport health care issues and may be better able to make judgments regarding participation status and follow-up treatment for conditions discovered during the PPE. The team physician, as medical director of the school's athletic program, may also be legally responsible for judging an athlete's participation status. On the other hand, the athlete's family physician may be more familiar with the athlete's personal and family history. This level of familiarity can be important in establishing the confidence that the athlete will need to confide in and be receptive to the physician. In some cases, the athletic setting may play a role in this decision. For example, in a college, university, or professional setting, a contracted team physician may have the ultimate say regarding an athlete's participation, whereas in a secondary school setting, it is not uncommon for individual athletes under the age of 18 to be cleared by their own physician. In a

TABLE 10.4 Strengths and Weaknesses of Office and Station PPEs

Strengths	Weaknesses
OFFICE-BASED PPE	
1. Greater privacy	1. Greater potential for breakdown in communication to school-based health care personnel
2. Easier access to patient records	2. Greater potential for lack of familiarity with specific sport demands
3. Easier access to medical supplies and equipment	3. Less efficient
4. More conducive to athlete counseling	4. Incorporation of fitness testing more difficult
5. Less personnel required	
STATION PPE	
1. Greater efficiency	1. Little to no privacy
2. Easier access to the whole sports medicine team	2. Difficult to counsel athletes
3. Easier to include fitness testing as part of the PPE	3. Can be noisy
4. Use of volunteers promotes the concept of shared responsibility for safety	4. Volunteers must be recruited and trained
	5. Facilities and transport of supplies must be arranged
	6. Athletes' records are usually not available

secondary school setting absent an identified contractually bound team physician, numerous physicians could ultimately serve in the decision-making role, making it a challenge for the athletic trainer to establish ideal relationships with all of them. Finally, many would argue that the technical skills required to perform an adequate PPE are commonplace enough that most primary care physicians have the competence required to provide this service.

In the final analysis, the nature of the patient will determine who is best suited to conduct the PPE. Personal physicians can effectively screen most young adolescents. As children grow older and routine visits to the family physician become less frequent, it may be more appropriate for the team physician to take over the administration of the PPE. Who, when all is said and done, is likely to provide athletes with the medical care they need if they become injured or ill during their seasons? For most junior and some senior high school students, this person will be the athlete's family physician. For many senior high school and most college and professional athletes, the team physician will provide medical care. Whoever is most likely to take care of the athletes during their seasons should probably conduct their PPEs. For the growing segment of the population without a family physician, the issue becomes more problematic. Similarly, the high school without a team physician faces difficulty in attempting to organize an effective PPE program.

Group PPEs and the Station Method

The preceding arguments in favor of office-based PPEs notwithstanding, the method that many schools employ involves screening many athletes at a common site using a variety of stations to collect information about their health. Although obtaining the privacy required for one-on-one counseling between a physician and an athlete in this setting is difficult, this method has proved successful in helping detect the more serious and common conditions that are likely to impair an athlete's ability to participate in sports with a relative degree of safety.

The answers to the questions on page 290 will determine the form that the **station PPE** takes. Many nonmedical volunteers can play an important role in helping conduct an organized, efficient mass PPE. The role of the athletic trainer is to identify the number of stations, recruit an adequate number of volunteers for each station, and, where appropriate, provide the training the volunteers will need to perform their duties. Parents, coaches, and students are capable of performing a variety of tasks, including checking height and weight, controlling flow through the various stations, collecting money (for those programs that charge a fee for the PPE—see Heinzman 1991), and checking to make sure that all the required forms have been completed before the athlete leaves the examination area. For PPEs that incorporate fitness testing, coaches who have training in the techniques are an excellent choice to operate these stations. See figure 10.2 for a schematic of a typical station approach to the PPE.

What Should Be Evaluated During the PPE

A surprising amount of disagreement exists among professionals regarding the content of the ideal PPE. Athletic trainers should consider the following factors when designing the PPE.

Factors to Consider in Designing the PPE

Athletic trainers should adjust the structure of the PPE based on the following factors:

■ **Athlete age and level of competition.** Obvious differences exist between a 30-year-old professional football player and a 12-year-old seventh grade basketball player. Although the elements of the PPE may be the same for both, the emphasis on those elements is likely to be different. The PPE for the 12-year-old, for example, should include a greater emphasis on developmental problems common to that age group. The National Football League (NFL) athlete will probably require a much more extensive orthopedic examination, perhaps even including magnetic resonance imaging and other imaging studies. Both athletes need an orthopedic screening, but the screening should be tailored to the athlete and will differ greatly for each.

■ **Sport.** Although the PPE should include certain aspects for all athletes, the exam should be as sport specific as possible. This is especially true in the part of the PPE designed to determine an athlete's physical fitness. For example, an isokinetic evaluation of a sprinter's hamstrings-to-quadriceps ratio may yield useful information that could help the athlete undertake an exercise program designed to prevent a hamstring strain while sprinting. To do the same test on a golfer would be interesting but not particularly useful. Similarly, the Wingate test of anaerobic power might be useful for an ice hockey player but not that important for a 10,000-meter runner on the track team, who would benefit more from a test of his $\dot{V}O_2$max. The biomechanical movements, joint flexibility, and muscle strength expectations of a field hockey player are vastly different from those of a fencer, yet both benefit from these findings as they relate to their specific screening.

■ **Follow-up.** The information collected during the PPE is valuable only if the problems discovered are acted on. Too often the PPE becomes a routine process that collects a massive amount of information but results in no follow-up (Briner 1993). Vision screening is useful only if athletes with problems are referred for follow-up evaluation by an optometrist or ophthalmologist. Strength and fitness screening is useful only if conditioning specialists are available to provide the athlete with feedback and advice for improvement. Questions on the medical history form designed to reveal the potential for disordered eating are useful only if the physician addresses them during the PPE and arranges appropriate referrals for the athlete. As part of the team that designs the PPE, the athletic trainer ought to ask the question "What will we do if . . . ?" for each component of the exam. If the institutional or community resources are so limited that the information collected cannot be acted on, a careful interdisciplinary review of that portion of the PPE ought to be undertaken.

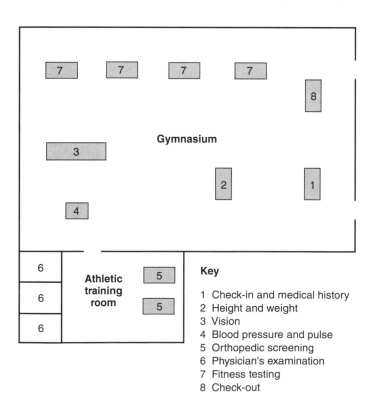

▶ **Figure 10.2** Station PPE schematic.

Examples of effective follow-up include single or group educational counseling for athletes identified as having sickle cell trait, asthma, diabetes, or other medical conditions that could affect their performance as well as their overall health status.

■ **Predictability of tests.** Unfortunately, the majority of the screening activities normally undertaken during the PPE are relatively weak and insensitive predictors of athletic injury (DuRant et al. 1992). The orthopedic exam, especially among athletes with no previous history of injury, is a surprisingly poor predictor of future athletic injury. However, for those with preexisting orthopedic conditions, such screens should continue to be performed and should be accompanied by a thorough history that specifically relates to their musculoskeletal status. A relatively small percent (14%) of the overall findings associated with a physical examination will require follow-up prior to clearance of the athlete for participation (Joy et al. 2004). Relatively sophisticated noninvasive tests for cardiac abnormalities, including two-dimensional echocardiography and 12-lead electrocardiogram, are not only prohibitively expensive to use on a routine basis but are unlikely to detect many problem cases (American Heart Association 1996). As part of the team charged with designing the PPE, the athletic trainer ought to ask "How likely is this test to uncover a problem?" for each element of the PPE.

Common Elements of the PPE

The preceding cautions notwithstanding, most practitioners agree that at least five elements should be part of the PPE.

■ **Health history.** The one portion of the PPE that seems to have the best predictive value is the medical history (Reed 2001). Most athletic injuries are, in fact, reinjuries (Lysens, Steverlynck, and van den Auweele 1984). The medical history, as recorded on a detailed questionnaire, constitutes the most important part of the PPE for most athletes. The answers provided on the questionnaire should guide the medical team in designing specific tests for each athlete to address his problems. See figure 6.1 on page 192 for an example of a **health history form**. A sense of confidentiality is an important aspect of this part of the PPE. If athletes think that the information they record on the health history form is likely to be shared too widely, they may not answer the questions truthfully and completely. Athletes need to be reassured that the information will be held in confidence and will not be shared with anyone outside the medical staff unless they specifically authorize such a release in writing. Despite the advances we have seen during the past decade with technology, few organizations currently utilize a web-based approach to collecting health history information in advance as a way to screen the information prior to the patient–practitioner interaction (Peltz et al. 1999). All questions on the PPE history form should have relevance to the evaluation, with a plan for addressing them if the athlete's response to a specific question is not favorable for clearance to participate.

■ **Physician's examination.** A physician should examine every athlete during the course of the PPE. In fact, in most states an athlete is not considered to have undergone a PPE unless a physician (or a nurse practitioner, physician assistant, or chiropractor in some states) has examined her and verified in writing that she is fit to participate. The major components of the physician's examination include a general review of systems, including examination of the head, eyes, ears, nose, throat, chest and abdomen, and genitalia (Kibler 1990). Every examination should include a general cardiac screening, including standing and supine precordial auscultation, brachial blood pressure in the sitting position, palpation of the femoral artery pulses, and screening for the physical stigmata of Marfan syndrome (American Heart Association 1996). Though it has its limitations, the preparticipation evaluation is the major instrument readily available for prevention of sudden cardiac death (Drezner 2000; Pfister et al. 2000). Some physicians (McKeag and Hough 1993) recommend **maturational assessment**, including **Tanner staging**, for junior and senior high school athletes, but little is known about the usefulness of this technique in preventing injuries (Smith 1994; American Academy of Family Physicians 2005; Tanner 1994).

For a helpful guide to Tanner staging, visit www.fpnotebook.com and search "Tanner staging."

■ **Orthopedic examination.** Although the orthopedic examination may not be a strong predictor of injury for athletes with no previous history of injury, it is an important part of the PPE for athletes who have suffered an injury. The orthopedic exam should focus on problems that the athlete identifies in the health history questionnaire using evaluation techniques specific to those body parts. McKeag and Hough (1993) recommend a quick general orthopedic examination for all athletes (see table 10.5), although the efficacy of this procedure in detecting problems that might lead to injury is unknown. Range of motion, flexibility, accessory joint motion, and muscle strength should be considered part of the orthopedic examination as each relates to the individual athlete's sport. Additionally, commonly performed orthopedic special tests should be included in the exam as they pertain to the more commonly involved anatomical structures for each individual and his sport. A physician need not perform the general orthopedic examination unless this is required by association rules. Athletic trainers, physical therapists, and physician assistants with the proper training can assume this responsibility.

■ **Special medical tests.** This portion of the PPE will vary greatly depending on the financial resources available and the philosophy of the physician. Common special tests include simple urinalysis to detect protein or sugar. Simple tests of visual acuity using a Snellen chart can also be performed at little cost. Routine X rays and cardiovascular or other assessments are not recommended unless warranted by the health history questionnaire or the physician's examination.

TABLE 10.5   Musculoskeletal Physical Examination

Athletic activity (instructions)	Observations
1. Stand facing examiner.	AC joints, general habitus
2. Look: at ceiling, at floor, over both shoulders. Touch ears to shoulders.	Cervical spine motion
3. Shrug shoulders (examiner resists).	Trapezius strength
4. Abduct shoulders 90° (examiner resists at 90°).	Deltoid strength
5. Full external rotation of arms.	Shoulder motion
6. Flex and extend elbows.	Elbow motion
7. Arms at sides, elbows at 90° flexed; pronate and supinate wrists.	Elbow and wrist motion
8. Spread fingers; make fist.	Hand/finger motion and deformities
9. Tighten (contract) quadriceps; relax quadriceps.	Symmetry and knee effusion
10. "Duck walk" four steps (away from examiner).	Hip, knee, and ankle motion
11. Back to examiner.	Shoulder symmetry; scoliosis
12. Knees straight, touch toes.	Scoliosis, hip motion, hamstring tightness
13. Raise up toes, heels.	Calf symmetry, leg strength

OR (shortened version)

1. Nod your head *yes;* shake your head *no.*	
2. Hands behind your head; hands behind your back.	
3. Slowly bend forward and touch your toes.	
4. Stand up straight; jump on your left foot, now on your right foot.	
5. Squat like a baseball player.	
6. Walk toward me like a duck.	

Reprinted, by permission, from D.B. McKeag and D.O. Hough, 1993, *Primary care sports medicine* (Dubuque, IA: Brown), 102. With permission of D.B. McKeag.

- **Physical fitness testing.** Many athletic programs use the PPE as an opportunity to establish a baseline for the athlete's physical fitness. Although this aspect of the PPE is usually not medically necessary to clear an athlete for participation, the information obtained can be useful to athletes and staff members in providing an assessment of the athlete's conditioning status. In particular, the strength and conditioning staff can benefit from these types of tests, and actually including the staff in the development and implementation of applicable fitness testing serves to strengthen the purpose of the exam overall. In all likelihood, the findings of the fitness performance conducted by the strength and conditioning staff will be thoroughly acted upon and incorporated into the athlete's ongoing conditioning program and goals. A variety of physical fitness tests are available; listing them is beyond the scope of this text. Two important points should be made regarding this portion of the PPE.

1. All physical fitness tests should be designed to provide data that are important to normal physiological function for a specific sport.

2. If fitness testing is to be included as part of the PPE, it should always be the last element completed. The athlete should always be subjected to the health history, physician's exam, and orthopedic exam before engaging in strenuous exercise so that any problems that might preclude such exercise can be identified first. Positioning the fitness tests at the end of the PPE also allows examination of the athlete in a resting state, which is an important factor in the collection of baseline cardiovascular data.

Legal Considerations

The legal precautions for conducting PPEs are similar to those of other aspects of medical and allied health care practice. Athletic trainers, physicians, and other health care professionals involved in the PPE will be held to the same standards of practice for this activity as they are for other aspects of their professional practice. Two areas are particularly important to emphasize.

Consent

As with any medical procedure, an athlete must consent to be examined during the PPE. For athletes to provide informed consent, they must be told what will happen to them during the PPE; they must understand what they were told; they should have the opportunity to ask questions; and they must sign a document indicating that they agree to submit to the procedure. The parents or guardians of minor children must provide informed consent on their behalf. Athletes past the age of majority can provide informed consent for themselves. See figure 10.3 for an example of an informed consent form for the PPE.

Waiver of Liability

The primary purpose of the PPE is to prevent athletes from participating when they have a medical condition that endangers their health or that of their teammates or opponents. From time to time, a team physician will decide that an athlete should not participate in a given sport. Unfortunately, this is often not the last word. Athletes and their parents frequently challenge the decision of the team physician and demand the right to participate, no matter the risk for permanent disability or death. Frequently, these athletes seek second, third, or even fourth opinions to justify their desire to participate. The actions of the medical staff, including the team physician and the athletic trainer, are important in cases like these, because they can involve litigation to resolve the matter.

One approach the medical team can take is to require athletes (and their parents in the case of minors) to sign waivers when they wish to participate against the advice of the physician. Such waivers must be tailored to each specific case and should include a full description of the medical condition; the findings of the PPE and other associated examinations connected to the condition; and a complete list of all the possible medical complications that could arise from

Statement of Informed Consent to a Preparticipation Physical Examination

It is the policy of Ohio Technological University that all students must undergo a preparticipation physical examination (PPE) by an OTU physician prior to the beginning of practice or competition in intercollegiate athletics. We insist that you undergo a PPE for the following reasons:

- We want to help you prevent injuries and illnesses.
- We want to make sure that you are ready for vigorous athletic participation.
- We want to establish a medical basis for your participation.
- We must comply with the NCAA requirement that all athletes be medically cleared for participation.
- We want to use the PPE to talk to you about your personal health issues.

The PPE has three parts:

- A health history questionnaire that you complete (please be honest and complete).
- Several special tests (vision, blood pressure, weight/height, etc.) performed by the athletic training or nursing staff.
- An examination by a physician.

Things you should know about your PPE:

- The information derived from the PPE is kept confidential. Only the medical staff will have access to the information unless you authorize its release to others in writing.
- You will be asked to partially undress for the physician's examination. The physician may have to touch you in private areas in order to complete the examination. If you would be more comfortable having a nurse or athletic trainer of your own gender in the room during the physician's exam, just ask and we'd be happy to do this.
- The physician may ask you a few questions that seem "personal" and not necessarily related to athletics. We want to use this opportunity to talk about your health, because illnesses and other nonathletic problems can interfere with your season as easily as an ankle sprain or a dislocated shoulder.

I, _____, have read the statement above and understand the reasons and components of the preparticipation physical examination. I freely consent to the examination. I have had an opportunity to ask questions regarding the preparticipation physical examination. All my questions have been answered.

_____
Student-athlete signature

_____
Parent or guardian signature

_____
Witness signature

_____
Date

▶ **Figure 10.3** Sample informed consent form for the PPE.

athletic participation, including permanent disability and death. If temporary or permanent disability is a potential outcome, the waiver should describe the financial implications of such a disability. If the athlete is married, the spouse should sign a similar document waiving her right to sue for **loss of consortium**. The waiver should be written in simple language, and all medical terms should be explained. Athletes, parents, and spouses should be offered the opportunity to ask questions regarding the contents of the waiver. The waiver should state that in signing it the athlete admits to having read the waiver, understanding it, and agreeing to hold the institution and its medical staff harmless for any future injuries associated with the condition in question. Although some courts have upheld waivers, they are often viewed as a violation of the public interest and are frequently not upheld, no matter how detailed or explicit.

The second approach the medical team should consider in these cases is simply to stick to their decision to deny medical clearance for participation and allow the athlete to bring suit. This approach forces the courts to make a decision as to the reasonableness of the physician's decision (Herbert 1997). Any orders that the court issues should be included in the athlete's medical file as a record of the facts of the case should an injury result from participation at a later date.

ORGANIZING DRUG-TESTING PROGRAMS

As Randy Tate in the opening case is now aware, even some high schools have implemented drug-testing programs. Regardless of the setting, all athletic trainers have the responsibility of educating the athletes in their care regarding the rules and mechanics of drug testing.

Why Drug Testing Should Be Performed

The reasons for drug testing are as varied as the number of people who have written about this controversial subject since it gained widespread attention in the 1980s. Some institutions envision drug testing as a means of promoting order and discipline on an athletic team. Others see it as a way to prevent or discourage potentially illegal activity. Yet others implement programs as a deterrent to unfair competitive performance. One would hope that most are genuinely concerned about instituting drug-testing programs as a means of helping those with chemical addictions come to grips with their problems.

The NCAA (2003) identified two overarching goals for its drug-testing program, which is generally viewed as the standard for collegiate sports in the United States. The first goal is to promote fair and equitable competition. At least two objectives can be inferred from this goal. First is the proposition that all athletes should compete on a "level playing field" where only the sum of their training and talent determines the outcome of a contest. The second part of this goal is the idea that no athlete should feel pressure to take drugs to have a chance to win. The design of the drug test should ensure that these two objectives are met. Unfortunately, so many athletes have been caught using drugs after world-record performances that athletes do not believe in the existence of a level playing field. The ability of athletes to keep technologically one step ahead of the drug-testing labs has greatly impaired the achievement of this goal (Thorland 1990).

The second goal that the NCAA identified is to safeguard the health and safety of athletes by discouraging drug use through drug testing. The potentially detrimental effects of drug use are well understood and universally acknowledged. The hope is that athletes who use drugs will be caught so that they may be counseled and, where appropriate, receive treatment for any problems their drug use may have engendered. Unfortunately, many, if not most, highly motivated athletes are willing to sacrifice their health for short-term glory on the athletic field. When asked if they would take performance-enhancing drugs even if they knew that they would suffer serious heart or liver disease as a result, a significant percentage of athletes said they would do so (NCAA 1988). Drug testing seems like weak ammunition in a fight in which such strong motivating forces are at work.

Athletic trainers in professional sports and NCAA Division I and II universities are often charged with development and implementation of drug-testing programs. These programs may occur year-round. Even athletic trainers in Division III settings should become familiar with the issues of organizing drug-testing programs because they may be asked to help administer postchampionship testing.

When Drug Testing Should Be Performed

Different models for the timing of drug testing account for most drug tests performed in collegiate, professional, and Olympic sports: postchampionship testing, preseason testing, and year-round testing.

■ **Postchampionship testing.** Many college athletes are exposed to drug testing after their teams participate in an NCAA championship event. Choice of which athletes to test at these events can be based on random selection, position of finish, playing position, or playing time. For testing that takes place at nonchampionship events like postseason football bowl games, financial aid status can be the basis for athlete selection.

■ **Preseason testing.** Professional athletes are frequently drug tested before their first season of competition. This test is usually part of the PPE and is considered a **preemployment test**. In the NFL, all rookies who are invited to attend the league combine are tested for anabolic steroids and drugs of abuse at the combine. Rookies who do not attend the combine are tested if they eventually sign a contract, which may be voided if they test positive.

■ **Year-round testing.** The NCAA requires athletes in Division I and II football and baseball and Division I indoor and outdoor track and field to submit to drug testing on a year-round basis. In addition, the NFL and several Olympic sports national governing bodies require year-round testing of athletes for a variety of performance-enhancing drugs, including anabolic steroids.

■ **In-house testing.** Many universities with large athletic programs also engage in year-round testing as a way of discouraging off-season drug use. More and more schools, both colleges and high schools, are implementing drug screening and education programs. In the high school setting, these may be state-mandated programs designed to curtail use of both performance-enhancing and street drugs. In any case, these programs are rather expensive to implement, require extensive organization skills and bookkeeping, and pose additional challenges when minors are being tested. Questions have arisen as to whether or not a child should be allowed to participate in state-sanctioned and -funded high school sports that require drug testing when the parent has not consented to allow the child to be tested.

How Drug Testing Should Be Conducted

Many important decisions regarding the mechanics of a drug-testing program will affect the eventual success or failure of the program. To implement the directive from his athletic director, Randy Tate will have to consider each of the following elements.

Consent

All athletes should sign a consent form agreeing to submit to drug testing. Although the language of the consent form indicates that this activity is voluntary, the sanction imposed when an athlete chooses not to sign is usually athletic ineligibility. Universities that conduct their own drug-testing programs besides those required by the NCAA should develop their own consent forms (see figure 10.4) in addition to those required by the NCAA. All programs should have established policies and procedures that are clearly outlined to inform those who consent to the testing.

Selection of Subjects

Few issues related to drug testing are more riddled with potential liability than selection of the athletes to be tested. Although most drug-testing programs associated with college, professional, and Olympic sports are purported to use **random selection**, definition of this term can take many forms. In some cases *random selection* means that the testing is random with regard to the subjects selected, and in other cases it means that the timing of testing is random (Elkouri and Elkouri 1993). Each category has several permutations, including the following:

■ **Random selection of subjects by sport.** The NCAA, some universities, and some high schools may randomly choose a sport to test during any given testing period. Under this system, athletes might be able to entirely avoid being tested during their college careers if their teams are never chosen or never participate in NCAA postseason championships.

■ **Random selection of subjects by position.** Some athletes are selected for testing based on the position they play on the team. For instance, Randy Tate may choose to test only the defensive players on the football team during any given testing period, saving the offensive players until another testing period.

> The NCAA drug-testing consent forms for Division I, II, and III can be found at www.ncaa.org; search "NCAA drug testing."

INDIANA UNIVERSITY DEPARTMENT OF INTERCOLLEGIATE ATHLETICS ALCOHOL AND DRUG SCREENING PROGRAM CONSENT FORM
READ CAREFULLY BEFORE SIGNING

PRINT NAME _____

SPORT _____

1. AGREEMENT

I have carefully read the *Indiana University Department of Intercollegiate Athletics Alcohol and Drug Screening Program and Policies* and know the contents thereof, and I understand that by my signature, I agree to abide by the policies and I acknowledge that I have received a copy of these policies. I also understand that failure to show for a substance-screening test may be treated as a positive test result.

Student-Athlete Signature _____ Date _____

2. CONSENT TO URINALYSIS

For the 2011-12 year (which includes the summer 2012 vacation period), I hereby consent to have a sample of my urine collected and tested during my annual physical examination and at other such times as necessary or required, for the presence of certain drugs or substances in accordance with the provisions of the *Indiana University Department of Intercollegiate Athletics Alcohol and Drug Screening Program and Policies.*

Student-Athlete Signature _____ Date _____

Parent/Guardian Signature _____ Date _____

3. AUTHORIZATION FOR RELEASE OF INFORMATION

I further authorize you to release to the head coach of any intercollegiate sport in which I am a participant, my parent(s) or legal guardian(s), the athletic director and the team physician at Indiana University all the information and records, including test results, you may have relating to the screening or testing of my urine sample(s) in accordance with the provisions of the *Indiana University Department of Intercollegiate Athletics Alcohol and Drug Screening Program and Policies.* To the extent set forth in this document, I waive any privilege I may have in connection with such information.

I understand that my urine sample will be sent to the Indiana University Medical Center, Indianapolis, Indiana, for actual testing.

Student-Athlete Signature _____ Date _____

Parent/Guardian Signature _____ Date _____

4. RELEASE OF LIABILITY

The trustees of Indiana University, its officers, employees, and agents are hereby released from legal responsibility or liability for the release of such information and records as authorized by this form.

Student-Athlete Signature _____ Date _____

Parent/Guardian Signature _____ Date _____

▶ **Figure 10.4** Institutional drug-testing consent form.

Reprinted with permission from the Indiana University Athletic Department.

- **Random selection of subjects by playing time or finish position.** The NCAA frequently chooses to test only within the group of athletes who contributed to the outcome of a particular contest by virtue of their playing time. A similar method involves selecting subjects who placed high in individual sport championships.

- **Random selection of subjects by financial aid status.** In some cases, especially those involving NCAA Division I sports, subjects for drug testing are drawn from the pool of athletes on athletic scholarship. Nonscholarship athletes are often eliminated from the pool.

- **Random timing—no notice.** One method frequently used in drug testing is to conduct unannounced spot checks at random intervals. This procedure often involves taking an athlete off the field to administer a drug test with no warning. Many experts believe that this is one of the only ways to discourage cheating the system, because athletes who know when they will be tested can often mask their drug use by abstaining for as little as a few days before the test.

- **Random timing—some notice.** The alternative to unannounced random testing is to provide subjects with some notice that they will be tested. The farther in advance an athlete knows about the test, however, the greater the chances that she will be able to manipulate the results. With some notice, individuals may attempt to dilute their samples by overhydrating in an effort to mask the test results.

To demonstrate that subjects were selected for testing at random, an athletic trainer must develop a system that equalizes the probability that one athlete has as much of a chance of being tested as any other athlete. Randomization can occur in many ways. Athletes are usually assigned a number. One can select their number either by consulting a table of random numbers or by generating a list of random numbers from a computer statistics program. In any case, the athletic trainer must document the method used so that she can withstand any challenge to the validity of the selection procedure.

Reasonable Suspicion

An alternative to random testing is to select subjects based on **reasonable suspicion**. Reasonable suspicion, also known as reasonable cause or probable cause, is based on specific signs of drug use in an individual. These signs are usually associated with observed behavior abnormalities that may or may not be related to the athlete's participation in sport. For example, an athlete may be asked to submit to a drug test after demonstrating rapid gains in muscle bulk and other signs of anabolic steroid use—a situation obviously related to the athlete's participation in sport. The same athlete may be asked to submit to drug testing after being involved in a traffic accident in which he was under the influence of drugs—an incident unrelated to the athlete's involvement in sport. Drug testing that involves reasonable suspicion as a selection criterion should be approached with great caution. What is reasonable to one person is often unreasonable to another, especially when sanctions may be involved. Suspicious behaviors must be carefully documented. Selection by reasonable suspicion is enhanced when more than one person observes the suspicious behavior on more than one occasion. Behaviors or qualities that are measurable (documented increases in size and strength, number of motor vehicle accidents, drop in grade point average) are particularly useful in defending the reasonableness of suspicion of drug use. With a clearly written policy, individuals can be tested without notice based on reasonable suspicion. It is imperative to base such suspicion on factual information, as such allegations are likely to incite a level of disagreement and possibly anger on the part of the athlete and potentially others she communicates closely with (coach, parents). A policy to allow for reasonable suspicion testing within an organization should clearly identify how information is gathered, how it is acted upon, and who will be made aware of the testing prior to its administration (e.g., coach, athletic director).

Drug-Testing Methods

The most common method for drug testing in sport is urinalysis. Tests involving blood, saliva, hair, and breath analysis are also available but are used with less frequency. A method frequently employed as a first-level screening for many drugs is the **enzyme multiplied immunoassay technique (EMIT)**. This method uses light absorption to establish the level of a drug in a subject's urine. The amount of light absorption is compared to norms for a variety of drugs commonly tested for in athletic settings. Although this method is relatively inexpensive, it may produce a high percentage of false-positive tests.

Because EMIT tests can indicate the presence of drugs in an athlete's urine at a level higher than is actually present, positive tests must be confirmed by a process known as **gas chromatography–mass spectrometry (GC-MS)**. This method, although more expensive, is widely regarded as the gold standard in urinalysis (Thorland 1990). This method is also the method of choice for determining the presence of anabolic steroids in the urine. The EMIT test is not sensitive to the presence of anabolic steroids. GC-MS works by separating the compounds found in the urine and developing "fingerprints" for each compound. These fingerprints can then be compared to those of known drugs. Although GC-MS is a sensitive method, athletes frequently beat the system by using "designer" drugs for which no reference fingerprints are available. **Liquid chromatography–mass spectrometry–mass spectrometry (LC/MS/MS)** is considered a more sensitive testing technology these days, as testing at lower thresholds can capture designer drugs.

Specimen Handling and Chain of Custody

Although observation is distasteful to all involved, the collection, labeling, and packaging of a urine sample must be observed by a reliable witness; otherwise the sample is of no value. Athletes should be observed while they deliver their urine samples. This obviously requires the presence of a toilet facility in the immediate vicinity of the drug-testing area. In the event that the athlete is having difficulty producing a specimen, caffeine-free and alcohol-free beverages from sealed containers should be provided. The athlete should be allowed to observe the handling of the sample until it has been transferred to an appropriate bottle provided by the testing lab. The athlete should also be allowed to observe as the bottle is being sealed and labeled. After the specimen has been labeled and sealed, the athlete should sign a form indicating that the specimen she provided was indeed her own, that she did not tamper with the specimen or any of the containers used to collect or store it, that she observed the transfer of the specimen to the storage bottle and the sealing thereof, and that the name on the storage bottle is hers.

Testing the Sample

Although simple immunoassay kits are available that athletic trainers can use to test urine samples in the athletic training room, this practice should be discouraged for several reasons. First, because of the potential loss of athletic eligibility and its associated social and financial consequences, a reliable, disinterested third party should test the samples. Ideally, the organization should contract with a laboratory experienced in athletic drug testing for every phase of the program, including subject selection, specimen collection, sample testing, and results reporting. The NCAA (2003) recommends that institutions contract only with labs that can provide information on **false-positive** and **false-negative** rates for the specific tests to be conducted. Utilizing federally certified labs is also highly recommended.

Reporting the Results

The results of positive drug tests should be reported only to those people with a legitimate need to have the information. This issue can become difficult, because denial of athletic eligibility is often the result of a positive drug test. How should Randy Tate respond to a reporter's question about why the star quarterback is on the bench even though he's been playing well this year? Is he injured? What happened? Institutions that choose to implement drug-testing programs must develop ironclad procedures regarding the dissemination of this information. People with a need to know might include the athlete, the team physician, the athletic trainer, the athletic director, and the head coach; this list will vary from institution to institution. Some may consider the strength and conditioning coaches from a safety perspective, as well

The following are examples of drug-testing agencies: National Center for Drug Free Sport, Inc. (www.drugfreesport.com/) and Aegis Sciences Corporation (www.aegislabs.com/).

as the academic advisors who may better understand a student's classroom performance as it relates to these social behaviors. Personnel who are included on the list should be warned of the potential negative consequences of releasing the information. The damage to an athlete's reputation and potential loss of income make this area especially ripe for litigation.

What to Test For

Which drugs should Randy Tate test for? On what basis should the list of banned drugs be developed? The two most common lists of banned drugs are those published by the NCAA and the list of drugs tested for in athletes who compete in the Olympic Games. The Olympic list is longer and more restrictive than the NCAA list. In general, drugs banned from use include certain kinds of stimulants (amphetamine, cocaine), anabolic agents (testosterone, clenbuterol), diuretics (acetazolamide, furosemide), street drugs (heroin, marijuana), and peptide hormones and analogs (human growth hormone, erythropoietin). In addition, some drugs are prohibited in certain sports but allowed in others. Interestingly, many institutional drug-testing programs do not test for alcohol, although this drug clearly has the greatest rate of abuse among high school and college-aged students.

Proceeding With Caution

Drug testing is a controversial subject. It has been widely litigated—a trend that will probably continue into the future. Legal counsel is an essential element of the drug-testing program. Athletic trainers asked to design a drug-testing program must be extremely careful to incorporate a number of elements to lend validity and reliability to the procedures as well as to protect the rights of those to be tested. When Randy Tate designs his program, he should be sure to build the following 10 elements into the process (Pickett 1986):

1. Develop written policies and procedures. The first step in instituting a drug-testing program is to codify the process in a written document that prescribes every step of the program. The process described in the NCAA *Drug-Testing Program 2009-10* booklet (NCAA 2009) (www.ncaapublications.com/productdownloads/DT10.pdf) is a useful template for institutions that wish to implement their own programs.

2. Clearly articulate the purpose of the program. Everyone associated with a drug-testing program must understand its purpose. If the purpose of the program is not clearly articulated, it can easily be manipulated and turned into something that its creators never intended it to be.

3. Make testing as sport-specific as possible. Defending a drug-testing program is easier if you can demonstrate that it is designed to prevent or detect problems clearly associated with a particular sport. Testing the entire cross country team for anabolic steroids and human growth hormone five times per year would be an example of testing for a problem that is unlikely to exist.

4. Use valid and reliable methods. You must be able to prove that each positive result is associated with a particular athlete's sample through a carefully documented chain of custody. The selected laboratory must confirm all positive results with GC-MS or LC/MS/MS technology.

5. Incorporate an appeal mechanism. If athletes have a property interest in retaining their athletic scholarship, eligibility, or position on a professional team, they must have access to due process before they can be sanctioned. All athletes who test positive should be allowed to appeal the results. The more severe the sanction, the more formal the process should be.

6. Protect the athlete's privacy. Only personnel with a legitimate need to know should be informed about positive drug tests. This list should be codified in written policies and procedures. Nobody else should have access to the information without the written permission of the athlete.

7. Obtain consent. Athletes may not be tested for drugs against their will. For the athlete's consent to be valid, the document he signs should include a detailed description of the drug-testing process and the sanctions associated with positive tests.

8. Inform potential athletes. Athletes being recruited to participate in an institution's athletic program should be informed that the institution has a drug-testing program to which they may be subjected. This information should be reiterated when the student enrolls. Such information helps establish the evidence required to prove informed consent.

9. Inform current athletes. All athletes with the potential to be tested should be informed, in writing, of the purposes of the program, the procedures for selection and testing, the sanctions associated with positive tests, and the appeal procedures. They should also be informed of the risk that information regarding positive tests may be accessible to third parties (through court order or other legal means).

10. Train and retrain personnel. All personnel associated with the drug-testing program should be thoroughly trained in their responsibilities. This training should occur regularly to ensure that personnel learn about changes in the program and are performing their duties correctly.

APPLICATIONS TO ATHLETIC TRAINING: THEORY INTO PRACTICE

Use the following two case studies to help apply the concepts in this chapter to real-life situations. The questions at the end of the studies have many possible correct solutions. The case studies can be used in class discussion or for homework or test questions.

■ Case Study 1

Glenda Hathaway's phone rang in her office at Northline Sports Medicine Clinic, where she was one of several certified athletic trainers. Her supervisor, James Jones, asked her if she would stop by his office later to discuss a new project he had in mind. When Glenda arrived 20 minutes later, James told her that the clinic would be offering a new service in the fall. "We want to expand our outreach services by offering to coordinate preparticipation physical examinations for the high schools we want to develop contracts with. We want you to pilot the program at Truman High in August. Here's the phone number of the athletic director at Truman. I've spoken with him already and he's really excited to have us doing this for him. Let me know how I can help."

Although Glenda was excited to get started on this project, she came away from her first meeting with Truman's athletic director a bit worried. The facilities were dark, in poor repair, and dirty. The athletic training room was a converted custodial closet. The boys' locker room was next to the gym, but the girls' locker room was down the hall in another wing of the building. Truman had a doctor—the parent of one of the student-athletes—but he came only to home football games on Friday nights. The athletic director told Glenda that he anticipated 500 students would need physical exams. The date was less than one month away.

QUESTIONS FOR ANALYSIS

1. What alternatives does Glenda have for the physical facilities she needs to conduct Truman's PPEs?

2. Of all the obstacles that Glenda faces, which are the most important? Why?

3. Assuming that Glenda can pull together a team of physicians for Truman's PPEs, who will decide the final participation status of each athlete? If an athlete challenges one of Glenda's physicians on a decision to deny clearance, how should Glenda handle it?

4. Put yourself in Glenda's position and develop a plan to organize and administer PPEs to Truman High's 500 student-athletes. Be sure to include a floor plan of whatever facility you plan to use, along with staffing and supply lists. Develop all the forms you'll need to document each step of the PPE.

Case Study 2

Mark Thomas, ATC, walked into the locker room to tell Bill Williams that his number had come up. "Bill," Mark began, "I know you're just a freshman on the football team, but everybody has to get drug tested if their number is drawn. Yours just came up, so I'll need a urine sample from you. Right now." "Mr. Thomas," responded Bill, "I've only been here five days, and besides, my religion doesn't permit me to do this. I think I should talk to my parents first." "Bill," Mark said, "you don't have a choice. You signed the drug-testing consent form when you arrived last week, so you should have known this was going to happen. I don't have all day to stand here and argue. Either fill the cup or I'll have to go to the coach." Bill reluctantly went into the bathroom where Mark watched him provide a specimen. After he was finished, Bill said to Mark, "Please don't let my folks know that I did this. They'd really be upset. They're pretty conservative." "If you don't test positive there's nothing to worry about," responded Mark. After that he turned and walked out of the locker room with Bill's specimen.

QUESTIONS FOR ANALYSIS

1. Based on what you read in this case, what potential flaws exist in Mark's drug-testing program? How could he correct these flaws?

2. Mark told Bill that he had no choice but to submit to the drug test. Is he right? Why or why not?

3. Assume that Bill's test was positive for the presence of anabolic steroids. Further assume that he was suspended for the season and that a story appeared in the newspaper reporting that Bill was being disciplined for "violating team rules." If Bill's parents called Mark wanting to know why their son was being suspended, how should Mark respond?

4. Would you challenge the results of this test and the resulting suspension if you were Bill? On what grounds?

5. Design a policies and procedures manual for a drug-testing program at an NCAA Division I university. Be sure to include a comprehensive list of procedures, including subject selection, drugs to be tested for, and sample collection and chain of custody. Develop a request for proposal to send to various laboratories that might do the testing. Develop an appeal process and a list of sanctions for positive tests.

SUMMARY

Preparticipation physical examinations are designed to assess an athlete's health status prior to vigorous participation. These should be performed six to eight weeks prior to the beginning of such activity, allowing for time to address concerns and complete further tests that may need to be performed. A thorough history form serves as the hallmark foundation in addition to a screening of the body's systems. The PPE can be performed in an office-based format, with assessment of one athlete at a time, or in a station-based format with multiple athletes and providers taking part in the process simultaneously. Both formats have strengths and weaknesses. Each assessment should also consider gender, sport, and level-specific needs. Athletic trainers are often involved with drug testing of student-athletes. This requires knowledge of consent procedures and the selection process. Testing may occur at random, postchampionship, or based on reasonable suspicion. Testing is performed at professional levels, for example in the National Football League, through the NCAA, and internally within school-specific programs administered under the supervision of a college or high school.

KEY CONCEPTS AND REVIEW

1. Understand and defend the rationale for administrating preparticipation physical examinations.

The preparticipation physical examination is the first step in injury prevention and a process that most athletic trainers eventually become involved with. Besides helping to prevent injury, the PPE allows institutions to comply with association rules, provides an opportunity for counseling and education, and helps improve compliance with standards of practice.

2. Understand the strengths and weaknesses of the various preparticipation physical examination models.

There are advantages and disadvantages to conducting PPEs in either the physician's office or in a station technique in a school setting. The option of using the family physician and the alternative of using the team physician both have advantages and disadvantages. Considerations for each setting include privacy, availability of equipment and supplies, and the thoroughness of the examination.

3. Organize and implement a comprehensive preparticipation physical examination program in a variety of settings.

PPEs should ideally be conducted six to eight weeks before the beginning of the season. The NCAA requires a comprehensive PPE only upon entry into the athletic program, whereas most state high school associations require an annual PPE. The content of the PPE should be based on the athlete's age and level of competition, the sport to be played, the level of follow-up available, and the predictability of the tests to be used. Common elements of the PPE include a comprehensive health history, physician's examination, orthopedic examination, special tests, and fitness tests. Athletes (or their parents) must give written informed consent to be examined during the PPE. Athletes who wish to challenge the judgment of the medical staff regarding their participation status should be required to sign a detailed waiver of liability. Even this, however, may not be enough to shield the medical staff from liability in the event of serious injury or illness. A more prudent approach may be to allow the courts to rule on the reasonableness of the physician's participation decision.

4. Understand and defend the rationale for administrating drug-testing programs in athletics.

Drug testing is intended to safeguard the athlete's health while providing a level playing field for equitable competition.

5. Understand the legal ramifications of drug testing in athletic programs.

Athletes should be observed as they provide the specimen, and they should be allowed to witness the handling of the specimen. Reporting of positive tests should be limited to those with a legitimate need to have the information. The NCAA list of banned drugs is not as extensive as that used for the Olympics but still contains a wide range of drugs of abuse and performance-enhancing drugs. Athletic trainers who are charged with developing drug-testing programs should always seek legal counsel and should comply with the 10 principles listed in the chapter.

6. Organize and implement a comprehensive drug-testing program.

Drug tests are normally conducted after championship games, as part of the PPE, or as part of a year-round program. Athletes must consent to be tested, but lack of consent usually results in ineligibility. Random selection of subjects for testing is the norm, but random selection can have several permutations based on timing of the test or characteristics of the athlete. Testing based on reasonable suspicion requires identification of objective signs of drug use, preferably by more than one observer on more than one occasion. Urinalysis is the usual method employed in athletic drug-testing programs. Initial positive tests conducted with immunoassay techniques should be confirmed with gas chromatography and mass spectrometry. To test the samples, the institution should use only reputable labs that can report their false-positive and false-negative rates.

APPENDIX A

WOTS UP Analysis for a Sports Medicine Program

The following nine worksheets comprise a WOTS UP analysis for a sports medicine program. This worksheet package has been adapted from material created by D.A. Campbell and Company for Hope College.

WORKSHEET 1:
Benefits and Concerns Relative to Strategic Planning

Instructions

1. List the benefits you expect from our strategic planning as well as any concerns.

2. Note possible ways to overcome each of your concerns. Circle the best ideas.

Benefits expected:

Concerns:

Ways to overcome concerns:

WORKSHEET 2: Organizing the Planning Process

Instructions

Indicate how each of the following issues should be handled. Outline the steps, responsibilities, and time lines for developing the strategic plan.

1. What are we developing a strategic plan for?

   The entire sports medicine program

   Only part of the sports medicine program (which part?)

   The entire sports medicine program and each of its subprograms

   Other

2. For what period of time should we plan?

Next 2 years	Next 5 years
Next 3 years	Next 6 years
Next 4 years	Other

3. What critical issues do you hope the planning will address?

4. How much time should we spend planning?

5. Should we use a consultant or other resource person in developing our plan?

   Yes

   No

   Unsure

   If so, what kind of help do we need?

6. Who should be part of the planning team? Circle all that apply.

Athletic trainers	Team physicians
Athletic administrators	Coaches
Consultants	Athletic training students
Patients	Others

7. How large should the planning team be?

   5-8

   9-12

   13-16

   17-20

   More than 20

8. Are there any others we should involve in the development of the plan? In the review of the plan?

9. Who should manage the overall planning effort?

10. Who should lead or chair the planning meetings?

11. By what date should we have the plan completed for approval?

12. Outline the steps you envision us using as we develop our plan.
  Steps
  Person(s) responsible
  Deadline

WORKSHEET 3:
History and Present Situation

Instructions

Review the history and present situation of the sports medicine program as they pertain to your area of responsibility. List any historical trends that will need attention as we plan for the future. Do not hesitate to comment on areas *outside* of your realm of responsibility if you so desire.

Historical trends

WORKSHEET 4:
Questions About Mission

1. Describe below what you understand the mission of the sports medicine program to be.

2. List any questions, ideas, or concerns you have about the present mission of the sports medicine program.

3. Do you envision any changes in the mission of the sports medicine program? If so, what do you want to accomplish? Who will be served by such a change?

WORKSHEET 5:
Client, Customer, and Stakeholder Needs

Instructions

1. List the needs of present or potential "customers" that the sports medicine program might address. Note ideas for how the sports medicine program might meet those needs.

2. List the significant groups who have a stake in what the sports medicine program does. How can the program meet their needs?

Clients and Customers

Describe existing or possible new target groups	
Their needs	Ways to meet those needs

Other stakeholders	
Their needs	Ways to meet those needs

WORKSHEET 6:
Competitors and Allies

Instructions

1. List present and potential new competitors, what the sports medicine program competes for, and our program's relative advantages and disadvantages (price, services, etc.).

2. List possible allies and how the sports medicine program might team up with each organization, person, or group.

Competitors

Existing:

New:

What we compete for

Our advantages	Our disadvantages

Allies of the sports medicine program	How can we team up with our allies?

WORKSHEET 7:
Opportunities and Threats

Instructions

1. List and rank the major opportunities and threats that you believe the sports medicine program will face in the next five years that will determine its success or failure.

2. Use the information from worksheets 5 and 6 to help provide a more detailed analysis of our clients and stakeholders.

3. Be sure to consider the social, cultural, economic, political, and technological forces that may affect the sports medicine program in the next five years.

Opportunities	Threats

WORKSHEET 8:
Strengths and Weaknesses

Instructions

List the major strengths and weaknesses of the sports medicine program as it looks toward the future.

Strengths and assets	Weaknesses and liabilities

WORKSHEET 9:
Critical Issues for the Future

Instructions

Review worksheets 3 through 8 and list critical issues or choices that the sports medicine program faces over the next five years.

Critical issues or choices

NATA Code of Ethics

Preamble

The National Athletic Trainers' Association Code of Ethics states the principles of ethical behavior that should be followed in the practice of athletic training. It is intended to establish and maintain high standards and professionalism for the athletic training profession.

The principles do not cover every situation encountered by the practicing athletic trainer, but are representative of the spirit with which athletic trainers should make decisions. The principles are written generally; the circumstances of a situation will determine the interpretation and application of a given principle and of the Code as a whole. When a conflict exists between the Code and the law, the law prevails.

Principle 1

Members shall respect the rights, welfare, and dignity of all.

1.1 Members shall not discriminate against any legally protected class.

1.2 Members shall be committed to providing competent care.

1.3 Members shall preserve the confidentiality of privileged information and shall not release such information to a third party not involved in the patient's care without a release unless required by law.

Principle 2

Members shall comply with the laws and regulations governing the practice of athletic training.

2.1 Members shall comply with applicable local, state, and federal laws and institutional guidelines.

2.2 Members shall be familiar with and abide by all National Athletic Trainers' Association standards, rules, and regulations.

2.3 Members shall report illegal or unethical practices related to athletic training to the appropriate person or authority.

2.4 Members shall avoid substance abuse and, when necessary, seek rehabilitation for chemical dependency.

Principle 3

Members shall maintain and promote high standards in their provision of services.

3.1 Members shall not misrepresent, either directly or indirectly, their skills, training, professional credentials, identity, or services.

3.2 Members shall provide only those services for which they are qualified through education or experience and which are allowed by their practice acts and other pertinent regulation.

3.3 Members shall provide services, make referrals, and seek compensation only for those services that are necessary.

3.4 Members shall recognize the need for continuing education and participate in educational activities that enhance their skills and knowledge.

3.5 Members shall educate those whom they supervise in the practice of athletic training about the Code of Ethics and stress the importance of adherence.

3.6 Members who are researchers or educators should maintain and promote ethical conduct in research and educational activities.

Principle 4

Members shall not engage in conduct that could be construed as a conflict of interest or that reflects negatively on the profession.

    4.1 Members should conduct themselves personally and professionally in a manner that does not compromise their professional responsibilities or the practice of athletic training.

    4.2 National Athletic Trainers' Association current or past volunteer leaders shall not use the NATA logo in the endorsement of products or services or exploit their affiliation with the NATA in a manner that reflects badly upon the profession.

    4.3 Members shall not place financial gain above the patient's welfare and shall not participate in any arrangement that exploits the patient.

    4.4 Members shall not, through direct or indirect means, use information obtained in the course of the practice of athletic training to try to influence the score or outcome of an athletic event, or attempt to induce financial gain through gambling.

GLOSSARY

90th-percentile fee—The fee below which 90% of all other medical vendors in a particular geographic area charge for a specific service.

abandonment—The desertion of a patient by the health care provider without the consent of the patient.

accreditation—Formal recognition provided to an organization or one of its programs indicating that it meets certain prescribed quality standards.

accuracy (standards)—Performance evaluation standards intended to improve the validity and reliability of the employee appraisal process.

actual cause—The degree to which a health care practitioner's actions are associated with the adverse outcomes of a patient's care.

adversaries—Persons who are unsupportive of both a program and a particular plan related to the program.

agreement–trust matrix—A model that identifies and types the most important people in developing support for a plan.

allies—Persons who exhibit a high level of support for a plan.

allocator of resources—A type of decisional role in which the leader exercises authority to determine how organizational assets will be deployed.

analytical listening—A type of listening approach in which one is open-minded despite listening for specific words or terms.

approved provider—A provider of continuing education for athletic trainers that has met all of the requirements of the BOC to offer CEUs to ATCs.

assumption of risk—A legal defense that attempts to claim that an injured plaintiff understood the risk of an activity and freely chose to undertake the activity regardless of the hazards associated with it.

athletic accident insurance—A type of insurance policy intended to reimburse medical vendors for the expenses associated with acute athletic accidents.

authority—The aspect of power, granted to either groups or individuals, that legitimizes the right of the group or individual to make decisions on behalf of others.

bedfellows—Persons who exhibit support for a particular plan but who have a history of untrustworthy behavior and vacillation.

bidding—A process whereby vendors provide cost quotations for goods and services they wish to sell.

bidding documents—The package of materials prepared by the architect and sent to contractors, including the invitation to bid, the bid form, and special bidding instructions.

breach of confidentiality—Violation of a commitment to privacy and protection of information or communications.

breach of contract—An unexcused failure to perform the services specified in a contract, either formal or informal.

bubble diagram—An abstract, graphic representation of the relationship of one function of a building to another based on the proximity factor established by the relationship chart.

budget—A type of operational plan for the coordination of resources and expenditures.

bulletin board—An electronic, online, interactive electronic database system, usually organized by topic or interest group.

business plan—Plan used by commercial loan officers to assess the viability of a business. Includes a written description of the activities the business will engage in, a market analysis, historical and projected financial statements, and other associated information.

capital campaign—A program, usually of fixed length, designed to raise funds for program creation, development, and improvement.

capitation—A system whereby medical vendors receive a fixed amount per patient.

carrier—Charge-based provider contracted by the federal government, charged with reviewing Medicare claims made by physicians or other health care providers.

catastrophic insurance—A type of accident insurance designed to provide lifelong medical, rehabilitation, and disability benefits for a victim of devastating injury.

certification—A form of title protection, established by state law or sponsored by professional associations, designed to ensure that practitioners have essential knowledge and skills sufficient to protect the public.

charting by exception—A type of medical record that notes only those patient responses that vary from predefined norms.

clinical practice guidelines (CPGs)—Systematic algorithm-like procedures that are universally followed in an effort to provide standardized clinical care and interventions.

clinical supervision—The process of direct observation of an employee's work, with emphasis on measurement of specific behaviors, and the subsequent development of plans to remediate deficiencies in performance.

CMS 1500—The form that private-practice clinics should use when filing a claim with an insurance company. Originally developed by the Health Care Financing Administration (now known as the Centers for Medicare and Medicaid Services) for Medicare claims.

code of ethics—A systematized set of standards or principles that defines ethical behavior appropriate for a profession. Moral values determine the standards and principles.

collegial culture—A type of organizational culture characterized by consensus, teamwork, and participatory decision making.

commercial loan—An amount of money, borrowed from a lending institution, for the purpose of establishing, improving, or maintaining a business.

commission—An action that violates a legal duty.

Commission on Accreditation of Rehabilitation Facilities (CARF)—A nonprofit agency that sets quality standards for rehabilitation services and facilities.

comparative negligence—A legal doctrine intended to determine the degree to which a plaintiff contributed to the harm caused by a defendant.

conflict of interest—Situation in which the interests of one individual or group are discordant or in competition with those of another individual or group.

construction documents—The highly detailed technical drawings that a contractor uses to determine building costs and guide construction.

construction management—A method that involves the general contractor as part of the design team from the beginning of the building process.

copayment—The percentage of a medical bill not paid for by the insurance company.

counterpower—The potential to influence the behavior of a superior.

criteria—Quantifiable measures used to determine whether a particular objective has been accomplished.

cultural awareness—A set of behaviors that an individual or group of individuals (organizations, businesses) possesses and implements through consistent actions that demonstrate appropriate behavior of diverse cultures.

culture—The shared values, beliefs, traditions, customs, and values of a particular group.

Current Procedural Terminology (CPT)—A coding system applied to medical procedures to standardize the language associated with third-party reimbursement.

data port—A dedicated phone line or network terminal used to connect computers in different locations.

decisional role—The portion of a manager's work that requires her to use authority to make decisions.

definers—People who use or receive the services of a program.

design-build—A method that uses only one firm both to design and to construct a new building.

developmental supervision—A supervisory model that emphasizes collaboration between supervisors and supervisees to help them solve problems and develop professionally.

diagnostic—Referring to a specific medical finding for the purposes of identification.

dictation—The act of orally recording, on a cassette tape or directly into a computer, the details of a health care assessment or treatment for later transcription and filing.

disability insurance—Insurance designed to protect an athlete against future loss of earnings because of a disabling injury or sickness.

disqualifying conditions—Injuries, illnesses, or other medical conditions that pose an undue risk to athletes, their teammates, or their competitors.

disseminator—An informational role that requires the leader to communicate with members of the group.

disturbance handler—A type of decisional role in which the leader manages conflict.

drug administration—Provision of a single dose of medication to a patient by order of a physician.

drug dispensing—Preparing and packaging medication for subsequent use by a patient.

elective—Referring to a surgical procedure that is not required but that one chooses to have performed.

electronic data interchange (EDI)—A system whereby insurance claims can be submitted electronically. Also known as paperless claims system.

emergency action plan (EAP)—A blueprint for handling emergencies that helps establish accountability for their management.

endowment—The portion of an institution's assets in cash and investments not normally used for operational purposes.

entrepreneurial role—A type of decisional role in which the leader initiates and designs controlled change within an organization.

enzyme multiplied immunoassay technique (EMIT)—A first-line screening procedure designed to detect abuse of drugs or the presence of performance-enhancing drugs by testing an athlete's urine.

ergonomics—The scientific study of human work.

ethics—The rules, standards, and principles that dictate right conduct among members of a society or profession. Ethics are based on moral values.

evidence-based medicine—The type of medicine that considers scientific findings, experience of the clinician, and considerations of the patient in an effort to provide the best care.

exclusions—Situations or circumstances specifically not covered by an insurance policy.

exclusive provider organization (EPO)—A type of preferred provider organization in which medical services are reimbursed only if the patient uses contracted providers.

exculpatory clause—A signed release from a patient or parents that waives all future legal claims against an athletic trainer or the employing institution.

excuse—A reason that is considered justifiable.

exemption—A legislative mechanism used to release members of one profession from the liability of violating another profession's practice act.

experimental treatments—Therapies not proved effective.

explanation of benefits form (EOB)—A summary prepared by an insurance company, and sent to a policyholder, that documents how the insurance policy covered the charges associated with a particular claim.

exploitation—Using another person for selfish purposes, particularly when it comes at the expense of that person or without the person's knowledge or full informed consent.

express warranty—An explicit statement specifying the conditions, circumstances, and terms under which a vendor will replace or repair a product if found to be faulty.

external chart audit—A patient records review technique, performed by an accreditation agency or a payer, intended to ensure that patient care is appropriate and meets certain minimum standards.

external evaluators—Experts not affiliated with an organization who are retained to assess the various programs within the organization.

false-negative—The results of a drug test that indicate either the absence of a banned compound or its presence below an acceptable level, when in fact the compound is present above acceptable levels.

false-positive—The results of a drug test that indicate the presence of a banned compound above an acceptable level, when in fact the compound is either absent or present below acceptable levels.

feasibility standards—Performance evaluation standards intended to help foster practicality in the employee appraisal process.

fee-for-service plan—Also known as an indemnity plan. A type of traditional medical insurance whereby patients are free to seek medical services from any provider. The plan covers a portion of the cost of covered procedures, and the patient is responsible for the balance.

FERPA (Family Educational Rights and Privacy Act)—Sometimes referred to as the Buckley Amendment. A 1974 federal law requiring student authorization to release educational records to a third party and ensuring access for students to their records.

figurehead role—An interpersonal role that requires the authority holder to represent the group, usually in a visible public capacity.

fixed budgeting—A method in which expenditures and revenues are projected on a monthly basis, thereby providing an estimate of cash flow.

FOB point—Freight-on-board point. The point at which the title for shipped goods passes from vendor to purchaser.

focus charting—A medical record that registers a patient's complaint data, the health care practitioner's actions, and the patient's response.

foot-pedal activator—A water-flow device, controlled by a foot pedal, used with hand-washing stations.

forbidden knowledge—Information about a situation that an athletic trainer is forbidden to act on.

forecast—A prediction of future conditions based on various statistics and indicators that describes an athletic training program's past and present situations.

foreseeability—The ability to project the likely outcome of an act.

formalistic culture—A type of organizational culture characterized by a clear chain of command and well-defined lines of formal authority.

formative evaluation—An assessment designed primarily for improvement of a program.

fraud—Criminal misrepresentation for the purpose of financial gain.

Gannt chart—A graphic planning and control technique that maps discrete tasks on a calendar.

gas chromatography–mass spectrometry (GC-MS)—A highly accurate method for detecting the presence of performance-enhancing and other drugs, including anabolic steroids, in an athlete's urine.

general contractor—The company responsible for coordinating the construction of a building.

goals—General statements of program intent.

Good Samaritan laws—Statutes intended to shield certain health care practitioners from certain types of legal liability when they voluntarily come to the aid of injured or ill persons under specific circumstances.

ground fault interrupter (GFI)—A highly sensitive device designed to discontinue the flow of electricity in an electrical circuit during a power surge.

guardian—A person who has legal responsibility for the care and decisions of someone who is incompetent to act for himself or who is a minor.

Hawthorne effect—Also known as the placebo effect. A phenomenon that occurs when the subjects in an experimental study alter their behavior simply because of the process of being studied, even when the independent variable produces no effect.

health history form—A detailed questionnaire designed to document an athlete's previous injuries, illnesses, and other medical conditions. This form often serves as the basis for additional medical follow-up and evaluation.

health history update—A brief questionnaire designed to determine whether an athlete suffered any injuries or developed any medical conditions since the last comprehensive PPE.

health insurance—A type of policy designed to reimburse the cost of preventive as well as corrective medical care.

health maintenance organization (HMO)—A type of health insurance plan that requires policyholders to use only those medical vendors approved by the company. All medical services are coordinated by a primary care physician, who acts as a gatekeeper to specialty services.

high-risk behaviors—Behaviors that expose a person to an unnecessarily high degree of physical or psychological jeopardy.

HIPAA—The Health Insurance Portability and Accountability Act of 1996; helps employees transfer their health insurance when they switch employers, ensures that their health information will remain private, and gives people more access to their own health care information.

honeymoon effect—The period of time, usually immediately after arriving in a new position, in which persons are more likely to be granted extra authority to make decisions.

implied warranty—An unstated understanding that a vendor will "make good" if a product is faulty.

individual practice association (IPA)—A managed care model whereby an HMO provides health care services through a network of individual medical practitioners. Care is provided in a physician's office as opposed to a large, multifunctional medical center.

informational role—Functions that require the manager to collect, use, and disseminate information.

inspection-production—A supervisory model that emphasizes the use of formal authority and managerial prerogatives to improve employee efficiency and efficacy.

insurance agent—A representative of an insurance company or an independent insurance agency who sells and services insurance policies.

insurance claim registry form—A worksheet that aids in tracking the progress of an insurance claim through the entire process.

interference—Anything, including environmental elements or characteristics of the communication medium, that distorts the message sent from the sender to the receiver.

intermediary—Cost-based provider contracted by the federal government and charged with reviewing Medicare claims made by hospitals.

internal chart audit—A patient records review technique performed by the sports medicine staff as part of a quality assurance program.

internal influencers—Organization decision makers.

International Classification of Diseases (ICD-10-CM)—A coding system applied to illnesses, injuries, and other medical conditions to standardize the language associated with third-party reimbursement.

interpersonal role—A managerial role, emanating from the possession of formal authority, that requires the manager to interact and form relationships with others in the organization.

inventory management—The process of controlling equipment and supply stocks so that services can be provided without interruption while the use of institutional resources is maximized.

job description—A written description of the specific responsibilities a position holder will be accountable for in an organization.

job specification—A written description of the requirements or qualifications a person should have to fill a particular role in an organization.

Joint Commission on Accreditation of Healthcare Organizations (JCAHO)—The oldest and largest health care standards organization in the country. JCAHO accredits ambulatory health care facilities.

laws—The rules and regulations governing the affairs of a community or society. Administrative authority and an established judicial system of the community enforce laws.

layered coverage—A method of using different insurance companies to underwrite different levels of coverage in a common policy.

leadership—A subset of power that involves influencing the behavior and attitudes of others to achieve intended outcomes.

legitimacy—The aspect of power that gives the leader the right to make a request and provides the obligation of the subordinate to comply.

liaison role—An interpersonal role that requires the leader to interact with others in the group, including superiors, subordinates, and coequals.

licensure—A form of state credentialing, established by statute and intended to protect the public, that regulates the practice of a trade or profession by specifying who may practice and what duties they may perform.

line-item budgeting—A method that allocates a fixed amount of money for each subfunction of a program.

liquid chromatography–mass spectrometry–mass spectrometry (LC/MS/MS)—A method of drug testing used to indicate the presence of drugs in an athlete's urine.

loss of consortium—A legal claim of damages for injuries to a spouse or for alienation of a spouse's affection.

lump-sum bidding—A process whereby general contractors provide cost quotations for the right to construct or renovate a building.

lump-sum budgeting—A method that allocates a fixed amount of money for an entire program without specifying how the money will be spent.

malpractice—Liability-generating conduct associated with the adverse outcome of patient treatment (Scott 1990, p. 6).

managed care—A growing concept in the insurance industry emphasizing cost control through coordination of medical services, for example with an HMO or PPO.

management—The element of leadership that involves planning, decision making, and coordination of the activities of a group.

manipulate—Shrewdly or deviously influence or control another person or a situation. When the influence or control is for self-interested purposes, it can be exploitative.

market analysis—Analysis that includes a written description of the competitive advantages of a business, analysis of the competition, pricing structure, and marketing plan.

mass screening—A preparticipation physical examination method whereby many athletes are screened simultaneously, usually in a school gymnasium or locker room.

master outline—A guide to the major sections of a filing system.

matrix structure—A type of chart that describes an organizational structure in terms of both functions and services.

maturational assessment—A medical screening procedure based on Tanner's stages of maturational development. It is often used to classify children and adolescents for the purpose of matching them with appropriate athletic opponents.

medical ethics—The process by which one determines right from wrong when medical care is involved.

medical insurance—A contract between a policyholder and an insurance company to reimburse a percentage of the cost of the policyholder's medical bills.

medical practice act—A state law regulating the practice of medicine, usually by specifying who may practice and under what circumstances.

medical record—Cumulative documentation of a person's medical history and health care interventions.

minor—A person under legal age to take on adult responsibilities and make adult decisions.

mission statement—A written expression of an organization's philosophy, purposes, and characteristics.

mixing valve—A type of plumbing fixture designed to blend hot and cold water, eliminating the need for separate hot- and cold-water controls.

monitor—A type of informational role that requires the leader to observe and keep abreast of changes that will affect the group and its activity.

narrative charting—A method of recording the details of a patient's assessments and treatments using a detailed, prose-based format.

natural lighting—Outside light used to illuminate indoor spaces, usually through windows or skylights.

need—The discrepancy between the present program status and the desired future state of one or more aspects of the program.

needs assessment—A systematic set of procedures undertaken to set organizational or programmatic priorities based on identified needs.

negligence—A type of tort in which an athletic trainer fails to act as a reasonably prudent athletic trainer would act under the circumstances.

negotiation—The process of bargaining.

negotiator—A type of decisional role in which the leader uses authority to bargain with members of the internal or external audience.

nonmedical correspondence—Letters and memoranda not associated with a specific patient's health status.

numeric analysis—The process of determining a staff member's workload by calculating and comparing the amount of time a person spends on certain tasks with the outputs that result from those tasks.

objectives—Specific statements of how a program intends to accomplish a particular goal.

omission—A failure to act when there was a legal duty to do so.

operational plan—A type of plan that defines organizational activities in the short term, usually no longer than two years.

opponents—Persons who support a particular program but dispute the implementation of a plan related to that program.

organizational chart—A graphic representation of an organization's structure, usually arranged by function, by service, or in a matrix format.

organizational culture—The values, beliefs, assumptions, and norms that form the infrastructure of the organizational ethos.

organizational structure—A model that defines the relationships among the members of an organization.

OSHA bloodborne pathogen standard—Federal government rules that require employers to protect employees against the accidental transmission of bloodborne pathogens, especially HIV and hepatitis B.

outcomes assessment—An evaluation method used in health care that seeks objective evidence that the care provided by the athletic trainer enhanced a patient's functional ability.

over-the-counter medication (OTC)—A medication that can be purchased without a physician's prescription.

performance budgeting—A method that allocates funds for discrete activities.

performance evaluation—The process of placing a value on the quality of an employee's work.

perpetrator—The person who is responsible for or has committed an act or both.

personalistic culture—A type of organizational culture characterized by autonomy in decision making and problem solving.

personal power—The potential to influence others by virtue of personal characteristics and personality attributes.

person specification—A specific delineation, based on the job specification, of the qualities, skills, and characteristics a person must have to fill a particular role.

PERT (program evaluation and review technique)—A method of graphically depicting the time line for and interrelationships of different stages of a program.

planning—A type of decision-making process in which a course of action is determined in order to bring about a future state of affairs.

planning committee—A group of institutional employees who work with an architect to develop the design of a building.

plumbing fixtures—The external hardware used to control the flow and temperature of water.

point-of-service plan (POS)—Managed care plans that are similar to PPOs except that primary care physicians are assigned to patients to coordinate their care.

¹policy—A type of plan that expresses an organization's intended behavior relative to a specific program subfunction.

²policy—A contract between an insurance company and an individual or organization.

pooled buying consortium—A group of similar institutions that merge resources to purchase goods in large quantities to receive volume discounts.

position description—A formal document that describes the qualifications, work content, accountability, and scope of a job.

position power—The power vested in people by virtue of the roles they play in an organization.

power—The potential to influence others.

practice—The action that takes place in response to administrative problems.

preemployment test—Any procedure (including a drug test) conducted on a potential employee that is used to determine the applicant's suitability for employment.

preferred provider organization (PPO)—A type of health insurance plan that provides financial incentives to encourage policyholders to use medical vendors approved by the company.

premium—The invoiced cost of an insurance policy.

preparticipation physical examination (PPE)—A medical screening procedure designed to determine an athlete's readiness for participation in a specific sport at a specific level of competition.

primary care provider—The physician, selected by an HMO member, who acts as the first source of medical service for the patient. Most HMOs require members to seek a referral from the primary care provider before seeking care from another medical vendor.

primary coverage—A type of health, medical, or accident insurance that begins to pay for covered expenses immediately after a deductible has been paid.

primary decision makers—Institutional members who have formal authority over large units or subunits of an organization.

primary party—A person directly involved as a participant in an activity.

problem-oriented medical record (POMR)—A system of medical record keeping that organizes information around a patient's specific complaints.

procedure—A type of operational plan that provides specific directions for members of an organization to follow.

proceedings—A book containing the abstracts or outlines of each speaker's presentation.

process—A collection of incremental and mutually dependent steps designed to direct the most important tasks of an organization.

process analysis—A technique for streamlining the number and complexity of steps needed to provide a service to a customer.

program administration records—Documentation of the activities of a program.

program evaluation—A systematic and comprehensive assessment of the worth of a particular program.

program statement—A document, prepared by the users, the architect, or both, that specifies the anticipated space requirements based on known work patterns provided by the users.

propriety standards—Performance evaluation standards intended to help ensure that a process is legal and fair.

proximate (legal) cause—The degree to which the harm caused by a health care practitioner was foreseeable.

purchase order—A document that formalizes the terms of a purchase and transmits the intentions of the buyer to purchase goods or services from a vendor.

purchasing—The process of acquiring goods and services.

random selection—A method for choosing subjects for drug testing based on permutations of timing, subject characteristics, or both. Implies an equal probability of choosing any subject within a given population for testing.

reason—The basis or explanation for an action.

reasonable suspicion—A basis for selecting subjects for drug testing taking into account observable signs of drug use. Also known as reasonable cause or probable cause.

receiving—The process of accepting delivery of goods purchased from a vendor.

recruitment—The process of planning for human resources needs and identifying potential candidates to meet those needs.

registration—A type of state credentialing that requires qualified members of a profession to register with the state in order to practice.

relationship chart—A table used to justify the placement of various rooms within a building.

relative value—The value of the overall cost of providing a service.

reliability (in staff selection)—Consistency of staff selection procedures.

request for quotation (RFQ)—A document that provides vendors with the specifications for bidding on the sale of goods and services.

requests for proposals (RFPs)—Notices from internal and external funding sources announcing the details of grant programs.

requisition—A type of formal or informal communication, usually written, used for requesting authorization to purchase goods or services.

rider—Additions to a standard insurance policy that provide coverage for conditions not normally covered.

right conduct—Behavior that is fitting or proper or conforms to legal or moral expectations.

rights—Moral or legal privileges inherent in being a member of a community or society.

risk management—A process designed to prevent losses of all kinds for everyone associated with an organization, including its directors, administrators, employees, and clients.

schematic drawings—A graphic representation, derived from the program statement, that illustrates the relationships among the principal functions of a building.

scientific management—A collection of management theories developed in the early 1900s whose emphasis is on the strict control of work in order to maximize production through increases in efficiency.

secondary coverage—A type of health, medical, or accident insurance that begins to pay for covered expenses only after all other sources of insurance coverage have been exhausted. Also known as excess insurance.

secondary decision makers—Professional staff members primarily responsible for delivering a program within an organization.

self-determination—Freedom to judge for oneself, to determine one's own course of action, and to manage one's own affairs.

SOAP note—Medical appraisal organized by subjective and objective evaluation, assessment of the patient's problem, and development of a plan for treatment.

sovereign (governmental) immunity—A legal doctrine that holds that neither governments nor their agents can be held liable for negligent actions.

span of control—The number of subordinates supervised by a particular individual in an organizational setting.

spending-ceiling model—A type of expenditure budgeting that requires justification only for expenses that exceed those of the previous budget cycle. Also known as the *incremental model*.

spending-reduction model—A type of budgeting used during periods of financial retrenchment that requires reallocation of institutional funds, resulting in reduced spending levels for some programs.

spokesperson—An informational role that requires communication with organizational influencers and members of the organization's public.

staff selection—The procedures used as the basis for any employment decision, including recruitment, hiring, promotion, demotion, retention, and performance evaluation.

standard of care—The legal duty to provide health care services consistent with what other health care practitioners of the same training, education, and credentialing would provide under the circumstances.

standards of practice—Widely accepted principles intended to guide the professional activities of a health care practitioner.

standpipe drain—A type of drain that is raised above floor level.

station PPE—A group screening process whereby information for individual athletes is collected at a variety of stations staffed by a combination of medical and nonmedical personnel, usually in the context of a school environment.

statutes of limitations—Laws that fix a certain length of time beyond which legal actions cannot be initiated.

strategic planning—A type of planning that involves critical self-examination to bring about organizational improvement.

subcontractor—A company hired by the general contractor to complete a particular portion of the building project. The subcontractor's work is usually devoted to a particular skilled trade, such as plumbing, electrical, or landscaping.

subpoena—The legal authority used to compel a person to provide testimony.

summative evaluation—An assessment designed primarily to describe the effectiveness or accomplishments of a program.

supervision—A process whereby authority holders observe the work activities of an employee to improve the outcomes of the employee's work or to improve the employee's professional development.

Tanner staging—A method for assessing physical maturation by categorizing the development of secondary sexual characteristics.

tax-exempt bonds—Bonds authorized and sold by governmental agencies to provide funding for construction projects.

testimony—Legally binding statements offered as evidence to the facts in a legal proceeding.

thermostat—A device that controls heating and cooling equipment.

[1]**third party**—A medical vendor with no binding interest in a particular insurance contract.

[2]**third party**—A party affected by, but not directly involved in, a situation. Professionals who simply have knowledge of an unethical act can be affected by it because they have a professional responsibility to act on such knowledge.

third-party reimbursement—The process by which medical vendors receive reimbursement from insurance companies for services provided to policyholders.

tort—A legal wrong, other than breach of contract, for which a remedy will be provided, usually in the form of monetary damages.

Total Quality Management (TQM)—Also known as continuous quality improvement. A management system that emphasizes continuous improvement in the process by which work is accomplished to create improvements in a product. A continuous focus on the needs and desires of clients is a major focus of TQM.

traffic patterns—The anticipated flow of people from one area of a building to another.

transactional leadership—The simple exchange between leaders and followers of one thing for another.

transformational leadership—The aspect of leadership that uses both change and conflict to elevate the standards of the social system.

UB-04 (also known as the CMS 1450)—Insurance claim form that hospitals should use.

unity of command—A principle of scientific management that requires a single supervisor to direct the work of an employee.

usual, customary, and reasonable (UCR)—The charge consistent with what other medical vendors would assess.

utility standards—Performance evaluation standards intended to help ensure that employee appraisal is useful to workers, employers, and others who need to use the information.

validity (in staff selection)—The employment of criteria that predict how well a candidate will perform in a role.

variable budgeting—A method requiring adjustment of monthly expenditures so that they do not exceed revenues.

vision statement—A concise statement that describes the ideal state to which an organization aspires.

WOTS UP analysis—A data collection and appraisal technique designed to determine an organization's strengths, weaknesses, opportunities, and threats in order to facilitate planning.

zero-based budgeting—A model that requires justification for every budget line item without reference to previous spending patterns.

zone of indifference—A hypothetical boundary of legitimacy outside of which requests or orders will be met with mere compliance or refusal.

BIBLIOGRAPHY

Abdenour, T.E. 1982. Computerized training room records. *Athletic Training* 17(3): 91.

Accreditation Association for Ambulatory Health Care. 2010. www.aaahc.org. Accessed February 15, 2010.

Acheson, K.A., and Gall, M.D. 1987. *Techniques in the clinical supervision of teachers.* 2nd Ed. New York: Longman.

Ackoff, R.L. 1970. *A concept of corporate planning.* New York: Wiley Interscience.

Agency for Health Care Research and Quality. 1995. *A press release: HIAA and AHCPR join forces to help consumers choose and use managed care plans,* August 28, 1995. http://archive.ahrq.gov/news/press/hiaa.htm. Accessed March 10, 2010.

Albohm, M.J., and Wilkerson, G.B. 1999. An outcomes assessment of care provided by certified athletic trainers. *Journal of Rehabilitation Outcomes Measurement* 3(3): 51-56.

Aldrich, J.W. 1985. Staffing concepts and principles. *Human resources management and development handbook,* edited by W. Tracy, 165-173. New York: AMACOM.

Alford, C.F. 2001. *Whistleblowers: Broken lives and organizational power.* Ithaca, NY: Cornell University Press.

Allan, J., and Englebright, J. 2000. Patient-centered documentation: An effective and efficient use of clinical information systems. *Journal of Nursing Administration* 30(2): 90-95.

American Academy of Family Physicians. 2005. *Preparticipation physical evaluation.* 2nd Ed. Minneapolis: McGraw-Hill and Physician and Sportsmedicine.

American Academy of Orthopaedic Surgeons. 2000. *Athletic training and sports medicine.* 3rd Ed. Park Ridge, IL: Author.

American Association of University Professors. 1995. *AAUP policy documents and reports: Statement on professional ethics.* Washington, DC: Author.

American Counseling Association. 1995. *Code of ethics.* Alexandria, VA: Author.

American Heart Association. 1996. Cardiovascular preparticipation screening of competitive athletes. *Circulation* 94: 850-856.

American Heart Association. 1998. Cardiovascular preparticipation screening of competitive athletes. *Circulation* 97: 2294.

American Hospital Association. 1992. *Ethical conduct for health care institutions.* Chicago: Author.

American Physical Therapy Association. 2010. *Code of ethics.* Alexandria, VA: Author.

American Psychological Association. 1992. *Ethical principles of psychologists and code of conduct.* Washington, DC: Author.

Ammer, C., and Ammer, D.S. 1984. *Dictionary of business and economics.* 2nd Ed. New York: The Free Press.

Andersen, J.C., Courson, R.W., Kleiner, D.M., and McLoda, T.A. 2002. National Athletic Trainers' Association position statement: Emergency planning in athletics. *Journal of Athletic Training* 37: 99-104.

Anderson, M.K., and Hall, S.J. 1995. *Sports injury management.* Media, PA: Williams & Wilkins.

Appelbaum, D., and Lawton, S.V. 1990. *Ethics and the professions.* Englewood Cliffs, NJ: Prentice Hall.

Arnheim, D.D., and Prentice, W.E. 1997. *Principles of athletic training.* 9th Ed. Dubuque, IA: Brown and Benchmark.

Arnheim, D.D., and Prentice, W.E. 2000. *Principles of athletic training.* 10th Ed. New York: McGraw-Hill.

Arnheim, D.D., and Prentice, W.E. 2002. *Essentials of athletic training.* 5th Ed. Boston: McGraw-Hill.

Baley, J.A., and Matthews, D.L. 1984. *Law and liability in athletics, physical education, and recreation.* Boston: Allyn & Bacon.

Barlow, C.W. 1982. *Negotiating skills for the purchasing agent.* New York: American Management Association Membership Publications Division.

Barnard, C.I. 1938. *The functions of the executive.* Cambridge, MA: Harvard University Press.

Barnes, R.P. 1997. Fiscal management. *Clinical athletic training,* edited by J. Konin, 77-86. Thorofare, NJ: Slack, Inc.

Bass, B.M. 1990. *Bass & Stogdill's handbook of leadership.* 3rd Ed. New York: Macmillan.

Belanger, A.Y. 2002. *Evidence-based guide to therapeutic physical agents.* Baltimore: Lippincott, Williams & Wilkins.

Benda, C. 1991. Sideline Samaritans. *The Physician and Sportsmedicine* 19(11): 132-142.

Bennis, W., and Nanus, B. 1985. *Leaders.* New York: Harper & Row.

Berni, R., and Readey, H. 1978. *Problem-oriented medical record implementation.* St. Louis: Mosby.

Biehle, J.T. 1982. Construction costs and the "oh my gosh!" syndrome. *American School and University* 54: C10-C14.

Bigby, J. 2003a. Advocating for health care systems that meet the needs of diverse populations. In *Cross-cultural medicine,* edited by J. Bigby, 269-275. Philadelphia, PA: American College of Physicians.

Bigby, J. 2003b. Beyond cultures: Strategies for caring for patients from diverse racial, ethnic, and cultural groups. In *Cross-cultural medicine,* edited by J. Bigby, 1-28. Philadelphia, PA: American College of Physicians.

Blake, R.R., and Mouton, J.S. 1984. *Solving costly organizational conflicts.* San Francisco: Jossey-Bass.

Block, P. 1987. *The empowered manager: Positive political skills at work.* San Francisco: Jossey-Bass.

Bok, S. 2004. Whistleblowing and professional responsibility. In *Taking sides: Clashing views on controversial issues in business ethics and society.* 8th Ed., edited by L.H. Newton and M.M. Ford, 174-181. Guilford, CT: McGraw-Hill and Dushkin.

Briner, W.W. 1993. Getting more out of athletic examinations. *American Family Physician* 48: 225.

Brown, D.C., Brown, D.A., and Yates, C.S. 2000. Controlling infectious hazards in the athletic environment. In *Athletic protective equipment: Care, selection and fitting*, edited by S.A. Street and D. Runkle, 13-25. Boston: McGraw-Hill.

Bruce, S.D. 1986. *Prewritten job descriptions.* Madison, CT: Business and Legal Reports.

Bureau of Nation Affairs. 1990. *The Americans with Disabilities Act: A practical and legal guide to impact, enforcement, and compliance.* Washington, DC: Author.

Burns, H.K., and Foley S. M. 2005. Building a foundation for an evidence-based approach to practice: Teaching basic concepts to undergraduate freshman students. *Journal of Professional Nursing* 21(6): 351-357.

Burns, J.M. 1978. *Leadership.* New York: Harper & Row.

Cady, C. 1979. A space saving taping table. *Athletic Training* 14(4): 224.

Callister, L.C. 2005. What has the literature taught us about culturally competent care of women and children. *MCN: The American Journal of Maternal Child Nursing* 30(6): 380-388.

Campbell, A.V., Gillett, G., and Jones, D.G. 2001. *Medical ethics.* 3rd Ed. Oxford, New York: Oxford University Press.

Campbell, D. 1999. Researchers update data from athletic training outcomes study. *NATA News* (April): 26-27.

Campinha-Bacote, J. 2003. *The process of cultural competence in the delivery of healthcare services: A culturally competent model of care.* 4th Ed. Cincinnati, OH: Transcultural C.A.R.E. Associates.

Cascio, W.F., and Bernardin, H.J. 1981. Implications of performance appraisal litigation for personnel decisions. *Personnel Psychology* 34: 211-226.

Cashmore, J. 2006. There's more than one way to effectively maintain equipment. *Materials Management in Health Care* 15(2): 60.

Castetter, W.B. 1986. *The personnel function in educational administration.* 4th Ed. New York: Macmillan.

Center for Evidence-Based Physiotherapy. 2006. PEDro – physiotherapy evidence database. www.pedro.org.au. Accessed December 19, 2009.

Centre for Review and Dissemination at York University. 2009. www.york.ac.uk/inst/crd. Accessed on December 29, 2009.

Chambers, D.W. 2004. The professions. *The Journal of the American College of Dentists* 71(4): 57-64.

Chambers, R.L., Ross, N.V., and Kozubowski, J. 1986. Insurance types and coverages: Knowledge to plan for the future (with a focus on motor skill activities and athletics). *Physical Educator* 44(1): 233-240.

Ciccolella, M. 1991. Caught in court. *College Athletic Management* 3(4): 10-13.

Cliska, D. 2005. Educating for evidence-based practice. *Journal of Professional Nursing* 21(6): 345-350.

Clover, J. 1997. Clinical marketing. *Clinical athletic training*, edited by J, Konin, 107-120. Thorofare, NJ: Slack Inc.

Cohen, A., and Cohen, E. 1979. *Designing and space planning for libraries.* New York: Bowker.

Cohen, J.J. 2006. Professionalism in medical education, an American perspective: From evidence to accountability. *Medical Education* 40(7): 607-617.

Cohn, B.M., Azzara, A.J., and Petrie, R. 1998. *Legal aspects of emergency medical services.* Philadelphia: W.B. Saunders.

Culp, B., Goemaere, N.D., and Miller, E. 1985. Risk management: An integral part of quality assurance. *Quality assurance: A complete guide to effective programs*, edited by C.G. Meisenheimer, 169-192. Rockville, MD: Aspen.

Dale, E. 1965. *Management: Theory and practice.* New York: McGraw-Hill.

Danzon, P.M. 1985. *Medical malpractice.* Cambridge, MA: Harvard University Press.

Davidoff, F. 2000. Changing the subject: Ethical principles for everyone in health care. *Annals of Internal Medicine* 133(5): 386-389.

DeCarlo, M.S. 1997. Reimbursement for health care services. In *Clinical athletic training,* edited by J. Konin, 89-104. Thorofare, NJ: Slack, Inc.

Dejnozka, E.L. 1983. *Educational administration glossary.* Westport, CT: Greenwood Press.

Denegar, C.R., and Hertel, J. 2002. Clinical education reform and evidence-based clinical practice guidelines. *Journal of Athletic Training* 37(2): 127-128.

Denegar, C.R., Saliba, E., and Saliba, S.F. 2006. *Therapeutic modalities for musculoskeletal injuries.* 2nd Ed. Champaign, IL: Human Kinetics.

DeRosa, G.P. 2006. Professionalism and virtues. *Clinical Orthopaedics and Related Research* 449: 28-33.

Dibner, D.R. 1982. *You and your architect.* Washington, DC: The American Institute of Architects.

Dobbins, G.H., and Russell, J.M. 1986. The biasing effects of subordinate likableness on the leaders' responses to poor performers: A laboratory and a field study. *Personnel Psychology* 39: 759-777.

Dorfman, P.W., Stephan, W.G., and Loveland, J. 1986. Performance appraisal behaviors: Supervisor perceptions and subordinate reactions. *Personnel Psychology* 39: 579-597.

Dougherty, N.J., and Bonanno, D. 1985. *Management service in sport and leisure services.* Minneapolis: Burgess International.

Drafke, M.W. 1994. *Working in health care: What you need to know to succeed.* Philadelphia: F.A. Davis.

Drake, J.D. 1982. *Interviewing for managers.* New York: AMACOM.

Drezner, J.A. 2000. Sudden cardiac death in young athletes: Causes, athlete's heart, and screening guidelines. *Postgraduate Medicine* 108(5): 37-44, 47-50.

Drowatzky, J.N. 1985. Legal duties and liability in athletic training. *Athletic Training* 20(1): 10-13.

Dunne, G.D. 2002. *The nursing job search.* Philadelphia: University of Pennsylvania Press.

DuRant, R.H., Pendergrast, R.A., Seymore, C., Gaillard, G., and Donner, J. 1992. Findings from the preparticipation athletic examination and athletic injuries. *American Journal of Diseases of Children* 146: 85-91.

Eder, L.B. 2000. *Managing healthcare information systems with Web-enabled technologies.* Hershey, PA: Idea Group Publishing.

Elkouri, F., and Elkouri, E.A. 1993. *Resolving drug issues.* Washington, DC: Bureau of National Affairs.

Equal Employment Opportunity Commission. 1978. *Uniform guidelines on employee selection procedures.* Washington, DC: Bureau of National Affairs.

Esposto, L. 1993. Applying functional outcome assessment to Medicare documentation. In *Documenting functional outcomes in physical therapy,* edited by D.L. Stewart and S.H. Abeln, 135-174. St. Louis: Mosby.

Fahey, T.D. 1986. *Athletic training: Principles and practice.* Palo Alto, CA: Mayfield.

Falcone, P. 1997. *96 great interview questions to ask before you hire.* New York: AMACOM.

Fayol, H. 1949. *General and industrial management.* London: Pitman & Sons.

Fein, R. 1986. *Medical care, medical costs.* Cambridge, MA: Harvard University Press.

Fineout-Overholt, E., Melnyk, B.M., and Schultz, A. 2005. Transforming health care from the inside out: Advancing evidence-based practice in the 21st century. *Journal of Professional Nursing* 21(6): 335-344.

Fitz-Gibbon, C.T., and Morris, L.L. 1987. *How to design a program evaluation.* Newbury Park, CA: Sage.

Fletcher, M.E., and Ranck, S.L. 1991. Building a committee. *Athletic Business* 15(8): 49-50.

Forseth, E.A. 1986. Consideration in planning small college athletic training facilities. *Athletic Training* 21(1): 22-25.

Fowler, A.R., and Bushardt, S.C. 1986. T.O.P.E.S.: Developing a task oriented performance evaluation system. *Advanced Management Journal* 51(4): 4-8.

Frankel, E. 1991. Handle with care. *College Athletic Management* 3(3): 11-13.

French, J.R.P., and Raven, B. 1959. The bases of social power. In *Studies in social power,* edited by D. Cartwright, 150-167. Ann Arbor, MI: Institute for Social Research.

Friedrich, C.J. 1963. *Man and his government: An empirical theory of politics.* New York: McGraw-Hill.

Fry, R. 1993. *Your first interview.* 2nd Ed. Hawthorne, NJ: Career Press.

Gabriel, A.J. 1981. Medical communications: Records for the professional athletic trainer. *Athletic Training* 16(1): 68-69.

Gallup, E.M. 1995. *Law and the team physician.* Champaign, IL: Human Kinetics.

Garofalo, M.J. 1989. How strategies can get lost in the translation. *Business Month* 134(10): 82-83.

Geisler, P.R. 2003. Multiculturalism and athletic training education: Implications for educational and professional progress. *Journal of Athletic Training* 38(2): 141-151.

Gibson, C.K., Newton, D.J., and Cochran, D.S. 1990. An empirical investigation of the nature of hospital mission statements. *Health Care Management Review* 15(3): 35-45.

Gibson, J.M. 2002. Deciding values. In *The tracks we leave: Ethics in healthcare management,* edited by F. Perry, 17-30. Chicago: Health Administration Press.

Gieck, J., Lowe, J., and Kenna, K. 1984. Trainer malpractice: A sleeping giant. *Athletic Training* 19(1): 41-46.

Gillies, D.A. 1994. *Nursing management: A systems approach.* 3rd Ed. Philadelphia: Saunders.

Glondys, B.A. 1988. *Today's challenge: Content of the health record.* Chicago: American Medical Records Association.

Godek, J.J. 1992. Sports rehabilitation in the '90s: Who's who? *Journal of Sport Rehabilitation* 1: 87-94.

Goldberg, B., Saratini, A., Witman, P., Gavin, M., and Nicholas, J. 1980. Preparticipation sports assessment: An objective evaluation. *Pediatrics* 67: 736-745.

Good, C.V., Ed. 1973. *Dictionary of education.* New York: McGraw-Hill.

Graham, J.D., and Rhomberg, L. 1996. How risks are identified and managed. The *annals of the American academy of political and social science,* edited by H. Kunreuter and P. Slovic, 545 (May 1996): 15-24.

Graham, L.S. 1985. Ten ways to dodge the malpractice bullet. *Athletic Training* 20(2): 117-119.

Griffin, L. 2005. The ethical health lawyer: Watch out for whistleblowers. *Journal of Law, Medicine & Ethics* 33(1): 160-163.

Gulick, L., and Urwick, L., Eds. 1977. *Papers on the science of administration.* Fairfield, NJ: Kelley.

Haddad, S.A. 1985. Compensation and benefits. In *Human resources management and development handbook,* edited by W. Tracy, 638-660. New York: AMACOM.

Hagerty, B.K., Chang, R.S., and Spengler, C.D. 1985. Work sampling: Analyzing nursing staff productivity. *Journal of Nursing Administration* 15(9): 9-14.

Hanak, M.P. 2004. *How to navigate a complex maze of opportunities within the federal government.* www.nata.org/sites/default/files/HowtoNavigateFederalGovernmentHanak2004.pdf. Accessed September 8, 2006.

Hart, P.M., and Cole, S.L. 1992. Subtracting insult from injury. *Athletic Business* 16(5): 39-42.

Hawkins, J. 1988. The legal status of athletic trainers. *The Sports, Parks and Recreation Law Reporter* 2(1): 6-9.

Hawkins, J.D. 1989. Sports medicine record keeping: The key to effective communication and documentation. *Sports Medicine Standards and Malpractice Reporter* 1(2): 31-35.

Haynes, B., and Haynes, A. 1998. Barriers and bridges to evidence based clinical practice. *British Medical Journal (Clinical Research Edition)* 317(7153): 273-276.

Health Insurance Association of America. 1999. *Health insurers' anti-fraud programs: Research findings 1999.* www.hiaa.org/search/content.cfm?ContentID=717. Accessed June 20, 2003.

Health Insurance Association of America. 2003a. *Guide to managed care: Choosing and using a health plan.* www.hiaa.org/consumer/choosing.cfm. Accessed June 20, 2003.

Health Insurance Association of America. 2003b. *2002-2009 data from CDC/NCHSs, National Health Interview Survey, 1997-2009, Family Care component.* www.cdc.gov/nchs/data/nhis/earlyrelease/201006_01.pdf.

Heinzman, S.E. 1991. Quality physicals that generate funds for the training room. *Athletic Training, JNATA* 26: 66-69.

Herbert, D.L. 1987. The use of prospective releases containing exculpatory language in exercise and fitness programs. The *Exercise Standards and Malpractice Reporter* 1(6): 89-90.

Herbert, D.L. 1990. *Legal aspects of sports medicine.* Canton, OH: Professional Reports Corporation.

Herbert, D.L. 1992. *The sports medicine standards book.* Canton, OH: Professional Reports Corporation.

Herbert, D.L. 1996. Athlete's exclusion from participation does not violate Federal Rehabilitation Act. *Sports Medicine Standards and Malpractice Reporter* 8: 40-43.

Herbert, D.L. 1997. Sports medicine physician has "final say" in exclusion of athlete from participation. *Sports Medicine Standards and Malpractice Reporter* 9(17): 20-23.

Herbert, D.L., and Herbert, W.G. 1989. *Legal aspects of preventative and rehabilitative exercise programs.* 2nd Ed. Canton, OH: Professional Reports Corporation.

Hertel, J. 2005. Research training for clinicians: The crucial link between evidence-based practice and third-party reimbursement. *Journal of Athletic Training* 40(2): 69-70.

Hollander, E.P. 1978. *Leadership dynamics: A practical guide to effective relationships.* New York: Macmillan.

Hootman, J.M. 2004. New section in JAT: Evidence-based practice. *Journal of Athletic Training* 39(1): 9.

Horine, L. 1991. *Administration of physical education and sport programs.* 2nd Ed. Dubuque, IA: Brown.

Horsley, J.E., and Carlova, J. 1983. *Testifying in court.* Oradell, NJ: Medical Economics.

Hrysomallis, C., and Morrison, W.E. 1997. Sports injury surveillance and protective equipment. *Sports Medicine* 24(3): 181-183.

Huber, V.L., Podsakoff, P.M., and Todor, W.D. 1986. An investigation of biasing factors in the attributions of subordinates and their supervisors. *Journal of Business Research* 14: 83-97.

Huff, P.S. 1998. Drug distribution in the training room. *Clinics in Sports Medicine* 17: 211-228.

Institute of Medicine. 2002. What health care system administrators need to know about racial and ethnic disparities in healthcare. www.iom.edu/CMS/3740/4475/14973.aspx. Accessed May 16, 2010.

Isear, J.A. 1997. Clinical professionalism. In *Clinical athletic training,* edited by J.G. Konin, 150-157. Thorofare, NJ: Slack, Inc.

Iyer, P.W. 1991a. New trends in charting. *Nursing 91* 21(1): 48-50.

Iyer, P.W. 1991b. *Nursing documentation: A nursing process approach.* St. Louis: Mosby Year Book.

Jacobs, T.O. 1970. *Leadership and exchange in formal organizations.* Alexandria, VA: Human Resources Research Organization.

Jette, D.U., and Portney, L.G. 2003. Construct validation of a model for professional behavior in physical therapist students. *Physical Therapy* 83(5): 432-443.

Johnson, R.L., Saha, S., Arbelaez, J.J., Beach, M.C., and Cooper, L.A. 2004. Racial and ethnic differences in patient perceptions of bias and cultural competence in health care. *Journal of General Internal Medicine* 19(2): 101-110.

Joint Committee on Standards for Educational Evaluation. 1981. *Standards for evaluations of educational programs, projects, and materials.* New York: McGraw-Hill.

Joint Committee on Standards for Educational Evaluation. 1988. *The personnel evaluation standards.* Beverly Hills, CA: Sage.

Jones, R.L., and Trentin, H.G. 1971. *Budgeting: Key to planning and control.* 2nd Ed. New York: American Management Association.

Joy, E.A., Paisley, T.S., Price Jr., R., Rassner, L., and Thiese, S.M. 2004. Optimizing the collegiate preparticipation physical evaluation. *Clinical Journal of Sports Medicine* 14(3):183-7.

Juckett, G. 2005. Cross-cultural medicine. *American Family Physician* 72(11): 2267-2274.

Kahn, R.F. 1968. A note on the concept of authority. In *Leadership and authority,* edited by G. Wijeyewardene, 6-14. Kuala Lumpur, Malaysia: University of Malaysia Press.

Kaiser Family Foundation. 2002. *Trends and indicators in the changing health care marketplace.* www.kff.org/insurance/3161-index.cfm. Accessed May 1, 2002.

Karelis, C.H. 1987. The limits of leadership. *Liberal Education* 73(2): 20-33.

Katz, D., and Kahn, R.L. 1966. *The social psychology of organizations.* New York: Wiley & Sons.

Kauffman, R., Rojas, A. M., and Mayer, H. 1993. *Needs assessment: A user's guide.* Englewood Cliffs, NJ: Educational Technology.

Keaveny, T.J., and McGann, A.F. 1980. Performance appraisal format: Role clarity and evaluation criteria. *Research in Higher Education* 13(3): 225-232.

Keirns, M.A., Knudsen, L., and Webster, K.J. 1997. Outcomes assessment in athletic training. In *Clinical athletic training,* edited by J.G. Konin, 245-253. Thorofare, NJ: Slack, Inc.

Kesler, S.P., and Fagan, D. 2005. Firm foundation, successful facility expansion is built on robust MEP master planning. *Health Facilities Management* 18(6): 31-33.

Kess, S., and Westlin, B. 1987. *Business strategies.* Chicago: Commerce Clearinghouse.

Kettenbach, G. 1995. *Writing S.O.A.P. notes.* 2nd Ed. Philadelphia: Davis.

Kibler, W.B. 1990. *The sport preparticipation fitness examination.* Champaign, IL: Human Kinetics.

King, A.A. 1987. *Power and communication.* Prospect Heights, IL: Waveland.

Knowles, J.M. 1997. Planning a new athletic therapy facility. In *Clinical athletic training,* edited by J.G. Konin, 55-66. Thorofare, NJ: Slack, Inc.

Koester, M.C. 1995. Refocusing the adolescent preparticipation physical evaluation toward preventive health care. *Journal of Athletic Training* 30: 352-360.

Kolodny, H.F. 1979. Evolution to a matrix organization. *Academy of Management Review* 4(4): 543-553.

Konin, J.G. 1997. *Clinical athletic training.* Thorofare NJ: Slack, Inc.

Konin, J.G., and Frederick, M. 2005. *Documentation for athletic training*. Thorofare, NJ: Slack Inc.

Kujawa, J.A., and Short, J.R. 2005. Six steps to managing service contracts effectively. *Biomedical Instrumentation & Technology* 39(3): 200-201.

Lasswell, H.D., and Kaplan, A. 1950. Power and society: A framework for political inquiry. *Yale Law School Studies* 2: 133.

Laster-Bradley, M., and Berger, B.A. 1991. Evaluation of drug distribution systems in university athletics programs: Development of a model or optimal drug distribution system for athletics programs. Unpublished report. (128 Miller Hall, Department of Pharmacy Care Systems, Auburn University, Auburn, AL 36849-5506).

Law, M. 2002a. Building evidence in practice. In *Evidence-based rehabilitation: A guide to practice,* edited by M. Law, 185-194. Thorofare, NJ: Slack, Inc.

Law, M. 2002b. Introduction to evidence based practice. In *Evidence-based rehabilitation: A guide to practice,* edited by M. Law, 3-12. Thorofare, NJ, Slack, Inc.

Lehr, C. 1992. Status of medical insurance provided to student-athletes at NCAA schools. *Journal of Legal Aspects of Sport* 2(1): 12-22.

Leiske, A.M. 1985. Standards: The basis of a quality assurance program. In *Quality assurance: A complete guide to effective programs,* edited by C.G. Meisenheimer, 45-72. Rockville, MD: Aspen.

Lencioni, P. 2002. *The five dysfunctions of a team*. San Francisco: Jossey-Bass.

Leverenz, L.J., and Helms, L.B. 1990a. Suing athletic trainers: Part I. *Athletic Training* 25(3): 212-216.

Leverenz, L.J., and Helms, L.B. 1990b. Suing athletic trainers: Part II. *Athletic Training* 25(3): 219-226.

Lipson, J.G. 1996. Culturally competent nursing care. *Culture and nursing care: A pocket guide,* edited by J.G. Lipson, S.L. Dibble, and P.A. Minarik, 1-6. San Francisco: UCSF Nursing Press.

Locke, L.F., Spirduso, W.W., and Silverman, S.J. 1993. *Proposals that work: A guide for planning dissertations and grant proposals*. 3rd Ed. Newbury Park, CA: Sage.

Lysens, R., Steverlynck, A., and van den Auweele, Y. 1984. The predictability of sports injuries. *Sports Medicine* 1: 6-10.

Magee, M. 2010. What ever happened to the Tavistock Principles and what is the consumer's role in defining professionalism? *Health Commentary*. http://healthcommentary. org/?page_id=1798. Accessed on March 25, 2010.

Maher, C.G., Sherrington, C., Elkins, M., Herbert, R.D., and Mosely, A.M. 2004. Challenges for evidence-based physical therapy: Accessing and interpreting high-quality evidence on therapy. *Physical Therapy* 84(7): 644-654.

Makarowski, L.M., and Rickell, J.B. 1993. Ethical and legal issues for sport professionals counseling injured athletes. In *Psychological bases of sport injuries,* edited by D. Pargman, 45-65. Morgantown, WV: Fitness Information Technology, Inc.

Makoul, G., Curry, R.H., and Tang, P.C. 2001. The use of electronic medical records: Communication patterns in outpatient encounters. *Journal of the American Medical Informatics Association* 8(6): 610-615.

Mangus, B.C., and Ingersoll, C.D. 1990. Approaches to ethical decision making in athletic training. *Athletic Training, JNATA* 25: 340-343.

Margolin, J.B. 1983. *The individual's guide to grants*. New York: Plenum.

Marrelli, T.M. 1992. *Nursing documentation handbook*. St. Louis: Mosby.

Martin, D.E. 1994. Emergency medicine and the underage athlete. *Journal of Athletic Training* 29(3): 200-202.

May, C.A., Schraeder, C., and Britt, T. 1996. *Managed care and case management: Roles for professional nursing*. Washington, DC: American Nurses Publishing.

Mayo, D., and Goodrich, J. 2002. *Staffing for results*. Chicago: American Library Association.

Mayo, H.B. 1978. *Basic finance*. Philadelphia: Saunders.

McCarthy, M.M. 1983. Discrimination in employment. In *Legal issues in public school employment,* edited by J. Beckham and P. Zirkel, 46-47. Bloomington, IN: Phi Delta Kappan.

McKeag, D.B., and Hough, D.O. 1993. *Primary care sports medicine*. Dubuque, IA: Brown.

Mehrabian, A. 1981. *Silent messages*. 2nd Ed. Belmont, CA: Wadsworth.

Miethe, T.D. 1999. *Whistleblowing at work*. Boulder, CO: Westview Press.

Miles, B.J. 1987. Injuries on the road: Good information reduces problems. *Athletic Training* 22(2): 127.

Mintzberg, H. 1973. *The nature of managerial work*. New York: Harper & Row.

Morris, L.L., and Fitz-Gibbon, C.T. 1978. *How to present an evaluation report*. Newbury Park, CA: Sage.

Moses, H., Dorsey E.R., Matheson, D.H., and Their, S.O. 2005. Financial anatomy of biomedical research. *Journal of the American Medical Association* 294(11): 1333-1342.

Mulder, S. 2003. Computer-aided planned maintenance system for medical equipment. *Journal of Medical Systems* 27(4): 393-398.

Murphy, J., and Burke, L.J. 1990. Charting by exception. *Nursing 90* 20(5): 65-69.

Muther, R., and Wheeler, J.D. 1994. *Simplified systematic layout planning*. Kansas City, MO: Management & Industrial Research Publications.

Myers, O.J. 1985. Myths concerning employees' performance appraisal. *Supervision* 47(12): 14-16.

Narayan, M.C. 2001. The national standards for culturally and linguistically appropriate services in health care. *Care Management Journals* 3(2): 77-83.

Nath, C., Schmidt, R., and Gunel, E. 2006. Perceptions of professionalism vary most with educational rank and age. *Journal of Dental Education* 70(8): 825-834.

National Athletic Trainers' Association. n.d. Internet job listings. www.nata.org/members1/CANWORC/military/ internetjobsites.pdf. Accessed September 8, 2006.

National Athletic Trainers' Association. 1995. *NATA code of ethics*. Dallas, TX: Author.

National Athletic Trainers' Association. 2004. *Role delineation study for the entry-level certified athletic trainer*. 5th Ed. Omaha, NE.

National Athletic Trainers' Association. 2006a. *Athletic training educational competencies.* 4th Ed. Dallas, TX: National Athletic Trainers' Association.

National Athletic Trainers' Association. 2006b. National outcomes research analysis. www.nata.org/members1/documents/nora/NORAcalltoaction_files/frame.htm. Accessed September 1, 2006.

National Athletic Trainers' Association. 2008. 2008 salary survey. www.nata.org/members1/salarysurvey2008/. Accessed February 9, 2010.

National Collegiate Athletic Association. 2002. *2002-2003 NCAA sports medicine handbook.* Overland Park, KS: Author.

National Collegiate Athletic Association. 2003. *Drug testing program.* www.ncaa.org/library/sports_sciences/drug_testing_program/2002-03/index.html. Accessed July 8, 2003.

National Collegiate Athletic Association. 2009. *Drug-testing program 2009-10.* www.ncaapublications.com/product-downloads/DT10.pdf. Accessed April 28, 2011.

National Collegiate Athletic Association, Committee on Competitive Safeguards and Medical Aspects of Sports. 1988. *Drugs and the intercollegiate athlete.* Indianapolis: Author.

National Collegiate Athletic Association. 2010. Catastrophic injury insurance program.www.ncaa.org/wps/portal/!ut/p/c5/04_SB8K8xLLM9MSSzPy8xBz9CP0os3gjX29XJydD-RwP_wGBDA08Df3Nzd1dXQwMDA_1wkA6zeGd3Rw8Tcx8DA3-jMAMDIz_T4ECD0GBjA09jiLwBDuBooO_nkZ-bqh-pH2WO0x53Y_3InNT0xORK_YLs7DTndEV-FAHpu34Y!/dl3/d3/L0lJSklna21BL0lKakFBTX1-BQkVSQ0pBISEvNEZHZ3NvMFZ2emE5SUFnIS83XzJNS0VCQjFBME9RUzEwSTBPNzdHRUUxMEczL0FLR0I3NDQ5MzAwMDM!/?WCM_PORTLET=PC_7_2MKEBB1A0OQS10I0O77GEE10G3_WCM&WCM_GLOBAL_CONTEXT=/wps/wcm/connect/ncaa/NCAA/About+The+NCAA/Budget+and+Finances/Insurance/sainsuranceprog. Accessed February 12, 2010.

Needy, J.R. 1974. *Filing systems.* Arlington, VA: National Recreation and Park Association.

Nelson, S., Altman, E., and Mayo, D. 2000. *Managing for results.* Chicago: American Library Association.

Newcomer, L.N. 1990. Defining experimental therapy: A third-party payer's dilemma. *The New England Journal of Medicine* 323(24): 1702-1704.

Newkirk, C. 2004. Overtime and the athletic trainer. *NATA News* 12: 16.

Nicholson, D. 2002. Practice guidelines, algorithms, and clinical pathways. In *Evidence-based rehabilitation,* edited by M. Law, 195-219. Thorofare, NJ, Slack Inc.

Nickell, R. 2006. Eight important principles for managing prescriptions in the athletic training room. *NATA News*: 30-32.

Occupational Safety and Health Administration. 1991. Occupational exposure to bloodborne pathogens. *Federal Register* 56(235): 64175-64182.

O'Leary, M.R. 1994. *Lexicon.* Oakbrook Terrace, IL: Joint Commission on Accreditation of Healthcare Organizations.

Organ, D.W., and Bateman, T. 1986. *Organizational behavior: An applied psychological approach.* Plano, TX: Business Publications.

Ouchi, W.G., and Dowling, J.B. 1974. Defining the span of control. *Administrative Science Quarterly* 19: 357-365.

Owens, R.G. 1987. *Organizational behavior in education.* 3rd Ed. Englewood Cliffs, NJ: Prentice Hall.

Oxford Centre for Evidence-Based medicine. CATmaker. www.cebm.net/catmaker.asp. Accessed September 5, 2006.

Panettieri, M. 2000. If it's not documented, you didn't do it: Documentation in school nursing practice. *School Nurse News* 17(1): 10.

Parks, J. 1977. Athletic trainer evaluation. *Athletic Training* 12(2): 92-93.

Parmet, W.E. 1993. Title III: Public accommodations. In *Implementing the Americans with disabilities act,* edited by L.O. Gostin and H.A. Beyer, 123-136. Baltimore: Paul H. Brookes.

Pearce, J.A. 1982. The company mission as a strategic tool. *Sloan Management Review* 23(2): 15-23.

Peltz, J.E., Haskell, W.L., Matheson, G.O. 1999. A comprehensive and cost-effective preparticipation exam implemented on the World Wide Web. *Medicine and Science in Sports and Exercise* 31(12):1727-40.

Penman, K.A. 1977. *Planning physical education and athletic facilities in schools.* New York: Wiley & Sons.

Penman, K.A., and Adams, S.H. 1980. *Assessing athletic and physical education programs.* Boston: Allyn & Bacon.

Penman, K.A., and Penman, T.M. 1982. Training rooms aren't just for colleges. *Athletic Purchasing and Facilities* 6(9): 34-37.

Penton/IPC Education Division. 1982. *Fundamentals of PERT.* Cleveland, OH: Author.

Perez, P.S., Hibbler, D.K., Cleary, M.A., and Eberman, L.E. 2006. Gender equity in athletic training. *Athletic Therapy Today* 11(2): 66-69.

Peter, L.J., and Hull, R. 1969. *The peter principle.* Cutchogue, NY: Buccaneer Books.

Pettigrew, A.M. 1972. Information control as a power source. *Sociology* 6: 187-204.

Pfister, G.C., Puffer, J.C., Maron, B.J. 2000. Preparticipation cardiovascular screening for US collegiate student-athletes. *Journal of the American Medical Association* 283(12):1597-1599.

Pheasant, S.T. 1991. *Ergonomics, work and health.* Gaithersburg, MD: Aspen.

Pickett, A.D. 1986. Drug testing: What are the rules? *Athletic Training* 21: 331-336.

Planning facilities for athletics, physical education, and recreation. 1979. North Palm Beach, FL: The Athletic Institute.

Porter, M.M., and Porter, J.W. 1981. Electrical safety in the training room. *Athletic Training* 16(4): 263-264.

Priest, S.L. 1989. *Understanding computer resources: A healthcare perspective.* Owings Mills, MD: National Health Publishing.

Randolph, W.A., and Posner, B.Z. 1988. What every manager needs to know about project management. *Sloan Management Review* 29(4): 65-73.

Rankin, J.M. 1992. Financial resources for conducting athletic training programs in the collegiate and high school settings. *Journal of Athletic Training* 27: 344-349.

Rankin, J.M., and Ingersoll, C. 2000. *Athletic training management: Concepts and applications.* 2nd Ed. New York: McGraw-Hill.

Ratanawongsa, N., Bolen, S., Howell, E.E., Sisson, S.D., and Larriviere, D. 2006. Residents' perceptions of professionalism in training and practice: Barriers, promoters, and duty hour requirements. *Journal of General Internal Medicine* 21(7): 758-763.

Ray, R.R. 1990. An injury-free budget. *College Athletic Management* 2(l): 42-45.

Ray, R.R. 1991a. Performance evaluation in athletic training: Perceptions of athletic trainers and their supervisors. *Dissertation Abstracts International* 51: 5053. (Doctoral dissertation, Western Michigan University, 1990).

Ray, R.R. 1991b. Training room efficiency. *Athletic Business* 15(l): 46-49.

Ray, R.R. 1996. Create your own HMO. *Athletic Therapy Today* 1(4): 11-12.

Ray, R.R. 1997. Technology in athletic therapy: Expectation or hope? *Athletic Therapy Today* 2(5): 5.

Reed, F.E. 2001. Improving the preparticipation exam process. *The Journal of the South Carolina Medical Association* 97(8): 342-346.

Reilly, T. 1981. Ergonomic aspects of sport and recreation. *Canadian Journal of Applied Sport Science* 6(1): 1-10.

Reinhardt, C. 1985. The state of performance appraisal: A literature review. *Human Resource Planning* 8(2): 105-110.

Ribaric, R.F. 1980. Taping/storage table. *Athletic Training* 15(1): 50.

Ribaric, R. 1982. The computer in sports medicine. *Athletic Training* 17(4): 309.

Ritter, H.T.M. 1990. Instrumentation considerations: Operating principles, purchase, management, and safety. In *Thermal agents in rehabilitation* (2nd Ed), edited by S. L. Michlovitz, 45-62. Philadelphia: F.A. Davis.

Rowell, J.C. 1989. *Understanding medical insurance reimbursement: A step-by-step guide.* Oradell, NJ: Medical Economics.

Rubin, R.H. 2002. Ethical issues in managed care. In *The tracks we leave: Ethics in healthcare management,* edited by F. Perry, 51-69. Chicago: Health Administration Press.

Sackett, D.L., Rosenberg, W.M., Gray, J.A., Haynes, R.B., and Richardson, W.S. 1996. Evidence based medicine: What it is and what it isn't. *British Medical Journal (Clinical Research Edition)* 312(7023): 71-72.

Salimbene, S. 2005. *What language does your patient hurt in? A practical guide to culturally competent patient care.* 2nd Ed. Amherst, MA: Diversity Resources.

Schlabach, G.A., and Peer, K.S. 2008. *Professional ethics in athletic training.* St. Louis, Missouri: Mosby/Elsevier Science.

Schneier, C.E., Beatty, R.W., and Baird, L.S. 1986. How to construct a successful performance appraisal system. *Training and Development Journal* 40(4): 38-42.

Schneller, T., and Godwin, C. 1983. *Writing skills for nurses.* Reston, VA: Reston.

Scholey, M., and Hair, M. 1989. Back pain in physiotherapists involved in back care education. *Ergonomics* 32(2): 179-190.

School Records. 1996. *Your school and the law* 26(5).

Scott, R.W. 1990. *Health care malpractice.* Thorofare, NJ: Slack, Inc.

Secor, M.R. 1984. Designing athletic training facilities or "Where do you want the outlets?" *Athletic Training* 19(l): 19-21.

Settle, S.M., and Spigelmyer, S. 1984. *Product liability: A multibillion-dollar dilemma.* New York: American Management Association.

Sikula, A.F. 1976. *Personnel administration and human resources management.* New York: Wiley & Sons.

Smith, D.M. 1994. Pre-participation physical evaluations: Development of uniform guidelines. *Sports Medicine* 18: 293-300.

Smith, E. 1975. Improving listening effectiveness. *Texas Medicine* 71:98-100.

Snider, S.W. 1982. Planning a new building? Consider design/build. *Athletic Purchasing and Facilities:* 50-51.

Spector, R.E. 2004. *Cultural diversity in health and illness.* 6th Ed. Upper Saddle River, New Jersey: Prentice Hall.

Standards of practice. 1987. Dallas: National Athletic Trainers' Association.

Steers, R.M., and Porter, L.W. 1987. *Motivation and work behavior.* 4th Ed. New York: McGraw-Hill.

Stein, J. 1996. *Source book of health insurance data.* Washington, DC: Health Insurance Association of America.

Steiner, G.A. 1979. *Strategic planning.* New York: The Free Press.

Steves, R., and Hootman, J.M. 2004. Evidence-based medicine: What is it and how does it apply to athletic training? *Journal of Athletic Training* 39(1): 83-87.

Stewart, D.L. 1993. Health care delivery system. In *Documenting functional outcomes in physical therapy,* edited by D.L. Stewart and S.H. Abeln, 1-31. St. Louis: Mosby.

Stiefel, R.H. 2002. Developing an effective inspection and preventive maintenance program. *Biomedical Instrumentation & Technology* 36(6): 405-408.

Stoner, J.A.F. 1982. *Management.* 2nd Ed. Englewood Cliffs, NJ: Prentice Hall.

Stovitz, S.D., and Satin, D.J. 2006. Professionalism and the ethics of the sideline physician. *Current Sports Medicine Reports* 5(3):120-124.

Streator, S., and Buckley, W.E. 2000. Clinical outcomes in sports medicine. *Athletic Therapy Today* 5(5): 57-61.

Swick, H.M. 2000. Toward a normal definition of medical professionalism. *Academic Medicine* 75(6): 612-616.

Tanner, D., and Tanner, L. 1987. *Supervision in education.* New York: Macmillan.

Tanner, S.M. 1994. Preparticipation exam targeted for the female athlete. *Clinics in Sports Medicine* 13(2): 337-353.

Taylor, S.L., and Lurie, N. 2004. The role of culturally competent communication in reducing ethnic and racial healthcare disparities. *The American Journal of Managed Care,* 10 Spec No. SP1-SP4.

The Foundation Center. 1997. *National guide to funding in health.* New York: Author.

Theunissen, W. 1978. Planning facilities: The role of the program specialist. *Journal of Physical Education and Recreation* 49(6): 27-29.

Thomas, K.W., and Kilmann, R.H. 1974. *The Thomas-Kilmann conflict mode instrument.* Tuxedo Park, NY: Xicom.

Thompson, R.A., and Sherman, R.T. 1993. *Helping athletes with eating disorders.* Champaign, IL: Human Kinetics.

Thorland, W. 1990. Drug detection. In *Substance abuse in sports: The realities* 71-75. Dubuque, IA: Kendall/Hunt.

Tropman, J.E. 1996. *Making meetings work: Achieving high quality group decisions.* Thousand Oaks, CA: Sage.

U.S. Department of Health and Human Services. *Healthy people 2010.* www.healthypeople.gov/. Accessed May 16, 2010.

U.S. Department of Health and Human Services Office of Minority Health. N*ational standards on culturally and linguistically appropriate services (CLAS).* www.omhrc. gov/. Accessed May 16, 2010.

U.S. Department of Labor Occupational Safety and Health Administration. *Medical screening and surveillance.* www. osha.gov/SLTC/medicalsurveillance/index.html. Accessed September 1, 2006.

U.S. Department of Labor Occupational Safety and Health Administration. *Safety and health topics: Medical and first aid.* www.osha.gov/SLTC/medicalfirstaid/index.html. Accessed September 6, 2006.

U.S. Small Business Administration. 1980a. *Business basics: Inventory management.* Washington, DC: U.S. Government Printing Office.

U.S. Small Business Administration. 1980b. *Job analysis, job specifications, and job descriptions.* Washington, DC: U.S. Government Printing Office.

U.S. Small Business Administration. 1981. *Risk management and insurance.* Washington, DC: U.S. Government Printing Office.

van der Smissen, B. 2001. Tort liability and risk management. In *The management of sport: Its foundation and application,* edited by B.L. Parkhouse, 177-198. New York: McGraw-Hill.

Varricchio, C.G. 1997. Culturally competent care: What is an administrator to do? In *Cultural diversity in nursing: Issues, strategies, and outcomes,* edited by J.A. Dienemann, 57-61. Washington, DC: American Academy of Nursing.

Wadlington, W., Waltz, J.R., and Dworkin, R.B. 1980. *Law and medicine.* Mineola, NY: Foundation Press.

Walsh, K.M., Bennett, B., Cooper, M., Holle, R.L., Kithill, R., and Lopez, R.E. 2000. National Athletic Trainers' Association position statement: Lightning safety for athletics and recreation. *Journal of Athletic Training* 35: 471-477.

Want, J.H. 1986. Corporate mission. *Management Review* 75(8): 46-50.

Watkins, P. 2003. A conference planner's 8 worst nightmares. www.gotkeynote.com/8_worst_nightmares.php. Last accessed May 30, 2003.

Watson, D. 2002. Evaluating the evidence: Economic analysis. In *Evidence-based rehabilitation: A guide to practice,* edited by M. Law, 171-182. Thorofare, NJ, Slack Inc.

Weber, M. 1962. *Basic concepts in sociology* (H.P. Secher, Trans.). Secaucus, NJ: Citadell.

Wildavsky, A. 1975. *Budgeting: A comparative theory of budgetary processes.* Boston: Little, Brown.

Witkin, B.R., and Altschuld, J.W. 1995. *Planning and conducting needs assessments: A practical guide.* Thousand Oaks, CA: Sage.

Worthen, B.R., and Sanders, J.R. 1973. *Educational evaluation: Theory and practice.* Worthington, OH: Charles A. Jones.

Wright, B.J. 1983. *Automated purchasing: Key to new potential.* New York: American Management Association Membership Publication Division.

Yate, M. 2002. *Knock 'em dead.* Avon, MA: Adams.

Yukl, G.A. 1981. *Leadership in organizations.* Englewood Cliffs, NJ: Prentice Hall.

INDEX

Note: The italicized *f* and *t* following page numbers refer to figures and tables, respectively.

ABOUT THE AUTHORS

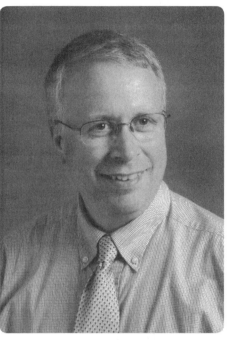

Courtesy of Richard Ray.

Richard Ray, EdD, ATC, is provost and professor of kinesiology at Hope College in Holland, Michigan. A recognized leader in the field of athletic training, he is a practicing administrator who is responsible for 400 employees and the author of the popular texts *Case Studies in Athletic Training Administration* and *Counseling in Sports Medicine.* He is also a former editor of the journal *Athletic Therapy Today* and associate editor of the *Journal of Athletic Training.*

Ray is a member of the NATA Research and Education Foundations Board of Directors. He was chair of the National Athletic Trainers' Association (NATA) Education Task Force and the Nomenclature Task Force. He is a member and former president of both the Great Lakes Athletic Trainers' Association (GLATA) and the Michigan Athletic Trainers' Society (MATS). Ray was named to the Educational Advisory Board of the Gatorade Sport Science Institute in 1993 and the MATS Hall of Fame in 1999. He was inducted into the NATA Hall of Fame in 2006 and received the 2004 Most Distinguished Athletic Trainer Award and the 2001 Sayers Miller Outstanding Educator Award from the NATA.

Ray received his EdD in educational leadership, as well as a master's degree in physical education, from Western Michigan University.

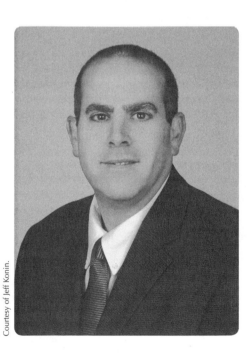

Courtesy of Jeff Konin.

Jeff Konin, PhD, ATC, PT, FACSM, FNATA, is associate professor and vice chair of the department of orthopaedics and sports medicine at the University of South Florida (USF). At USF, he also serves as the executive director of the Sports Medicine & Athletic Related Trauma (SMART) Institute, a community outreach program with a mission of promoting safety in sports. Konin is a founder and partner of the Rehberg Konin Group, which provides scientific investigation, research, and litigation support services for incidents involving sports and physical activity. He is the author of textbooks including *Clinical Athletic Training*, *Special Tests for Orthopedic Examination*, *Documentation for Athletic Training*, and *Reimbursement for Athletic Training.*

Konin is a fellow of both the National Athletic Trainers' Association (NATA) and the American College of Sports Medicine (ACSM). He is a recipient of the NATA Service Award (2008), the NATA Continuing Education Excellence Award (2008), the Southeast Athletic Trainers' Association Education/Administration Athletic Trainer of the Year Award (2010), and the NATA Most Distinguished Athlete Trainer Award (2011).

Konin received his PhD in physical therapy from Nova Southeastern University, a master of physical therapy from the University of Delaware, master of education from the University of Virginia, and a bachelor of science from Eastern Connecticut State University.

Athletic Training Education Series

Human Kinetics' Athletic Training Education Series contains six textbooks, each with its own supporting instructional resources. Featuring the work of respected athletic training authorities, the series parallels and expounds on the content areas established by the NATA Executive Committee for Education. To learn more about the books in this series, visit the Athletic Training Education Series website at **www.HumanKinetics.com/AthleticTrainingEducationSeries**.

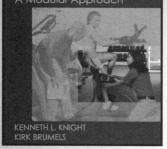

Fourth Edition

DEVELOPING CLINICAL PROFICIENCY IN ATHLETIC TRAINING
A Modular Approach

KENNETH L. KNIGHT
KIRK BRUMELS

Kenneth L. Knight, PhD, and Kirk Brumels, PhD
©2010 • Spiral-bound
352 pp
ISBN 978-0-7360-8361-4

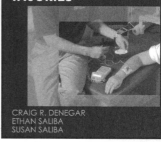

Third Edition

THERAPEUTIC MODALITIES FOR MUSCULOSKELETAL INJURIES

CRAIG R. DENEGAR
ETHAN SALIBA
SUSAN SALIBA

Craig R. Denegar, PhD, ATC, PT, Ethan Saliba, PhD, ATC, PT, and Susan Saliba, PhD, ATC, PT
©2010 • Hardback • 304 pp
Print: ISBN 978-0-7360-7891-7
E-book: ISBN 978-0-7360-8558-8

Ancillaries: instructor guide, test package, image bank
www.HumanKinetics.com/ TherapeuticModalitiesFor MusculoskeletalInjuries

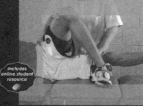

Third Edition

EXAMINATION OF MUSCULOSKELETAL INJURIES

includes online student resource

SANDRA J. SHULTZ
PEGGY A. HOUGLUM
DAVID H. PERRIN

Sandy J. Shultz, PhD, ATC, CSCS, Peggy A. Houglum, PhD, ATC, PT, and David H. Perrin, PhD, ATC
©2010 • Hardback • 720 pp
Print: ISBN 978-0-7360-7622-7
E-book: ISBN 978-0-7360-8694-3

Ancillaries: instructor guide, test package, image bank
Online Student Resource: examination checklists, tables, full-color photos
www.HumanKinetics.com/ ExaminationOfMusculoskeletalInjuries

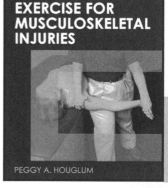

Third Edition

THERAPEUTIC EXERCISE FOR MUSCULOSKELETAL INJURIES

PEGGY A. HOUGLUM

Peggy A. Houglum, PhD, ATC, PT
©2010 • Hardback • 1040 pp
Print: ISBN 978-0-7360-7595-4
E-book: ISBN 978-0-7360-8560-1

Ancillaries: instructor guide, test package, presentation package plus image bank
www.HumanKinetics.com/ TherapeuticExerciseFor MusculoskeletalInjuries

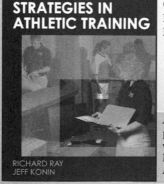

Fourth Edition

MANAGEMENT STRATEGIES IN ATHLETIC TRAINING

RICHARD RAY
JEFF KONIN

Richard Ray, EdD, ATC, and Jeff Konin, PhD, ATC, PT, FACSM, FNATA
©2011 • Hardback • 360 pp
Print: ISBN 978-0-7360-7738-5
E-book: ISBN 978-1-4504-1623-8

Ancillaries: instructor guide, test package, image bank
www.HumanKinetics.com/ ManagementStrategiesIn AthleticTraining

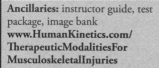

CORE CONCEPTS IN ATHLETIC TRAINING AND THERAPY

Includes a web resource with 41 clinical modules

SUSAN KAY HILLMAN
EDITOR

Susan Kay Hilllman, ATC, PT
©2012 • Hardback • 640 pp
Print: ISBN 978-0-7360-8285-3
E-book: ISBN 978-1-4504-2355-7

Ancillaries: instructor guide, test package, image bank, web resource
www.HumanKinetics.com/ CoreConceptsInAthleticTraining AndTherapy

HUMAN KINETICS
The Information Leader in Physical Activity & Health

For more information:
(800) 747-4457 US • (800) 465-7301 CDN • 44 (0) 113-255-5665 UK
(08) 8372-0999 AUS • 0800 222 062 NZ • (217) 351-5076 International
Or visit **www.HumanKinetics.com**

Q002